# PSYCHOTHERAPY AFTER BRAIN INJURY

# Psychotherapy
## after Brain Injury

**PRINCIPLES AND TECHNIQUES**

**Pamela S. Klonoff**

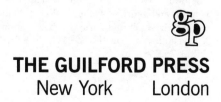

**THE GUILFORD PRESS**
New York    London

**Library of Congress Cataloging-in-Publication Data**

Klonoff, Pamela S.
  Psychotherapy after brain injury : principles and techniques / Pamela S. Klonoff.
    p. ; cm.
  Includes bibliographical references and index.
  ISBN 978-1-60623-861-5 (hardcover: alk. paper)
  1. Brain—Wounds and injuries—Patients—Mental health services.  2. Brain—
Wounds and injuries—Patients—Rehabilitation.  3. Psychotherapy.  I. Title.
  [DNLM: 1. Brain Injuries—rehabilitation.  2. Brain Injuries—psychology.
3. Psychotherapy—methods.  WL 354 K66p 2010]
  RC387.5.K56 2010
  617.4'81044—dc22

                                                                2010014395

# About the Author

**Pamela S. Klonoff, PhD, ABPP-CN,** is a faculty neuropsychologist and (since 1993) Clinical Director of the Center for Transitional NeuroRehabilitation, Barrow Neurological Institute of St. Joseph's Hospital and Medical Center, Phoenix, Arizona. She has been affiliated with the program since 1986. Dr. Klonoff is board certified in Clinical Neuropsychology by the American Board of Professional Psychology. She specializes in outpatient milieu-oriented neurorehabilitation, with a particular interest in psychotherapy with patients and their families after brain injury. Dr. Klonoff has published many articles and presented theoretical and clinical papers around the world; her expertise and research focus on holistic neurorehabilitation, including psychotherapy and cognitive retraining after traumatic and other acquired brain injury.

# Preface

My devotion to psychotherapy began when I was a naïve yet keen graduate student collecting dissertation data. I interviewed young adults with traumatic brain injuries and evaluated their quality of life 2–4 years postinjury. Preeminent in that sobering experience were their pervasive despair, social isolation, and unproductive existences. As the focus of neuropsychology at that time was on assessment rather than treatment, none of these patients had had the luxury of psychotherapeutic interventions, or even a "listening ear." At that juncture, I decided to commit my professional career to providing psychotherapy and neurorehabilitation for such patients.

After finishing graduate school, I completed a postdoctoral residency at Presbyterian Hospital in Oklahoma City under the tutelage of George Prigatano, PhD, and Mary Pepping, PhD. From then on, my professional vantage point became holistic neurorehabilitation. Many of the psychotherapeutic treatment principles and techniques presented in this book emanate from my 24 years (at this writing) of clinical experience as a psychotherapist/neuropsychologist and 16 years as Clinical Director of a holistic neurorehabilitation program (the Center for Transitional NeuroRehabilitation, Barrow Neurological Institute). This milieu-oriented treatment approach addresses patients' multiple treatment needs through the interventions of an interdisciplinary team composed of neuropsychologists, occupational therapists, physical therapists, speech–language pathologists, and recreational therapists, as well as a neurorehabilitation technician, dietician, rehabilitation physician, and psychiatrist. The team works together in an integrated and cohesive manner to maximize patients' community independence and productivity. The nurturing and healing aspects of this environment are palpable, and patients experience compassionate care in a setting imbued with the indispensable ingredients of collaboration, structure, accountability, and hope.

My favorite professional endeavor is psychotherapy with patients and their families after brain injury. This passion was deepened by the extraordinary mentorship, empathy, and skills training proffered over a 15-year period by Dr. Gustavo Lage, psychiatrist and psychoanalyst. In my setting, the psychotherapeutic interventions start with individual psychotherapy for both patients and families; family therapy; group psychotherapy for patients; family groups; and postdischarge aftercare groups for patients and families. Because psychotherapy after brain injury requires such a strong psychoeducational focus, I have included in this book a number of adjunct treatment options from which psychotherapists can choose. I consider these "collaborative evidentiary techniques"; by wearing other "clinical hats," a psychotherapist enters a patient's phenomenological world, and together they derive vital and diverse information that ultimately enhances the patient's awareness, acceptance, and realism. This process includes cognitive retraining exercises and group treatment experiences, which afford a multidimensional perspective and an expanded knowledge base about each patient. Patients can benefit from the versatility of their psychotherapists as they receive direct feedback from multiple treatment types and venues.

This book describes principles and techniques of psychotherapy for patients and their families in the postacute phase of the patients' neurological recovery. To accomplish this, theoretical and pragmatic treatment approaches are integrated and presented. The focus is on progression from psychotherapeutic phenomena to interventions for patients and their families. Case study material is interwoven throughout to illustrate specific concepts and interventions.

Even though I believe that the psychotherapeutic process can unfold best within a milieu treatment environment, I recognize that such an environment often cannot be replicated, for a variety of reasons. Therefore, this book is designed and intended to cover a broad spectrum of applications. For example, it provides an array of free-standing ideas and approaches that can readily be incorporated into a solo practice. A solo therapist can utilize "talk therapy" in combination with other treatment interventions (e.g., cognitive retraining) as conduits to help a patient attain awareness, acceptance, and realism after brain injury. The solo practitioner can also gather several such patients and create a group psychotherapy or aftercare experience, in which the patients thrive on peer support and mentoring relationships.

Psychotherapists who work in other sites, such as outpatient settings, can enhance their repertoires by collaborating with members of other neurorehabilitation disciplines (e.g., occupational therapists and speech–language pathologists). Sample groups (e.g., psychoeducational group, communication pragmatics group), with associated protocols, are also described in this book, for the purposes of partnership with other disciplines. The intent is to give psychotherapists treating patients and families after brain injury the flexibility and fluidity of choosing from assorted treatment elements, based on their own preferences and access to resources. Each reader can pluck from a smorgasbord of therapeutic possibilities and creatively concoct a personalized model and eclectic style that is most suitable for his or her neurological population and vocational circumstances.

PAMELA S. KLONOFF

# Acknowledgments

Countless individuals helped to fashion and nurture this project. First, I would like to deeply thank my family—Irwin, Zachary, Jeremy, and Aaron—for their unwavering love, support, and patience. They made many accommodations for this endeavor and were an enduring source of emotional sustenance. Thank you as well to the rest of my family and friends who cheered me on past each milestone.

I have been fortunate to have many professional mentors, including Louis Costa, Otfried Spreen, Esther Strauss, William Gary Snow, George Prigatano, and Mary Pepping. I appreciate the support from my administrators at Barrow Neurological Institute, where scholarly endeavors are actively promoted. I have huge gratitude to all of the readers of earlier drafts, including Melanie Talley, Karen Olson, Barbara Gruner, Susan Rumble, Maura Rynn, Pamela McNamara, Jennifer Lutton, and Irwin Altman.

I am appreciative of the editorial prowess and guidance from The Guilford Press, and I am also indebted to Edward Koberstein. His steadfast confidence in the merit of this undertaking manifested in innumerable hours of administrative assistance. I am grateful to both him and Stephen Myles for their coauthorships.

My "CTN family" is the foundation of my professional growth, and I am eternally grateful for their unflagging dedication to patient care. They are a testament to the power of collaborative strivings for ideals. I am in awe of the many patients and families who have the courage to undertake a new life journey; they have served as my empathy compass and professional inspiration. I so appreciate those who granted permission for original case study material, art, and poetry as a way to convey content in an authentic and creative manner in the book. Last, I dedicate this book to Gustavo Lage and Laya Braemer for their life wisdom and unconditional empathic responsiveness.

# Contents

# PSYCHOTHERAPY AFTER BRAIN INJURY

# CHAPTER 1

# Introduction and Overview

Incorporation of psychotherapy as a treatment modality in neurorehabilitation is recent, multifarious, and evolving. Originally psychotherapy was thought to be contraindicated, as brain-injured patients were considered incapable of benefiting from such interventions because of poor self-awareness; their deficits in the areas of attention, memory, and comprehension; and their emotional dysregulation (for reviews of this earlier literature, see Coetzer, 2007; Prigatano et al., 1986). Pioneers in the field of psychotherapy after brain injury include Kurt Goldstein (1952, 1954), who described the effects of brain damage on personality—including impaired abstract thought capacity, "catastrophic reactions" (i.e., strong emotional reactions to difficulties in task accomplishment and other postinjury challenges), transference, and protective mechanisms (e.g., denial). Cicerone and colleagues (Cicerone, 1989; Cicerone, Levin, Malec, Stuss, & White, 2006) have emphasized the psychotherapeutic interventions of education and concrete feedback to reduce denial and improve self-observation and self-assessment after brain injury, especially in the aftermath of executive function deficits. Lisa Lewis (1999; Lewis & Rosenberg, 1990), and Karen Langer (1999) have described the benefits of psychodynamically oriented psychotherapy, also incorporating premorbid personality variables. Other visionaries in this area include Yehuda Ben-Yishay (1996), Anne-Lise Christensen (Christensen, Pinner, Moller Pedersen, Teasdale, & Trexler, 1992), and George Prigatano (Prigatano et al., 1986; Prigatano, 1999), with their emphases on psychotherapeutic interventions as part of holistic treatment to improve patients' awareness and self-acceptance, as well as to help them find meaning in life. Finally, Gustavo Lage has enriched the field of psychotherapy after brain injury through incorporating concepts of self psychology (Klonoff & Lage, 1991; Klonoff, Lage, & Chiapello, 1993).

## THE COLLABORATIVE MODEL OF PSYCHOTHERAPY AFTER BRAIN INJURY

### Definition of Psychotherapy

"Psychotherapy after brain injury" can be defined as the collaborative working relationship between a psychotherapist and a brain-injured patient, with the goals of increasing the patient's awareness of, acceptance of, and realism about his or her predicament. At the same time, the psychotherapist educates and supports the patient's family and community connections, so as to facilitate the patient's renewed sense of identity, hope, and meaning.

This book addresses the process of psychotherapy for older teen/adult patients and their families in the postacute phase of the patients' neurological recovery. The emphasis of psychotherapy with this patient population is on psychoeducation, coping, and adjustment. A "hands-on," practical, systematic approach incorporating explicit treatment principles and techniques is presented.

### Brief Description of the Collaborative Model

There is a dearth of psychotherapy models for treating acquired brain injury, especially ones that incorporate an integrated theoretical and multidimensional approach (Ben-Yishay & Lakin, 1989; Coetzer, 2006). Recently Coetzer (2007) has applied the generic model of psychotherapy (Orlinsky & Howard, 1995) to the field of brain injury. He emphasizes six facets: the therapeutic contract, operations, and bond; self-relatedness; in-session impacts; and phases of treatment.

Figure 1.1 depicts an adapted multifactorial model that helps guide and articulate the psychotherapy process for patients with brain injury (Klonoff, 2004). In this integrated model, a patient and psychotherapist are engaged in a collaborative approach to change. This collaboration includes each partner's perception of the other and of their relationship, as well as meaningful therapeutic interventions that involve active sharing and willing participation (Bachelor, Laverdiere, Gamache, & Bordeleau, 2007; Klonoff, 1997; Lewis, 1999; Mateer, 2005; Sutherland & Couture, 2007). The underpinning—indeed, the essence—of the collaborative process is the working alliance between the psychotherapist and patient, in conjunction with his or her family and/or primary support network.

In this model, the psychotherapist functions as a facilitator of change. He or she is equipped with an armamentarium of knowledge, which serves as the theoretical and conceptual framework within which he or she understands and interprets the patients' cognitive, emotional, and interpersonal status. As the psychotherapist evolves, his or her knowledge base and techniques also mature. The next section of this chapter describes some major theoretical and conceptual areas from which principles for treating patients with brain injuries are abstracted. This core knowledge is coupled with specific treatment techniques, as described in the remainder of the book.

The patient's postinjury recovery and adjustment are affected by a multiplicity of factors—primarily the nature and extent of the brain injury and its effects on cognition, emotions, and behaviors. Patients with brain injuries expe-

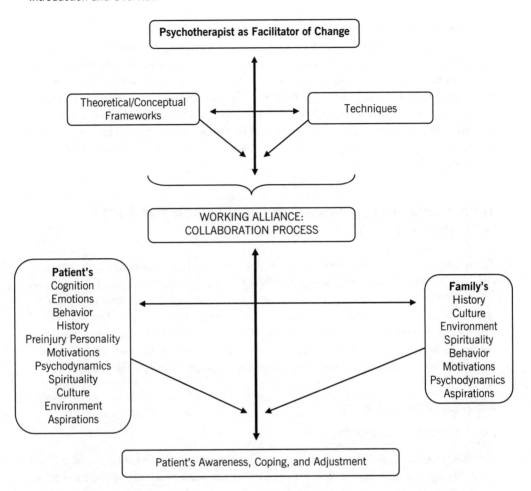

**FIGURE 1.1.** A collaborative model of psychotherapy after brain injury. Adapted from Klonoff (2004).

rience emotional changes emanating from two sources. The first set of changes is a direct result of damage to areas of the brain that subserve emotions, such as the amygdala, cingulate gyrus, insula, globus pallidus, temporal lobe, and orbitofrontal cortices (Critchley, 2005; Filley, 2008; Murphy, Nimmo-Smith, & Lawrence, 2003; Tantam, 2003; Vaishnavi, Rao, & Fann, 2009). Patients with damage to any of these areas may have difficulty modulating and titrating emotions (Miller, 1999). Second, patients' emotional status after brain injury is affected by their multifaceted reactions to the changes in their life circumstances, including heightened states of anxiety and emotional turmoil (Lewis & Rosenberg, 1990). A strategic role of the psychotherapist is to assist his or her patients in accessing, defining, expressing, and integrating their emotions, in the context of an often perplexing and startling reality. This is crucial, because a patient's troublesome coping can undermine rehabilitation and alienate family members and helping professionals.

The effects of the brain injury manifest themselves in the context of each patient's background history, including his or her characterological attributes, motivations, psychodynamics, spirituality, culture, environment, and aspirations. The patient is also embedded in a social milieu with his or her family. The family's history, culture, environment, spiritual beliefs, behaviors, motivations, psychodynamics, and aspirations will all influence the patient's awareness, coping, recovery, and ultimately his or her adjustment. The collaborative model thus takes into account the full complexity of the process and components involved in effective psychotherapy.

## THEORETICAL FRAMEWORKS APPLICABLE FOR PATIENTS WITH BRAIN INJURY

The therapist working with brain-injured patients can draw from an eclectic range of conceptual frameworks, including psychodynamic, self-psychological, existential, cognitive, and behavioral approaches. In addition to individual therapy, patients with brain injury may also participate in group psychotherapy, psychoeducational groups, milieu therapy, and family therapy, and may benefit from psychopharmacology as well. The following discussion reviews some of the salient theoretical frameworks and concepts applicable to psychotherapy after brain injury.

### Individual Psychotherapy

#### Psychodynamic Constructs

Psychodynamic constructs that are applicable to psychotherapy for acquired brain injury include ego development and separation–individuation, as well as feelings of inferiority secondary to family dynamics (e.g., maternal and paternal reactions to the disability) (Jureidini, 1988). Transference reactions are inherent in the working alliance and to the psychotherapeutic process as a whole. "Transference" refers to the fact that patients' current relationships (including that with the psychotherapist) are perceived and experienced in the context of past significant relationships and the ways these relationships have affected personality development (Lewis, 1999). These prior attitudes, values, and behaviors can become entrenched and create stereotyped ways of thinking, feeling, and behaving (Wolberg, 1967). Psychotherapeutic interventions should incorporate transference interpretations, which assist patients in understanding the connections between their here-and-now interactions with the psychotherapist and their past circumstances (Hobson & Kapur, 2005; Waska, 2006). This process is particularly important in situations where past relationships have been troubled or problematic, as a patient can unconsciously displace unresolved issues onto current relationships (Lewis, 1999). The intensity and coherence of transference reactions are related to ego organization, which in turn is affected by experiential, developmental, and neurological factors, specifically emotional regulation and executive functions (Lewis, 1999).

Transference reactions often incorporate inappropriate expectations and misperceptions derived from these past experiences (Lomas, 1993). Similarly, patients with neurological damage may misperceive or distort input because of the nature and location of their brain injuries. Therefore, the psychotherapist must differentiate the underlying sources of emotional turmoil and relationship upheaval, incorporating transference reactions without an exclusive focus on neurological interpretations. In essence, the complex juxtaposition of current life alterations against the backdrop of historical relationships becomes potent material and a compass for the psychotherapeutic dialogue and resolution of maladaptive coping styles.

## Self Psychology

"Self psychology" has been defined as the psychology of the vicissitudes of the self—its emergence and development, cohesion, boundaries, structure, functions, and disorders (Wolf, 1988). Central to the theory of self psychology is the concept of "self objects," defined as objects or persons who in the real world are separate and distinct, but who in the psychic world are experienced as part of the self, performing certain functions (e.g., soothing, calming, and organizing) (Kohut, 1984a). Beginning with parents as the earliest and most important selfobjects, selfobject experiences are instrumental in the emergence, maintenance, and completion of the self (Wolf, 1988). Another primary concept in self psychology is "self-cohesion," or the ego strength that enables stress tolerance, emotional stability, psychological well-being, and self-esteem (Wolf, 1988).

Injured self-esteem can result in the experience of "narcissistic rage," which is the reaction of the self when it experiences a sense of shame, vulnerability, helplessness, and loss of integrity (Klonoff, 2005). Prior publications have noted parallels between narcissistic rage and catastrophic reactions after brain injury, as both represent the damaging effects of perceived failure on the integrity of the self (Klonoff & Lage, 1991; Klonoff, Lage, & Chiapello, 1993). Empathic responsiveness is critical for the development and maintenance of self-cohesion and for the amelioration of catastrophic reactions, and has been characterized as "subjective listening," "vicarious introspection," and "affect attunement" (Kohut, 1984a; D. Stern, 1985; Wolf, 1988).

## Existential Psychotherapy

"Existential psychotherapy" is a dynamic approach to therapy that focuses on concerns rooted in every individual's existence, including death, freedom, existential isolation, and meaninglessness (Frankl, 1984; Yalom, 1980). It presupposes that suffering is a universal part of the human condition (Yalom, 1980). Existential psychotherapy espouses antideterminism, self-actualization, freedom, meaning, choice, purpose, values, responsibility, and appreciation of the unique experiential world of each individual (Yalom, 1980). These theoretical constructs are used to inspire patients to transform personal despair and suffering into meaningful fulfillment as better human beings (Frankl, 1984; Yalom, 1980). The relevance of existential psychotherapy to patients with acquired brain injury is enormous, given their anguish and the uncertainty of their postinjury existence.

## Behavior Therapy

Behavior therapy is based on learning theory (Yamagami, 1998). It identifies those antecedent factors and consequences that reinforce self-defeating behavior. Clear contingencies are employed to reduce problematic behaviors (via extinction and defusion techniques), while increasing self-enhancing behaviors (via positive reinforcement and rewards) (Borgaro, Caples, & Prigatano, 2003; Giles & Manchester, 2006; Gregory, 2007; Persel & Persel, 2004). Behavior therapy is well suited for some patients with acquired brain injury, as it is problem-oriented and emphasizes cognitive skills, including problem solving. Incorporating principles of behavior analysis, behavior plans can be instituted to modify undesirable behaviors after brain injury, including aggression, disinhibited behavior, and self-injury (Corrigan & Bach, 2005; Persel & Persel, 2004; Rothwell, LaVigna, & Willis, 1999; Ylvisaker, Jacobs, & Feeney, 2003). The psychotherapist identifies relevant stimulus cues and then develops specific reinforcement contingencies by incorporating active listening, limit setting, redirection, shaping, and withdrawal of attention, as well as relevant cues, prompts, checklists, and contracts (Corrigan & Bach, 2005; Mateer & Sira, 2006; Persel & Persel, 2004). Other components include positive programming (e.g., teaching adaptive behaviors); ecological change (modifying the environment to correspond with the patient's cognitive status); focused treatment (using behavioral contingencies to achieve a reduction in target behaviors); reactive strategies (identifying actions to gain immediate control over challenging behavior); and generalization (transferring learned behaviors to other settings) (Persel & Persel, 2004; Rothwell et al., 1999). As such, behavior therapy is practical and emphasizes the use of concrete interventions to develop real-life survival skills (Yamagami, 1998).

## Cognitive-Behavioral Therapy

Cognitive-behavioral therapy (CBT) is based on the hypothesis that emotions and behavior are influenced by preexisting cognitive schemas. CBT assists patients in understanding the links among their beliefs, thinking, and behavior. It identifies cognitive distortions and negative automatic thoughts, and helps patients replace these with more adaptive and balanced cognitive attitudes (Beck, 2005; Demark & Gemeinhardt, 2002; Gregory, 2007). The patients gain an understanding of how thoughts influence mood and behavior, and learn to identify cognitive distortions such as catastrophizing, dichotomous thinking, and absolute thinking (Freeman, Pretzer, Fleming, & Simon, 2004), which are common consequences of acquired brain injury. CBT techniques to help patients stop and think before acting (Gregory, 2007) include homework, lists of pros and cons, self-talk, and thought records, as well as the setting of attainable goals with specific subgoals (Demark & Gemeinhardt, 2002; Gregory, 2007). Its structured and concrete techniques involve written aids, prompts, and repetition, which also make CBT efficacious for patients with acquired brain injury (Anson & Ponsford, 2006a; Mateer, Sira, & O'Connell, 2005).

Specific applications include the treatment of depression, anxiety, anger, psychosocial functioning, coping skills, and self-esteem (Anson & Ponsford, 2006a, 2006b; Bradbury et al., 2008; Demark & Gemeinhardt, 2002; Mateer & Sira, 2006). CBT is also effective in building self-regulatory skills and promoting management of postinjury stress and frustration (Mateer & Sira, 2006). It has been used to help patients with executive function deficits improve their problem-solving skills, skill acquisition, internal initiation, and goal-directed behavior, and thus to enhance their functionality in daily life (Anson & Ponsford, 2006a; Gordon, Cantor, Ashman, & Brown, 2006; see McDonald, Flashman, & Saykin, 2002, for a review).

### Psychoeducation and Skills Training

Psychoeducation and skills training are fundamental components of cognitive rehabilitation after brain injury. Psychoeducation provides patients with information to improve their understanding of their neurological sequelae; it is therefore a precursor to instilling awareness after brain injury (Klonoff, 1997; Mateer et al., 2005; Prigatano et al., 1986). Relevant topics include the definition and nature of cognitive, language, physical, and functional deficits, and their anatomical correlates (Klonoff, Lamb, Henderson, Reichert, & Tully, 2000). Skills training interventions are designed to remediate and ameliorate functional deficits, such as those in memory and attention (Mateer & Sira, 2008; Mateer et al., 2005). Techniques include multiple forms of compensations and external cueing systems (e.g., checklists, datebooks, calendars, Datalink watches, personal digital assistants), repetitive drills and exercises, cognitive remediation techniques, and so forth (Klonoff et al., 1997; Mateer & Sira, 2008; Mateer et al., 2005). Restorative exercises and compensation training can be conducted within the treatment environment, or generalized to the home, the community, and other functional contexts (Klonoff et al., 1997; Mateer & Sira, 2008; Prigatano, 2008a; Ylvisaker, Hanks, & Johnson-Greene, 2002).

### Group Psychotherapy

Group psychotherapy provides psychotherapeutic support and education for patients with acquired brain injury (Anson & Ponsford, 2006a; Delmonico, Hanley-Peterson, & Englander, 1998; Forman, Vesey, & Lincoln, 2006; Forssmann-Falck & Christian, 1989; Klonoff, 1997; Klonoff, Lamb, Henderson, Reichert, et al., 2000; Prigatano et al., 1986). The format for group psychotherapy after acquired brain injury is generally quite structured (Demark & Gemeinhardt, 2002; Klonoff, 1997; Langenbahn, Sherr, Simon, & Hanig, 1999; Prigatano et al., 1986), in order to help psychotherapists manage group members' challenges related to emotionality (e.g., depression, frustration, and anger), behavior (e.g., self-regulation), and cognitive deficits (e.g., memory, divided attention). This form of therapy incorporates the invaluable dimensions of peer input and mentorship in order to improve patients' insight and psychological adjustment. Furthermore, the group process facilitates acquisition of hope; recognition of the universality of experience; altruism and socialization; learning of social skills and coping techniques; and development of self-esteem, awareness, acceptance, and adaptation (Delmonico et al., 1998; Forssmann-Falck & Christian, 1989; Forssmann-Falck, Christian, & O'Shanick, 1989; Klonoff, 1997; Klonoff, Lamb, Henderson, Reichert, et al., 2000; Langenbahn et al., 1999; Prigatano et al., 1986; Yalom, 1975). Ancillary techniques include art and music therapy; discussion of relevant movies, books, and poetry; appearances by patient "graduates" as guest speakers; and structured exercises, such as defining life values (Klonoff, Lamb, Henderson, Reichert, et al., 2000).

### Holistic Milieu Treatment

Milieu treatment emphasizes the power of the healing environment. Each patient is part of a therapeutic community where the emphasis is holistic—that is, geared toward the needs of the whole person, rather than partitioned deficits (Ben-Yishay, 1996; Klonoff, Lamb, Henderson, Reichert, et al., 2000; Prigatano et al., 1986). As such, holistic treatment emphasizes metacognition, emotional regulation, interpersonal functioning, and community reintegration (Cicerone et al., 2008). Critical ingredients in the milieu are concern and commitment to the community at large, including mutual respect and compassion. Ideally, clear parameters, expectations, and goals are delineated for the therapeutic endeavors, in the context of an ambience that is nurturing and supportive. Humor and camaraderie are also inherent components of effective milieu treatment; they are powerful healing tools that promote an atmosphere of joy and instill a sense of togetherness.

The key element of the healing process within the holistic treatment milieu is empathic responsiveness (Klonoff, 1997). Every interaction with patients and families, therapeutic intervention, and recommendation is rooted in empathic relatedness. All milieu members mentor and encourage one another; nurturance and genuine caring and concern are deeply embedded and palpable within the setting. Patients (and therapists) feel respected, safe, and protected. The ambience has been described as "luvfesty" (L. K. Dawson, personal communication, n.d.) For example, one day a week in a milieu session, patients can participate in a "circle of positives," in which they relate areas of progress and happiness to one another and the therapists. Birthdays and graduations are celebrated in milieu sessions with songs and a cake, most often prepared by other patients. Patients who fall ill receive get-well cards from the entire milieu. Empathy creates a curative Gestalt whereby all patients are transported to greater accomplishments and places of psychological well-being, just by being part of a group whose members truly matter to one another.

The psychotherapist plays a unique and vital role in the holistic milieu treatment environment. Most often it is his or her mission to "blaze the psychological trail" in this environment for a patient and family. The psychotherapist will be the emissary for the awareness, acceptance, and realism process, helping to expose and ameliorate the understandable distress and resistance reactions, so that the remainder of the interdisciplinary team members can better dedicate their energies to their multiple interventions without psychological hindrances. This united and integrated approach provides patients (and their families) with the fundamental educational and psychological tools they will need to alter their lifestyle and adopt and adapt to integral compensatory strategies.

## Psychopharmacology

Psychopharmacological treatment is often an adjunct to psychotherapy after brain injury, especially for patients suffering from mood disorders (including depression and anxiety), affect dysregulation (Fann et al., 2009; Mateer & Sira, 2008; Silver, Arciniegas, & Yudofsky, 2005; Turner-Stokes & MacWalter, 2005), and catastrophic reactions. Psychotropic medications can help a patient attain the requisite level of psychological resources and stability necessary to tolerate and benefit from psychotherapeutic interventions. Such medications include selective serotonin reuptake inhibitors (SSRIs), selective serotonin–norepinephrine reuptake inhibitors (SSNRIs), and mood stabilizers (Ghaffar & Feinstein, 2008; Jorge & Robinson, 2003; Lee et al., 2005; Mynatt & Cunningham, 2007; Silver et al., 2005; Vaishnavi et al., 2009; Zafonte, Cullen, & Lexell, 2002). Anticonvulsants, antidepressants, anxiolytics, and antipsychotics have also been utilized to treat anger, agitation, and aggression problems after brain injury (Demark & Gemeinhardt, 2002; Lombard & Zafonte, 2005; Vaishnavi et al., 2009). Secondary problems with sleep related to mood disorders or neurological factors can be ameliorated with various medications as well, including antihistamines, melatonin, trazodone, and mirtazapine (Thaxton & Myers, 2002; Vaishnavi et al., 2009; Zafonte et al., 2002).

## Family Therapy

Intrinsic to the psychotherapy process with a patient after brain injury is intervention with the family, for the benefit of both the patient and the family unit (Gan, Campbell, Gemeinhardt, & McFadden, 2006; Klonoff, Lamb, & Henderson, 2001; Klonoff, Lamb, Henderson, & Shepherd, 1998; Mauss-Clum & Ryan, 1981; Sander et al., 2002; Sohlberg, McLaughlin, Todis, Larsen, & Glang, 2001). Family systems theory proposes that the patient and family members constitute a complex system, including relationship patterns, norms, rules, communication styles, and roles (Gan et al., 2006; Laroi, 2003; Palmer & Glass, 2003). From a family systems perspective, a primary goal of psychotherapy after brain injury is to help the family system accommodate to the patient's functional and social changes, while simultaneously meeting the psychosocial needs of the other members; this ensures the continuity of meaningful family relationships (Palmer & Glass, 2003). Therapy formats vary, but they include psychotherapy for family members (with and without the patient), couple therapy, group therapy, bibliotherapy, and support groups (Gan et al., 2006; Klonoff, Koberstein, Talley, & Dawson, 2008; Klonoff & Prigatano, 1987; Kreutzer, Kolakowsky-Hayner, Demm, & Meade, 2002; Laroi, 2003; Palmer & Glass, 2003). Goals of therapy are multifocal, including psychoeducation, skills training, emotional support, and coping techniques (Gan et al., 2006; Klonoff et al., 2008; Klonoff & Prigatano, 1987; Kreutzer et al., 2002; Laroi, 2003).

## THE WORKING ALLIANCE

Regardless of the mode of therapy employed, the development and maintenance of the working alliance between a patient and his or her psychotherapist are intrinsic to effective psychotherapy. The patient and psychotherapist search for insight and interpretation together, and foster a relationship built on trust and collaboration (Ackerman & Hilsenroth, 2003; Bachelor et al., 2007; Goldstein, 1954; Horvath & Luborsky, 1993; Judd & Wilson, 2005; Lewis & Rosenberg, 1990; Newman, 2002; Weiner, 1997). Recent research indicates that better patient outcomes and higher patient satisfaction are related to stronger therapist–patient alliances (Baldwin, Wampold, & Imel, 2007; Kim, Kim, & Boren, 2008; Klonoff et al., 2001, 2007).

The working alliance with a patient after brain injury can be conceptualized as integrating three processes. The first is a process of understanding: The psychotherapist's emotional attunement, in combination with his or her clinical acumen, enables him or her to achieve new insights into the patient's predicament. In the second process, the therapist interprets the gathered insights and educates the patient about them. The third is an implementation process: The patient willingly undertakes active and concerted efforts to modify his or her behavior because of the potency of the revelations and the working alliance. Of course, alliance ruptures are unavoidable within the treatment process; these are related to difficulties in establishing, or fluctuations in the quality of, the therapeutic relationship (Ackerman & Hilsenroth, 2001). Restoration and enhancement of a positive working alliance are predicated on the psychotherapist's recognizing and remediating negative processes (Ackerman & Hilsenroth, 2001, 2003). Further exploration of this topic can be found in Chapter 10 as part of the discussion of countertransference.

## Understanding: Therapists' Attunement + Acumen = Insight

Attunement with patients requires psychotherapists to sense the patients' level of psychic pain and resiliency, so as to help them reach their genuine capacities without overburdening them psychologically (Lewis & Rosenberg, 1990). It requires as a foundation a "relational climate of security," where a patient feels safe and protected (J. M. Stern, 1985, as cited in Lewis & Rosenberg, 1990, p. 70). Through clinical perceptiveness, the psychotherapist is able to "understand" or to grasp empathically on some level what the patient is experiencing (Kohut, 1984a). The basis of this understanding process is the therapist's capacity for empathy, as well as attentive and reflective listening.

## Interpretation/Education

Productive movement in the therapeutic process requires the therapist to interpret the insights gathered and use these to educate the patient, particularly about the "whys" of his or her behavior (Bachelor et al., 2007; Pepping, 1993). The "whys" are particularly salient after brain injury, due to patients' organic unawareness and defense mechanisms; a psychotherapist's awareness and insights foreshadow the assimilation process for a patient. After brain injury, this process unearths patients' emerging awareness and they can begin to acquire insights, while at the same time they can freely express their emotions, ideas, and needs. This is a dynamic process, with often rapid oscillations between the understanding and interpreting phases (Kohut, 1984a; Luborsky, 1976). Overall, patients are helped to be more self-observant and to integrate correct interpretations through observation, synthesis, and acceptance (Rawn, 1991).

The interplay of understanding/insight and interpretation/education is a complex and fluid one. Yalom (2002) postulates that effective therapy should be "relationship-driven, not theory-driven" (p. xviii). He describes an alternating sequence of evocation and experiencing of affect, followed by its analysis and integration. The therapist's role is to guide the patient and assist him or her in analyzing and resolving conflicts, not to control or mandate changes in the patient. In other words, psychotherapists guide patients toward decisions whereby they act in their own best self-interest (Prigatano et al., 1986). The process of "educating, stimulating, and encouraging patients to broaden and deepen their awareness allows them to expand their repertoire of behaviors, feelings, and cognitions" (Newman, 2002, p. 174). After brain injury, this process of interpreting and educating evolves the awareness process in patients and deepens their level of insight, while at the same time preparing them psychologically for the practical process of change and adjustment.

## Implementation: Change and Adjustment

The outgrowths of the mutual insight and interpretation/education processes are change and adjustment in a patient's behavior and goals. This implementation process represents the final transformation and manifestation of the working alliance. A patient who has improved his or her level of self-understanding can work collaboratively with the psychotherapist to problem solve and to plan a course for adaptive behavior (Lewis & Rosenberg, 1990). Real-life manifestations of change and adjustment are necessary at this stage, including the incorporation of new techniques and compensatory strategies. Therefore, the emotional bond between the psychotherapist and the patient with a brain injury facilitates acquisition of awareness and overall treatment compliance, and is a sign of the solidity of the working alliance (Schönberger, Humle, & Teasdale, 2006a; Schönberger, Humle, Zeeman, & Teasdale, 2006).

It is worth emphasizing that the three processes embedded in the working alliance with patients after brain injury are interactive, dynamic (Kim et al., 2008), and cyclical. As the therapeutic process unfolds, new insights, interpretations, behavioral changes, and ultimately personal growth ensue.

An effective, "user-friendly" working model for defining the specific subcomponents of the working alliance for patients has been proposed by Bordin (1979). Its components include the "bonds," or the relationship between the patient and therapist, founded on rapport, trust, and respect. The "tasks" are the substance of the counseling process, including specific therapeutic activities (e.g., the use of a datebook and the Home Independence Checklist, described in Chapter 6). The "goals" are the outcomes and targets of the therapy (e.g., achieving independence in the home, returning to work or school, etc.). Progress in and potential barriers to the therapeutic process can be categorized in terms of this model, so the patient and family understand where their efforts need to be targeted.

## CHARACTERISTICS OF PSYCHOTHERAPISTS AND PATIENTS

### Educational Background of Psychotherapists Treating Patients with Brain Injury

Psychotherapists who work with brain-injured patients come from several backgrounds. In the United States and Canada, these include neuropsychologists who develop an interest and specialty in psychotherapy during their academic studies, or as part of their residency training; or, alternatively, clinical psychologists who later specialize in neuropsychology, usually during their postdoctoral residency training. Either form of training is appropriate for this field, as long as the individual has a sufficient academic knowledge of brain–behavior relationships, in combination with a broad range of psychotherapy skills. Content areas include functional neuroanatomy; neuroimaging and neurodiagnostic techniques; neuropsychological evaluation (including personality testing) of multiple neurological etiologies across the lifespan; interview and consultation skills; and intervention techniques (e.g., psychoeducation, cognitive retraining, and datebook training). Specialization within the field of neuropsychology and rehabilitation also exists in the form of board certification (e.g., by the American Board of Professional Psychology) (Warschausky, Kaufman, & Stiers, 2008).

Some rehabilitation psychologists, psychiatrists, behavioral/mental health counselors, and clinical social workers also provide psychotherapy for patients with brain injuries. The challenge for therapists is finding appropriate training opportunities that address the multiplicity of their patients' needs and the complex interplay of organic and preexisting factors from which these needs arise. Clinicians must also obtain training and learn therapeutic techniques for helping their patients' families and/or other support systems (Jackson & Manchester, 2001; Klonoff et al., 2008).

### Psychotherapist Qualities

The psychotherapist working with patients requires specialized skills and abilities, given the nature and challenges of the work. These qualities include substantial empathy, patience, kindness, and supportiveness, due to the magnitude and pervasiveness of patients' deficits and the laboriousness of the recovery process. When the therapist is working with a team of other professionals, he or she will also need qualities of collegiality, as well as the capability to weigh opinions and to compromise. Given these patients' deficits in executive functions, the psychotherapist needs to have particularly strong executive function capacities, including analytical thinking, organizational skills, planning, problem solving, and goal setting (Klonoff, 1997; Lewis & Rosenberg, 1990). Often a psychotherapist must function as a patient's "auxiliary ego" or "alter ego" and guide the patient in the arenas of decision making, flexible thinking, and "seeing the big picture" (Freed, 2002; Klonoff, 1997; Klonoff & Lage, 1991). Given the enormity, and frequently the chronicity, of the losses that these patients experience, the psychotherapist will also need the emotional resources and hardiness to tolerate extended and extensive contact with patients' deep psychic pain and sorrow.

Psychotherapists helping patients cope with brain injury can develop the capacity to embrace the vulnerabilities and fragility of life, and to cherish and respect their position and influence. The attitude they take toward unavoidable suffering can inspire patients to "transform a personal tragedy into a triumph, to turn [their] predicament into a human achievement" (Frankl, 1984, p. 135). Strivings for altruism and self-transcendence can sustain psychotherapists in their mission of ministering to others (Yalom, 1980). Ultimately it is our capacity as psychotherapists to have enthusiasm, be visionary and hopeful, feel inspired, and embrace life's pleasures and values that transmits willingness, openness, and belief in a better future to our patients (Aniskiewicz, 2007; Ben-Yishay et al., 1985; Klonoff, 1997; Strozier, 2001).

## Patient Characteristics

The techniques of psychotherapy after brain injury described in this book are considered most appropriate for older adolescents and adult patients being treated on an outpatient basis. Patients with brain injury from diverse etiologies—including traumatic brain injuries, cerebrovascular accidents, aneurysms, arteriovenous malformations, seizure disorders, encephalitis, anoxia, and low-grade brain tumors—can benefit. The patient population discussed in this book includes those who have sustained moderate to severe acquired brain injuries, characterized by some combination of the following: Glasgow Coma Scale scores of 3–12; loss of consciousness of at least 24 hours; a period of posttraumatic amnesia of at least 1 week; positive radiological scans, often including neurosurgical intervention; and an array of physical, language, cognitive, emotional, and psychosocial sequelae. The approaches and goals of psychotherapy are relevant for the postacute population; the treatment interval can range from weeks or months postinjury to many years after the event. More important than the etiology or chronicity of injuries are the perceptions of the psychotherapist, patient, and family that there are potential benefits to embarking on a psychotherapeutic relationship.

Insight-oriented psychotherapy is not appropriate for all patients with acquired brain injury. For example, patients with severe disorientation and confusion, and/or severe behavioral problems requiring behavior modification plans, are generally not ideal candidates. They lack the necessary cognitive abilities and emotional resources to confront and cope with their neurological sequelae. Although patients suffering from a postconcussion syndrome (McAllister, 2005; McCrea, 2007) or posttraumatic stress disorder (Warden & Labbate, 2005) may benefit from psychotherapy that furthers their psychological adjustment, these clusters of symptoms are complex and outside the scope of this book. Potential psychiatric disturbances may also preclude the self-exploration process. Examples of problematic behavioral and psychiatric conditions include paranoia, severe agitation, and violent behavior, especially when a patient is therapeutically confronted with insight-oriented material. Caution should also be exercised in embarking on psychotherapy with patients who have active substance use problems (see Chapter 8). Patients require the cognitive and emotional capabilities to improve their levels of awareness, acceptance, and realism about the effects of their injuries, including a capacity for at least basic self-introspection (Ben-Yishay & Lakin, 1989; Klonoff, 1997). Other core considerations include the patient's overall level of functionality and general neurological prognosis, as well as the degree of cognitive reserve (Kesler, Adams, Blasey, & Bigler, 2003). These are critical parameters that a clinician must include in his or her assessment of any patient's compatibility for insight-oriented psychotherapy.

Better candidates are those patients who have, at a minimum, the functional aptitude to eventually attain unsupervised status in the home and community. That is, they should eventually be capable of independently managing activities of daily living and personal care (e.g., medication management, household chores and responsibilities, transportation needs), and of participating in meaningful hobbies and socialization opportunities within the family unit and in society. Patients eligible for higher-order goals, including the potential to return to some form of productive school or work status, are also very suitable for this type of psychotherapy. The ultimate outcome can be quite variable, depending on the nature and extent of the brain injury. Some patients return to gainful employment at their preinjury levels; others return to a modified job status; still others are unable to maintain gainful employment because of the severity of their injury sequelae, so they pursue meaningful volunteer placements.

## UNDERSTANDING THE PATIENT'S EXPERIENCE AFTER BRAIN INJURY

Patients' awareness of their deficits, and their ability to accept and cope realistically with those deficits, are central to the overall recovery process after brain injury. Psychotherapy helps to guide the patient adaptively through this complex journey. An overview of the process is depicted in Figure 1.2, through the patient experiential model (PEM) of recovery after brain injury. The model depicts the recovery and rehabilitation process for patients after moderate to severe brain injuries who participate in holistic milieu-oriented therapies and/or insight-oriented treatment. I consider the Figure 1.2 chart integral to the psychoeducational process after brain injury, and it is a pivotal reference and resource for my patients and their families. The chart is written in the first person, to emphasize the importance of personal ownership of the rehabilitation and recovery process. A similar model of the family's experience is discussed in Chapter 7.

The PEM groups the recovery process into seven phases emanating from a preinjury reference point (Phase 0). Each phase has distinct events and experiences, as described in Figure 1.2. As patients move forward in time, they may revisit phases, rotating again through Phase 3 (Seeks Help) or 4 (Starts Outpatient Therapy) to Phase 6 (Therapy Transition) or 7 (Future), based on new insights and life lessons. The dotted lines between columns in Figure 1.2 indicate that these rotations are possible. The psychotherapeutic tasks of increasing patients' awareness, acceptance of deficits, and realism in future planning are most prominent in Phases 4, 5, and 6.

In Phases 1 and 2, patients are not yet capable of insight-oriented psychotherapy, due to the acuteness of the injury and its associated cognitive sequelae of disorientation and confusion. In Phases 3 through 7, however, patients may cope adaptively or problematically. The patients' possible coping styles are represented in the bottom three rows of the figure. Color-coded like a traffic light, these rows represent a healthy, more adaptive coping zone ("green" = light gray); a warning zone ("yellow" = darker gray), signifying prevalent coping difficulties; and a crisis zone ("red" = darkest gray). The ("red") crisis zone represents a period of disintegration, when a patient is either unable and/or unwilling to cope with the realities of his or her injury and deteriorates into a state of turmoil and crisis. For patients, this zone illustrates the perils associated with either ignoring or rejecting the therapeutic process anywhere within Phases 3 through 7. Refusal to improve their awareness, acceptance, and realism can result in work failures, financial ruin, alienation, and/or fragmentation of family life. Ultimately, patients may be consumed by intense rage, despair, hopelessness, and helplessness. Life can implode; goals and aspirations can be obstructed or ruined. Over time, there are understandable fluctuations in patients' coping skills and adjustment, represented by dotted lines and arrows between the horizontal zones. Patients can meander through these coping zones, depending on the complex and often daunting obstacles they encounter.

In Phase 3, patients recognize that problems associated with the brain injury have become overwhelming for themselves and their families, resulting in life upheaval. This eventually leads to the search for treatment resources. Patients who are coping well in Phase 3 are tentative, yet have basic trust in the treatment recommendations of their support system. On the other hand, patients in the warning zone of Phase 3 dismiss their problems, underestimate them, or attribute their difficulties to external factors. They are convinced that they will make a full recovery on their own, and are skeptical of the possible benefits of treatment.

In Phase 4, patients are immersed in the *awareness* development process; they are confronting reality. The evaluation and early treatment process (detailed in the next two chapters) begin to teach them about their strengths and difficulties. Generally there is a "honeymoon period," when patients are enthusiastic about their therapies. However, as awareness grows and the nature and extent of their deficits become more apparent, patients often experience catastrophic reactions ("CRs" in the figure and in "rehab lingo"). They may find the rehabilitation process stressful and demanding. The emphasis of the treatment process on structure and accountability can feel like "rehab boot camp." Patients with adaptive coping tend to enjoy the predictable regimen and nurturing atmosphere, and feel empowered by their acquisition of knowledge. They are able to manage their understandable emotional reactions to their awareness of losses, and are buoyed by their trust in the treatment process. Patients in the warning zone are much less able to cope with feedback, and they generally respond to it with intense and extended emotional distress. These patients want to "kill the messenger," and target their therapists as the causes of their unhappy predicaments. There may be rejection, denial, and/or disavowal of the education process. Ultimately, these reactions produce strained relationships with the family and therapists. Chapter 3 discusses the awareness process in more detail.

In Phase 5, the emphasis is on *acceptance,* typified by the development and implementation of compensatory strategies. Patients practice with work or school

Discharge

| PHASE 0 | PHASE 1 | PHASE 2 | PHASE 3 | PHASE 4 | PHASE 5 | PHASE 6 | PHASE 7 |
|---|---|---|---|---|---|---|---|
| Preinjury | Time of Brain Injury | Early Adjustment | Seeks Help | Starts Outpatient Therapy | Retraining | Therapy Transition | Future ∞ |
| | | | | *AWARENESS* | *ACCEPTANCE* | *REALISM* | |
| **Reference Point** Life as it was. | **Sudden Impact** • Intensive care unit/acute care. • Different types of brain injuries. • Coma duration. • Agitated, combative, disoriented. →↓→↓→ • Subacute setting. | **Initial Problems** • Inpatient neurorehabilitation. • Posttraumatic amnesia; confusion. • Organic unawareness—I see my physical problems, but not my cognitive or emotional difficulties. • Primary focus is on my basic activities of daily living. | **Can't Cope** • I refuse or can't get the treatment. • Life upheaval and financial setbacks; problems escalate. • My family is stressed out and overloaded, so we intensify the treatment search. | **Confronting Reality** • I may experience a "honeymoon period." • Holistic approach teaches individualized strengths and difficulties. • The process is demanding/stressful and evokes "CRs." • "Rehab boot camp." | **Compensations** • Psychological introspection of injury aftermath. • I develop and implement compensations. • I gain perspective on the spectrum of injury types and severities. • I begin work and/or school. • "Dress rehearsal" for my new life. • Opportunity for "second chance." | **Approaching Discharge** • I set attainable goals in the outside world, using new insights, skills, and compensations. • I am exposed to new freedoms, independence, and meaningful activities. • "Dignity of risk." **Cake Day** | **The Real World** • I have my tools to function independently and productively. • My new reality sets in. • Life is ever-changing and evolving. • Things aren't the same, but everyone can live a meaningful and productive life. |
| | | | • I am tentative, but trust that the physician and family have my best interest at heart. • I am open to considering further outpatient rehabilitation to improve my circumstances. | • I have increased awareness of the effects of my injury. • I enjoy the structure and feel empowered by my new knowledge. • I constructively manage my anxiety, anger, frustration, and/or sadness. • I become less overwhelmed, and I develop better coping techniques. • I develop trust in holistic therapies. | • I mourn the losses. • I adjust expectations and accept myself for who I am now. • I embrace compensations with a "just do it!" attitude. • I implement feedback and strategies everywhere. • improved communication pragmatics enhances my interpersonal relationships. • I realize that "things take time," but I am invested in compensation training. | • I collaborate with therapists and my family toward community reintegration. • I am realistic about my level of independence, productivity, and socialization skills. • I constructively manage my fears and trepidations about my discharge. • I develop self-confidence in my skill attainment. • I expand my support system. | • I maintain a collaborative dialogue with significant others about my compensations and life decisions. • I consistently use my compensations, both at home and at work/school. • I modify my compensations when home/job demands change. • I am successful in establishing and maintaining a "two-way street" in relationships in and outside of the home. |

F A M I L Y 'S

↕ (Fluctuation)

**LEGEND**

☐ Phases

▢ Coping Zone

▨ Warning Zone

▩ Crisis Zone

----- Rotation

↕ Fluctuation

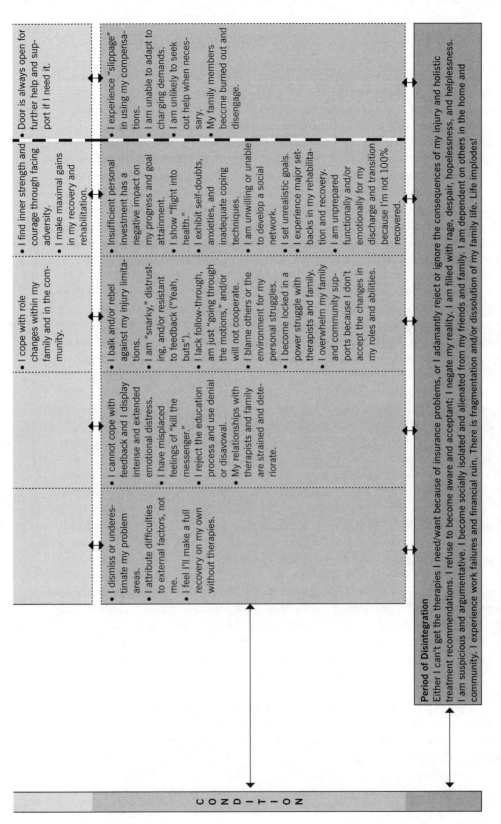

**FIGURE 1.2.** Patient experiential model (PEM) of recovery after brain injury.

Adapted from Prigatano (1999). Copyright 1999 by Oxford University Press. Adapted by permission in *Psychotherapy after Brain Injury* by Pamela S. Klonoff (Guilford Press, 2010). Permission to photocopy this figure is granted to purchasers of this book for personal use only (see copyright page for details).

tasks and situations as a "dress rehearsal" for their new life. They have a vision of a future and a focus on a "second chance." In Phase 5, adaptively coping patients also actively mourn their losses, culminating in an adjustment of their expectations. They take a "just do it" attitude about their use of compensations, along with the realization that "things take time" (Hein, 2004) in the recovery process. Patients in the warning zone of Phase 5 are characterized by rebellion and resistance, which compromise their progress and overtax their community supports. Interactions are characterized by a "snarky" (i.e., irritable; see Chapter 5) and distrusting attitude. A hallmark of this problematic coping style is the response "Yeah, but," which is perceived by others as making excuses and externalizing blame. Often patients are "just going through the motions," and/or become locked in a power struggle with their therapists. Chapter 5 describes the acceptance process for patients.

In Phase 6, patients are striving for *realism* or attainable goals, based on their new insights and skill sets. The patients are "spreading their wings" from the clinic setting into the community, and are enjoying new freedoms, greater independence, and more meaningful activities. Adaptively coping patients embrace the spirit of collaboration and realism, and make maximum gains in their recovery. Although they feel some trepidation about their impending discharge, they take pride in their skill attainment. New courage and inner strength emerge from facing and overcoming adversity. Chapters 6 and 8 address how to help patients improve their life skills and social reintegration.

Patients in the warning zone of Phase 6 are unprepared—functionally, emotionally, or both—for their community reintegration because of insufficient personal investment and unrealistic goal setting. Patients may display self-doubts, anxieties, and disappointments because they have not recovered 100%. Alternatively, some enter a "flight into health," characterized by ignoring or minimizing the realities of their condition. This scenario is discussed more fully in Chapter 9.

In Phase 7, the patients are out in the real world, armed with their compensatory tools. Life is different and ever-changing, but the patients (and their families) can live a meaningful and productive life. Adaptively coping patients successfully modify their compensations. They accept and function within the centrality of "two-way street" relationships, in and out of the home. They also recognize that the door is always open for further treatment, if needed. Patients in the warning zone of Phase 7 cannot adapt to the demands of their environment; there is "slippage" away from, or complete abandonment of, the tools essential for their success. They reject further treatment, and their behavior and attitudes burn out their support systems.

As depicted by the Family's Condition column in the left half of the figure, there are interconnections and reverberations between patients and their families throughout all phases of recovery. The patients' current challenges and/or triumphs in their physical, cognitive, functional, psychological, and interpersonal domains are mirrored in their families' stress load and sense of well-being, and vice versa. Families experience a recovery process of their own, which is explored further in Chapter 7.

The role of the psychotherapist is to encourage patients (and families) to move adaptively through their difficult postinjury experiences. The key instrument in facilitating this process is the collaborative working relationship between the psychotherapist and the patient.

The remainder of this book describes in more detail the psychotherapeutic process for patients, as well as their families. The emphasis is on the patients' personal, professional, family, societal, and existential adjustment; "talk therapy" and multiple psychoeducational techniques are used. Each chapter addresses a specific component of the psychotherapeutic continuum, with an emphasis on awareness, acceptance, and realism. Chapter 2 offers detailed theoretical and practical guidelines for the initial and early psychotherapy sessions, as well as an overview of effective treatment tools and techniques. Chapter 3 discusses organic unawareness and therapeutic interventions for increasing self-awareness. Here and throughout the book, interventions include not only individual psychotherapy, but also such modalities as group psychotherapy, cognitive retraining, and psychoeducational group. With emerging awareness, patients experience loss and grief; they begin to question who they are postinjury. Chapter 4 addresses the recalibration of patients' sense of self, identity, values, and social roles. Chapter 5 explores the process of patients' acceptance of their limitations, which is essential if they are to compensate, adjust, and functionally recover from their challenges. Chapter 6 describes how to encourage and train patients to use specialized compensatory systems to maximize life skills. Patients' families are vital participants in the rehabilitation process; they too undergo a recovery process that mirrors their loved ones' journey. This process is depicted in Chapter 7 on family life. Because brain injury can result in impaired communication and social skills, such skills must be relearned if patients are to be successfully and happily reintegrated into their communities; this process is discussed in Chapter 8. Optimal adjustment following brain injury requires patients to develop realistic expectations and productive goals. Chapter 9 discusses how to foster realism in patients, as well as how to help them attain meaning, quality of life, self-actualization, and hope. Treatment termination and aftercare are also addressed. The final chapter explores self-care for psychotherapists and offers strategies for avoiding burnout, to enhance professional longevity and fulfillment.

# CHAPTER 2

# Guidelines for Early Psychotherapy Sessions and General Treatment Considerations

This chapter offers detailed guidelines for the initial consultation and the early psychotherapy sessions. It then describes some important general treatment parameters and techniques for effecting meaningful change with brain-injured patients. A few comments on care coordination and the reimbursement process, together with a brief case study, conclude the chapter.

## THE INITIAL CONSULTATION

The initial consultation emanates from Phase 3 of the PEM (see Chapter 1, Figure 1.2). A key determinant for referral of a brain-injured patient to psychotherapy is that the patient has struggled and often failed to achieve independence in the home and community, and/or has been unable to reintegrate successfully to work or school. Alternatively, patients may be referred by their physicians immediately after discharge from an inpatient rehabilitation setting, so as to avoid potential posthospitalization adjustment problems. Of note, patients themselves are often not the ones seeking psychotherapy; distressed and overwhelmed family members or astute health care professionals are usually the ones who recognize that the patients need psychotherapy, with an emphasis on psychoeducation, coping, and adjustment to their deficits. Therefore, a psychotherapist should not assume that a patient is motivated (at least initially) for psychotherapy.

Typically, a patient being considered for psychotherapy will need a physician's referral. This facilitates the acquisition of relevant medical records, which are necessary for determining the patient's appropriateness for therapy and anticipating possible psychotherapeutic needs and challenges. Records should be obtained and reviewed in advance of the initial consultation. Helpful medical records should include the background neurological findings and associated medical history; radiographic reports; neurosurgical reports; consultations by neurologists and neuro-ophthalmologists; and summary reports from other rehabilitation settings (both inpatient and outpatient). If available, prior neuropsychological reports are very informative—especially when they contain pertinent preinjury social history, including drug and alcohol use, employment history, and the psychosocial adjustment of the patient and family members. For a student, prior grades and standardized test scores are very beneficial in establishing the individual's academic and behavioral history.

This volume does not address how to do a neuropsychological evaluation (see Lezak, Howieson, Loring, Hannay, & Fischer, 2004; Strauss, Sherman, & Spreen, 2006; Snyder, Nussbaum, & Robins, 2006; Uomoto, 2004). However, an up-to-date neuropsychological evaluation will provide essential quantitative and qualitative data about the patient's neuropsychological and emotional status, and will delineate specific cognitive strengths and difficulties; therefore, it will guide the consultation (and treatment) process (Erickson, 1995; Prigatano & Klonoff, 1988). For example, the intake interview approach will need to be modified to fit the patient's memory capacity, abstract reasoning skills, language abilities, and speed of information processing. In some situations, the psychotherapist may also be the neuropsychologist who performs the neuropsychological examination. This can be useful, as clinical observations and other data obtained by the neuropsychologist/psychotherapist during the evaluation process typically provide an excellent starting point for the psychotherapeutic and alliance-building process. Table 2.1 lists assessment domains and sample neuropsychological tests for each domain. This list is not exhaustive and can be modified according to the preferences of the examiner, the requirements of the treatment setting, and the nature and extent of the patient's neurological injury. Note that symptom validity testing should be included, in order to be sure that the patient has the necessary motivation to embrace the psychotherapeutic process, with a goal of improving independence and functionality.

The purpose of an initial 1-hour consultation is to make a formal determination of the patient's "fit" for a psychotherapeutic relationship, as well as the potential for meaningful change. It is recommended that family members be included for at least a portion of the consultation. This gives the clinician the opportunity to preview not only the family members' unique emotional resources and psychodynamics, but also the dynamics, interaction styles, and behavior patterns between family members and the patient. All parties are asked in advance for permission (and the patient is asked to sign a release form) to discuss the patient's and family members' perceptions about the patient's deficits. Also, when the first appointment is set, the patient and attending support system members are told that the consultation precedes formal initiation of psychotherapy services, and that as part of the appointment, all parties will be asked about their willingness to proceed with treatment sessions.

**TABLE 2.1. Sample Neuropsychological Domains and Tests**

| Neuropsychological domain | Sample tests |
| --- | --- |
| Effort/motivation | • Number Memory Test (Hiscock & Hiscock, 1989)<br>• Letter Memory Test (Inman et al., 1998)<br>• Victoria Symptom Validity Test (Slick, Hopp, Strauss, & Thompson, 2005)<br>• Test of Memory Malingering (Tombaugh, 1996)<br>• California Verbal Learning Test—Second Edition, Adult Version (CVLT-II) Long-Delay Forced-Choice Recognition (Delis, Kramer, Kaplan, & Ober, 2000) |
| Attention/ concentration | • Wechsler Adult Intelligence Test—Fourth Edition (WAIS-IV) Digit Span (Wechsler, 2008)<br>• WAIS-IV Arithmetic (Wechsler, 2008)<br>• WAIS-IV Letter–Number Sequencing (Wechsler, 2008)<br>• WAIS-IV Cancellation (Wechsler, 2008)<br>• Trail Making Test, Part A (Heaton, Grant, & Matthews, 2004)<br>• Wechsler Memory Test—Fourth Edition (WMS-IV) Spatial Addition (Wechsler, 2009) |
| Speed of information processing | • WAIS-IV Symbol Search (Wechsler, 2008)<br>• WAIS-IV Coding (Wechsler, 2008)<br>• WAIS-IV Cancellation (Wechsler, 2008)<br>• WAIS-IV Processing Speed Index (Wechsler, 2008)<br>• Symbol Digits Modalities Test (Lezak, Howieson, Loring, Hannay, & Fischer, 2004) |
| Motor functioning | • Rey Complex Figure Test—Copy (Meyers & Meyers, 1995)<br>• Bicycle Drawing Test (Lezak et al., 2004)<br>• Porteus Mazes (Porteus, 1965)<br>• WAIS-IV Block Design (Wechsler, 2008)<br>• Finger Tapping Test (Heaton, Grant, et al., 2004)<br>• Grooved Pegboard Test (Heaton, Grant, et al., 2004) |
| Verbal functioning | • Expression<br>  • WAIS-IV Vocabulary (Wechsler, 2008)<br>  • Controlled Oral Word Association (COWA) (Heaton, Miller, Taylor, & Grant, 2004)<br>  • Boston Naming Test (Goodglass & Kaplan, 2000)<br>• Comprehension<br>  • WAIS-IV Verbal Comprehension Index (Wechsler, 2008) |
| Visuospatial functioning | • WAIS-IV Block Design (Wechsler, 2008)<br>• WAIS-IV Perceptual Reasoning Index (Wechsler, 2008)<br>• Rey Complex Figure Test—Copy (Meyers & Meyers, 1995)<br>• Bicycle Drawing Test (Lezak et al., 2004) |
| Memory | • Working memory<br>  • WAIS-IV Arithmetic (Wechsler, 2008)<br>  • WAIS-IV Letter–Number Sequencing (Wechsler, 2008)<br>  • WAIS-IV Digit Span (Wechsler, 2008)<br>  • WAIS-IV Coding (Wechsler, 2008)<br>  • WAIS-IV Working Memory Index (Wechsler, 2008)<br>  • WMS-IV Spatial Addition (Wechsler, 2009)<br>  • WMS-IV Visual Working Memory Index (Wechsler, 2009) |

*(cont.)*

**TABLE 2.1.** *(cont.)*

| Neuropsychological domain | Sample tests |
|---|---|
| | • Verbal memory<br>  • WAIS-IV Information (Wechsler, 2008)<br>  • CVLT-II (Delis et al., 2000)<br>  • WMS-IV Auditory Memory Index (Wechsler, 2009)<br>• Visual memory<br>  • Rey Complex Figure Test—Delayed Recognition and Recall (Meyers & Meyers, 1995)<br>  • Subtest 7 of the Category Test (Heaton, Grant, et al., 2004)<br>  • WMS-IV Visual Memory Index (Wechsler, 2009) |
| Concept formation | • Verbal<br>  • WAIS-IV Similarities (Wechsler, 2008)<br>  • CVLT-II Semantic Clustering (Delis et al., 2000)<br>• Visual<br>  • Wisconsin Card Sorting Test (WCST) (Heaton, 2003)<br>  • Category Test (Heaton, Grant, et al., 2004) |
| Reasoning | • Verbal<br>  • WAIS-IV Comprehension (Wechsler, 2008)<br>• Visuoperceptual<br>  • WAIS-IV Picture Completion (Wechsler, 2008)<br>  • WAIS-IV Block Design (Wechsler, 2008)<br>  • WAIS-IV Figure Weights (Wechsler, 2008)<br>  • WAIS-IV Visual Puzzles (Wechsler, 2008)<br>  • WAIS-IV Matrix Reasoning (Wechsler, 2008)<br>• Mathematical<br>  • WAIS-IV Arithmetic (Wechsler, 2008) |
| Executive functioning | • Organization/planning<br>  • Porteus mazes (Porteus, 1965)<br>  • Rey Complex Figure Test (Meyers & Meyers, 1995)<br>• Flexible problem solving<br>  • Trail Making Test, Part B (Heaton, Grant, et al., 2004)<br>  • COWA (Heaton, Miller, et al., 2004)<br>  • Ruff Figural Fluency Test (RFFT) (Ruff, 1996)<br>  • Tower of London (Culbertson & Zillmer, 2005)<br>• Effective performance<br>  • WCST (Heaton, 2003)<br>  • CVLT-II (Delis et al., 2000)<br>  • RFFT (Ruff, 1996)<br>  • Category test (Heaton, Grant, et al., 2004) |
| Awareness | • Patient Competency Rating Scale (Patient and Relatives' Forms) (Prigatano et al., 1986) |
| Personality composition and psychological distress | • Minnesota Multiphasic Personality Inventory–2 (MMPI-2; Butcher, 2005)<br>• Millon Clinical Multiaxial Inventory–III (MCMI-III; Millon, 2005) |
| Estimate of premorbid intelligence | • American National Adult Reading Test (Gladsjo, Heaton, Palmer, Taylor, & Jeste, 1999) |

The initial consultation provides a critical opportunity to assess the patient's neuropsychological and emotional status in order to make cogent recommendations, including possible goals of the psychotherapy process. If psychotherapy is to occur in the context of other treatment modalities, this consultation often provides valuable input regarding the patient's potential to benefit from other therapies.

Table 2.2 lists the relevant domains for inquiry during the initial consultation. These include demographics, social and medical history, injury-related data, subjective report of present status, and current medical treatment. Other key areas to assess are the patient's overall psychological/psychiatric status and the family's involvement.

---

### TABLE 2.2. Topics for the Initial Consultation

Demographics

- Age
- Gender
- Date and place of birth
- Educational history (grade/degree completed and academic status)
- Marital status (current and past) and current family composition
- Occupational history (overview of current and past jobs)
- Living situation and activities of daily living with level of independence

Social history

- Preinjury and current alcohol and drug use
- Preinjury legal problems (e.g., arrests)

Medical history

- Previous brain injury or disease (e.g., loss of consciousness, seizures, high fever)
- General medical history (systemic illness, comorbid disease)
- Prior medical and psychological treatments
- Prior medications

Injury-related data

- Circumstances of injury (date, location, and surrounding events; mechanism of injury; presence–absence of paramedics and/or hospitalization/surgery)
- Absence–presence of loss of consciousness and length of time
- Estimated period of posttraumatic amnesia
- Glasgow Coma Scale score
- Radiographic findings (computed tomography [CT] and/or magnetic resonance imaging [MRI])

Subjective report of post-injury status

- Current cognitive, language, and physical status
- Emotional status (e.g., anxiety, depression, self-harm)
- Sleep, appetite, and libido
- Driving status
- Use of strategies or compensations (e.g., datebook, pillbox)
- Presence–absence of litigation or financial disincentives

Current medical treatment

- Rehabilitation (overview and perception of proposed needs)
- Medical management (other medical services/practitioners involved)
- Medications, including psychotropics
- Medical complications (e.g., pain, seizures)

### *Preliminary Inquiry into Awareness, Acceptance, and Realism*

A primary goal of the initial consultation is to begin to ascertain the patient's current level of awareness, acceptance, and realism in regard to the injury sequelae. "Level of *awareness*" refers to the patient's understanding of deficit areas (see Chapter 3). Awareness affects the degree of motivation for psychotherapy and other treatment interventions. A preliminary overview of the patient's level of awareness of his or her difficulties is accomplished by asking open-ended questions about current problems in the physical/perceptual, cognitive/language, and emotional domains. During the discussion, the patient is asked to rate items in these three domains on a 10-point Deficit Rating Scale, with 0 representing no problem and 10 indicating a severe problem (see Figure 2.1). For patients who experience an absence of self-reported changes, specific questions can be asked (e.g., "Do you notice changes in your speed of thinking? How about your memory?"), followed by cautious inquiry into self-ratings. In order to encourage a sense of autonomy, the patient is asked first for his or her perceptions. Family members are then included in the exploration process, with an eye to evaluating the concordance versus dissimilarity of perceptions, as well as the patient's responsiveness (or lack thereof) to his or her family's input. Family members' ratings may differ significantly from the patient's, often ascribing greater degrees of impairment. In order for the patient not to feel "ambushed," the purpose of asking family members for their input is explained beforehand, including a proviso that their ratings may be different.

A rough index of *acceptance* is obtained by asking the patient about his or her willingness to employ new compensatory strategies, such as a detailed datebook system or procedural checklists (see Chapter 5). This also yields prognostic information about his or her "coachability" in acquiring new skills. A preliminary and general overview of the patient's level of *realism* is obtained by inquiring about career aspirations, driving status, and the capability to be unsupervised in the home and community (see Chapter 9). Family input on these topics is also beneficial.

The clinician must be astute to the particular distinctions between patients with more acute versus more chronic injuries. An acutely injured patient often struggles primarily with organic unawareness, convinced that he or she does not need intensive treatment and can simply return to his or her preinjury existence. A benchmark of readiness for change is a patient's voluntary identification of at least one area of nonphysical deficit that he or she will even tentatively consent to address (e.g., memory, depression). The combination of dawning awareness with the patient's voiced trust and motivation for the ensuing treatment process bodes well for a positive outcome.

Patients with more chronic injuries have generally encountered multiple "hard knocks" in attempts to successfully regain their former independence and quality of life. They are more aware, at least on a basic level, of some of their deficits and the potential advantages of treatment. However, these individuals tend to struggle more in the domain of acceptance and realism. Their life aspirations tend to be a poor match with their neurological status. They have also often developed entrenched inefficient or otherwise unhelpful ways of compensating for their deficits, which need to be supplanted with more efficient compensations. In this

Ask the patient, followed by a significant other, to provide *oral* ratings of the domains below. Use the following scale: 0 = no problem; 1 = small (mild) problem; 5 = medium (moderate) problem; 10 = large (severe) problem.

| Domain | Patient | Significant Other |
|---|---|---|
| **Physical/perceptual** | | |
| Weakness | | |
| Coordination | | |
| Visual neglect | | |
| Double vision | | |
| Headaches | | |
| **Cognitive/language** | | |
| Memory | | |
| Attention and concentration | | |
| Speed of thinking | | |
| Reasoning and problem solving | | |
| Organization | | |
| Multitasking | | |
| Impulsivity | | |
| Language comprehension | | |
| Language expression | | |
| Reading | | |
| Writing | | |
| Spelling | | |
| Arithmetic | | |
| **Emotional** | | |
| Frustration | | |
| Depression | | |
| Feeling overwhelmed | | |
| Irritability | | |
| Distrust | | |

**FIGURE 2.1.** Deficit Rating Scale.

case, the psychotherapist will explore the patient's openness to trying new compensations (e.g., a datebook). It is a positive sign for effective collaboration when these patients express even cautious receptivity to new interventions. Therefore, the clinician must gain an overall appreciation of the patient's capacity for change, regardless of the multitude of areas to be addressed.

## Overall Psychological and Psychiatric Status

During the initial consultation, the clinician is on a discovery course to gain an initial sense of the patient's general pre- and postinjury psychological and psychosocial status. This is accomplished by empathic inquiry, with "clinical eyes" on how the individual tolerates preliminary questioning, including the extent to which he or she can disclose pertinent and personal information. For example, does the individual become annoyed or defensive early in the interview when asked about preinjury individual and family psychiatric history, work performance, or problems with the law? Guardedness, evasiveness, suspiciousness, or irritability in regard to this type of inquiry constitutes a potential warning sign that the patient may be too easily overwhelmed or emotionally brittle to tolerate or benefit from an insight-oriented, psychoeducational approach. However, even when encountering preliminary trepidations or resistance (i.e., PEM "yellow" [warning zone] behavior; see Figure 1.2), the psychotherapist should try to develop rapport with the patient and not make too quick a presumption that the patient cannot benefit from psychotherapy. Over time, the commitment to the psychotherapy process can evolve (i.e., PEM "green" [coping zone] behavior).

Often patients arrive at the initial consultation interview in considerable emotional distress, or even, in crisis. Possible symptoms of depression should be explored, such as feelings of helplessness, hopelessness, and joylessness. It is essential to inquire into such a patient's current (and past) intentions of self-harm. Access to firearms should be determined. The psychotherapist must have a protocol for immediate intervention, should the patient present with either overt or covert signs of suicidal risk. Preferably, the therapist should have a professional relationship with a psychiatrist who can intervene or provide appropriate consultation, as well as a list of appropriate emergency treatment options or settings.

Patients should also be asked directly about preexisting substance use patterns. Total abstinence from alcohol and street drugs is a requirement for psychotherapy in my practice. These substances directly interfere with active rehabilitation and neurological recovery; they also increase the likelihood of medical complications, such as seizure disorders (see Lezak et al., 2004, for a review; see also Sparadeo, 1993). Alcohol and street drugs also cloud judgment and affect other capacities (e.g., impulse control, problem solving, and balance) that are important to the patient's safety. Furthermore, postinjury problems with depression, anxiety, suicidality, and psychosocial adjustment are increased in patients with substance abuse histories (Felde, Westermeyer, & Thuras, 2006; Klonoff & Lage, 1995; MacMillan, Hart, Martelli, & Zasler, 2002; Mainio et al., 2007; Wagner, Hammond, Sasser, & Wiercisiewski, 2002). Because the psychotherapist has reviewed the medical records in advance, he or she will generally be aware of preexisting problems. The patient's and family's candid disclosure of this information demonstrates the willingness for honest dialogue and personal ownership. Patients with a preexisting substance abuse history must agree to random urinalyses as part of their psychotherapy, be open to psychiatric treatment and/or concurrent substance abuse counseling, and commit to disclosing possible relapses.

The psychotherapist should also be alert to a patient's possible attempts to consciously exaggerate symptomatology for purposes of secondary gain (Millis, 2008; Rogers, 2005). Motivational problems will undermine progress within a psychotherapeutic relationship founded on improving the patient's adjustment, especially when a goal of therapy is working toward gainful employment (Klonoff & Lamb, 1998).

In general, the initial consultation is aimed at helping the psychotherapist begin to differentiate the patient's underlying neurobehavioral difficulties, preinjury psychiatric status, and postinjury motivations and emotional reactions. This differentiation provides a basis for developing meaningful psychotherapeutic interventions (Prigatano et al., 1986).

### *Family Involvement*

Family members (or the members of a patient's support network) often experience overwhelming bewilderment and anguish about their loved one's condition and prognosis. In this context, part of the initial consultation is to evaluate the psychological status of the family members and their capacity to collaborate with the psychotherapist and patient. Considerations include their commitment to physically attend regular family sessions and/or a family group (see Chapter 7). Active involvement is the foundation for necessary psychoeducation and emotional support, without which their loved one will flounder. The family members' demeanor, verbalizations, and style of interaction with the patient during the consultation will also provide a preliminary indication of their general psychological health and aptitude for developing a positive working alliance, including comfort and frankness in sharing. This sets the stage for later progress in setting and achieving psychotherapeutic goals, and for improving family adjustment and harmony.

At the end of the initial consultation with the patient and family, all parties decide on the advisability of continuing the dialogue process. Typically, the next step is to agree to a finite number of sessions (e.g., two to six) to further explore the patient's (and family's) psychological status and needs, and to gain a better appreciation for the patient's and family's capacity to develop a working alliance. For a variety of reasons, the parties may decide not to continue with treatment, and the psychotherapist should then provide information about other appropriate treatment resources in the community. If psychotherapy seems feasible, the psychotherapist arranges one or more follow-up appointments to conduct a more in-depth interview.

## THE IN-DEPTH INTERVIEW PROCESS

When a patient is a likely candidate for psychotherapy, the therapist conducts a more in-depth interview, with an emphasis on gaining a more holistic perspective of the patient. This process may take a few sessions, which constitute the beginning of the psychotherapy. These sessions should further the collaboration. There are three components to this process: a preinjury psychosocial history; a comprehensive exploration of the patient's impressions of his or her current neurological/neurobehavioral status; and early goal setting.

## The Preinjury Psychosocial History

The psychosocial history is integral to further exploring the patient's preinjury behaviors, interests, psychological constructs, and interpersonal relationships. It is often striking how much suffering patients have experienced prior to their neurological event. Discovering their prior life events allows interpretation of present feelings and behaviors in the context of these events and gives insight into the preinjury coping style. The latter is a predictor of psychological readiness for the psychoeducation process and eventual postinjury adjustment (Lewis & Rosenberg, 1990). Taking a psychosocial history also facilitates clinical observations of a patient's capacity for trust—a fundamental precursor to any substantive progress in the psychotherapeutic process.

There are various approaches to taking a psychosocial history. Some psychotherapists prefer structured interviews for increased reliability and validity (Groth-Marnat, 2003; Karg & Wiens, 2005). The disadvantages are that these may constrain the flow and spontaneity of the interview process, and may make patients feel that they are being interrogated, or that the psychotherapist is merely on a fact-finding mission. Likewise, some psychotherapists have patients complete a lengthy questionnaire prior to the first appointment. This can seem impersonal or even intrusive, especially when patients are asked to recount in writing troubling personal history, outside of an empathic treatment ambience.

I prefer to take a semistructured approach—that is, to cover a list of topic areas by asking open-ended questions (see Table 2.3). This approach offers flexibility, encourages patients to tell their stories, and heightens rapport (Groth-Marnat, 2003; Roter, Cole, Kern, Barker, & Grayson, 1990). The open-ended questions also allow a psychotherapist to walk in a patient's shoes. Yalom (2002) describes the process of taking a history as intuitive and automatic—as *part of* therapy, not *preceding* therapy. Helpful adjunct approaches include comments to encourage the flow of conversation and asking for more specifics (Groth-Marnat, 2003).

It is worth noting that exploration of the patient's past often happens over time, and that the past may well be revisited intermittently as part of the psychotherapy process. Often only later in therapy do patients reveal personal details of their lives that heretofore they were ashamed or frightened to share. This only serves to empower the working alliance. For example, a male patient who suffered a traumatic brain injury felt depressed and emotionally detached from his teenage sons. Once the working alliance solidified, he shared a long-kept secret: He had been the victim of severe beatings and horrifying sexual abuse by his father, which had always interfered with his ability to become emotionally involved with and attuned to his own sons. This history was a powerful declaration, which enhanced the course of treatment by bridging the neurological, historical, and interpersonal realms.

**TABLE 2.3. Topics for a Detailed Psychosocial History**

Social history

*Topics*
1. Family history (including parents' and siblings' occupational, medical, and psychiatric health)
2. Childhood experiences and traumas
3. Preinjury psychiatric diagnoses and treatment
4. Preinjury financial status
5. Preinjury hobbies and interests

*Sample inquiries*
1. Which parent are/were you closer to and why?
2. How would you describe your home life while you were growing up?
3. How did your childhood experiences/traumas affect you while you were growing up? How do they affect you currently?
4. How was your experience of any prior psychiatric/psychological counseling? Did it help (and if so, how)?
5. How did any prior financial burdens affect you?
6. Why did you choose to get involved in certain hobbies?
7. What was your favorite pasttime and why?

Developmental and educational history

*Topics*
1. Developmental history (prenatal or postnatal complications; developmental delays in walking, talking, etc.)
2. Academic strengths and difficulties; learning and/or behavioral problems in school

*Sample inquiries*
1. How did any early health problems affect you and your family?
2. Did you like school? Why or why not?
3. What was your favorite/least favorite class and why?
4. How did you behave in school?

Occupational history

*Topics*
1. Occupational history (including major job fields, job transiency, and occupational problems)

*Sample inquiries*
1. Why did you choose this (these) occupation(s)?
2. What was your favorite job and why?
3. What was the most difficult aspect of your job?
4. How did you get along with your supervisors and coworkers?
5. How were your performance evaluations and why?
6. Were you ever terminated from a job? If so, why?

Subjective report of postinjury status

*Topics*
1. More detailed exploration of cognitive, physical, language, emotional, and interpersonal problems
2. Perception of course of recovery—improvement versus deterioration
3. Family relationships
4. Hobbies, interests, and socialization
5. Perception of work capacity
6. Goals and aspirations for the future

*(cont.)*

**TABLE 2.3.** *(cont.)*

*Sample inquiries*
 1. How do your (cognitive, physical, etc.) problems manifest themselves from day to day?
 2. Do you ever feel hopeless about the future, as if there is no reason to go on?
 3. How do you feel about your recovery—its pace and timing?
 4. How is your family reacting to/handling your circumstances?
 5. Are you happy with your current involvement in hobbies?
 6. How is your social life going and why?
 7. What do you miss most currently?
 8. What is your current impression of your work abilities?
 9. What occupation do you want to pursue and when?
10. How do you see yourself in the next 6 to 12 months?

Table 2.3 lists the areas to be explored in taking a detailed psychosocial history. These include social history, developmental and educational history, and past occupational history. Some sample questions are included; however, the clinician is cautioned to follow the flow of the unfolding process, rather than adhere to a predetermined script. Overall, these early sessions signal the patient's capacity to share information.

## Patients' Impressions of Their Current Neurological/Neurobehavioral Status

Exploration of patients' current frustrations, desires, and ambitions is central to the early sessions. The therapist should query patients in more depth about their impressions of cognitive, physical, language, emotional, and interpersonal problems, including their perceived course and pace of recovery. Other topics include assets and challenges within a patient's family and support network; the presence or absence of meaningful postinjury hobbies and outlets; and the patient's ideas about work. Table 2.3 also contains some sample questions for these domains. This inquiry is in part a precursor to a more in-depth evaluation of the patient's degree of awareness, which is discussed further in Chapter 3.

## Early Goal Setting

In collaboration, the psychotherapist and patient identify initial treatment goals; again, this is a gradual process. The therapist should note that patients' (and families') current levels of awareness, acceptance, and realism are further revealed by inquiry into their expected time frames for goal completion. In general, the benefits of psychotherapy often take many months to manifest themselves, and patients (as well as families) often underestimate the amount of time and energy that they will need.

Preliminary goal setting can generate the necessary commitment and momentum for change. It is recommended that the agreed-upon goals be explicit and concrete (e.g., 12 sessions to address catastrophic reactions and improve awareness). The patient needs to have an unambiguous understanding of the purpose of the psychotherapy. This is particularly crucial with this population, given the influence of memory, language, and executive function deficits, and the prevalence of organic unawareness. The family members should be included in the dialogue about initial goal setting, to maximize their "buy-in."

The initial goals of therapy should be made realistically attainable, to avoid creating undue frustration and disenchantment in the patient. This requires the psychotherapist to have a sufficient working knowledge of the nature and extent of the patient's organically based deficits. Specific subgoals with anticipated time frames should also be developed. For example, if a patient is adjusting to a new work environment, it is helpful to propose a 6- to 8-week period to monitor mood and adjustment. Specific markers should be identified, including positive work reviews and self-ratings of psychological well-being. These mutually chosen benchmarks of progress will help the therapist and patient determine whether psychotherapy is succeeding. Later chapters explore the distinctive approaches and techniques for goal setting in the context of awareness, acceptance, self-identity, realism, and social reintegration.

Overall, the above-described interview techniques and clinical observations provide a mechanism for contemplating and embarking upon the psychotherapy process.

## GENERAL TREATMENT CONSIDERATIONS

The following treatment considerations are recommended for accommodating the common cognitive, psychological, and interpersonal sequelae after acquired brain injury. These recommendations should be tailored to the needs of each patient, of course.

### Structure, Regimen, and Accountability

The broader goals of psychotherapy with brain-injured patients are improved relationships and a return to productive status. Therefore, the context of therapy should emulate the context of healthy real-world relationships. It is most effectual to impose a level of structure (Judd & Wilson, 2005), regimen, and accountability within the psychotherapeutic relationship. Given patients' memory, auditory processing, and comprehension problems, therapy expectations and their rationale should be introduced in a written contract format along with in-session explanations (see Figure 2.2). The contract should be reviewed with the patient prior to the formal initiation of treatment. For example, the patient should be informed in writing about the purposes, risks, and benefits of psychotherapy; the frequency, length, and location of appointments; expectations regarding homework; fees, insurance reimbursement, and payment requirements; limits of confidentiality; record-keeping protocols; cancellation policies; and ways to contact the psychotherapist after hours in case of an emotional crisis or other emergency. It is advisable to have the patient sign this document, indicating that he or she has read and understands this information. The family members involved in the treatment process should also be aware of this information, to avoid confusion about the nature and purpose of the psychotherapy process.

[Insert your professional name,
address,
phone,
fax,
and e-mail address]

## Outpatient Services Contract

Welcome to my practice. This document contains very important information about how I conduct my professional practice and business policies. Please read it carefully and make notes on any questions you might have, so that we can discuss them. Once you sign this document, it will reflect that you have read and fully understood the contents, and that it will constitute a binding agreement between us.

## Psychological Services

The process of psychotherapy is not easily defined or described. The nature of the process varies, depending on a number of factors—including the training and experience of the therapist, the personalities of all parties involved, and the particular problems that a patient brings forth to work on. It is not like visiting a medical doctor, because it requires you to take a very active, participating role. To gain the most benefit from psychotherapy, you will need to work both during the sessions and at home.

Psychotherapy involves both risks and benefits. The risks include possibly experiencing uncomfortably strong feelings, such as sadness, frustration, guilt, anger, anxiety, loneliness, and helplessness. To be successful, psychotherapy also often requires recalling and talking about unpleasant events in the past. However, psychotherapy has also been shown to benefit those who undertake it: There is often a reduction in feelings of distress, resolution of specific problems, or an improvement in significant relationships. However, these are not guarantees about what will happen.

Entering into a psychotherapeutic relationship is a decision that requires serious thought and commitment. Therapy involves a great amount of time, money, and energy, so you should be very careful about the therapist you decide to work with. I would ask that you commit to coming in for two sessions, during which we will have the opportunity to evaluate one another and make an informed decision about continuing further with psychotherapy. At the end of that evaluation period, I will be able to provide you with some initial impressions of what our therapy should include and a beginning treatment plan, if you should decide to continue and enter into a professional relationship. If you have questions about my approach or procedures, we should discuss them whenever they arise. At the end of the evaluation or at any time thereafter, if you should have significant doubts or wish to discontinue treatment, I will be happy to help you obtain an appropriate consultation with another mental health professional.

## Meetings

If we both agree to begin psychotherapy, I typically schedule one 45-minute session each week at a mutually agreed-upon time. Sometimes sessions will be longer or more frequent, as your needs dictate and as we agree upon. Once this appointment hour is scheduled, you will be expected to pay for it unless you provide 24 hours' notice of cancellation, or unless we agree that you were unable to attend because of circumstances beyond your control.

*(cont.)*

**FIGURE 2.2.** Outpatient services contract.

## Professional Fees

My fee is _____ per 45-minute treatment session. In addition to weekly appointments, it is my practice to charge this amount on a prorated basis for other required professional services (such as report writing or telephone conversations) that last longer than 10 minutes; attendance at meetings or consultations with other professionals that you have authorized; preparation of records or treatment summaries; or time required to perform any other service that you may request of me. At times, patients become involved in legal proceedings that may require my participation. If this should occur, you will be expected to pay for the professional time required to prepare for such an event, even if I am compelled to testify by another party. Because of the complexity and difficulty of litigation, I charge _____ per hour in preparation for and attendance at any legal proceedings.

## Billing and Payments

You will be expected to pay for each session at the time it is held, unless we agree otherwise or you have insurance coverage that requires another arrangement. Payment schedules for other professional services will be agreed upon at the time the services are requested. In circumstances of financial hardship, you have the option to fill out our Sliding Scale Fee Reduction Application, in which my billing company will review and set a fee based upon the U.S. Department of Health and Human Services poverty guidelines.

    If you are using insurance to reimburse me for my professional services, once we have all the information concerning your insurance coverage, we will discuss what we can expect to accomplish with the available benefits and what will happen if those benefits run out before you feel ready to end our sessions. You should also remember that you always have the right to pay for the services yourself and avoid the complexities involved with many insurance claims. If your account is more than 60 days past due and suitable payment arrangements have not been agreed upon, I have the option of using legal means to secure payment, including collection agencies or small-claims court. In such cases, usually the only information I release about a client's treatment would be the client's name, the nature of services provided, and the amount due. Even if this circumstance should come about, I will provide you with referral sources to deal with your treatment needs.

## Insurance Reimbursement

In order to set realistic treatment goals and priorities, it is important to evaluate what resources are available to pay for your treatment. If you have a health benefits policy, it will usually provide some coverage for psychotherapy through mental health benefits. You should carefully read the section in your insurance coverage booklet that describes mental health services. If you have any questions, please call your plan and inquire. Of course, I will provide you with whatever information I can, based on my experience, and will be happy to try to help you understand the information you receive from your carrier. I am willing to call the carrier on your behalf, if this is necessary to resolve any confusion. I will also provide assistance in filling out any necessary forms, as appropriate. However, you, and not your insurance company, are responsible for full payment of the fee to which we have agreed. Therefore, it is very important that you find out exactly what mental health services your insurance policy covers.

    The increasing concern and debate over the cost of health care have resulted in increasing levels of complexity in insurance benefit programs, to the point that it is sometimes difficult to determine exactly how much mental health coverage is available. Managed health care plans, such as health maintenance organizations (HMOs) and preferred provider organizations (PPOs), often require advance authorization before providing reimbursement for mental health services. Such plans are often oriented toward a short-term treatment approach that is designed to resolve specific problems interfering with a person's overall level of functioning. In my experience, while much can

*(cont.)*

**FIGURE 2.2.** *(page 2 of 4)*

be accomplished in such short-term therapy, many clients feel that more services are necessary after insurance benefits expire. It may therefore be necessary to seek additional approval for a certain number of sessions. Be aware that some HMOs and PPOs do not allow for additional services once your benefits are no longer available.

You must also realize that most insurance agreements require you to authorize me to provide them with a clinical diagnosis and, at times, additional clinical information (such as a treatment plan or summary). In rare cases, such agreements require them to obtain a copy of the entire treatment record. This information will become part of the insurance company's files, and in all probability some of it will be computerized. All insurance companies claim to keep such information confidential, but once it is in their hands, I have no control over what they do with it. In some cases, they may share the information with a national medical information databank. If you request it, I will provide you with a copy of any report that I submit to them.

## Contacting Me

I am often not immediately available by phone. Although I am usually at work between 8 A.M. and 5 P.M., the bulk of this time is spent in treatment with patients, and I usually will not answer the phone when in a treatment session. However, during those hours someone is almost always available to take a message at (000) 000-0000. Outside of the above-mentioned hours, there is an answering machine available at this number, and the messages are checked every workday morning. If you are difficult to reach, please leave times when you will be available, so that I can return your call as promptly as possible. In case of an emergency, call the hospital operator at (000) 000-0000 and inform them that it is an emergency. The operator will then page me. If you cannot reach me, and you feel you cannot wait for me to return your call, you should call your family physician or go to the nearest emergency room and ask for the psychiatrist who is on call. If I am unavailable for an extended time, I will provide you with a name of a trusted colleague whom you may contact if necessary.

## Professional Records

Both the law and the ethical code of my profession require that I maintain appropriate treatment records. You are entitled to receive a copy of these records. However, because they are professional records and may be misinterpreted and/or can be upsetting, if you wish I can prepare an appropriate summary that will provide the level of detail necessary for your purposes. If you wish to see your records, I recommend that we view them together, so that we will have the opportunity to discuss what they contain. There will be an appropriate fee charged for any preparation time required to comply with any information requests.

## Minors

If you are under 18 years of age, please be aware that the law provides your parents with the right to examine your treatment records. It is my policy to request an agreement from parents for their consent to give up access to your records. If they agree, I only provide general information on how your treatment is proceeding, unless I feel there is a legitimate reason to do otherwise. For example, if there is a high risk that you will seriously harm yourself or another person, or I learn of child abuse, pregnancy, or serious drug use, I will notify them of these concerns. I will also provide them with a summary of your treatment when it is complete. Before giving them any information, I will discuss the matter with you and do my best to resolve any objections you may have about what I am prepared to discuss with them.

*(cont.)*

**FIGURE 2.2.** *(page 3 of 4)*

## Confidentiality

In general, the confidentiality of all communications between a client and a psychologist is protected by law, and I can only release information about our work to others with your written permission. However, there are some exceptions.

In most judicial proceedings, you have the right to prevent me from providing any information about your treatment. However, in some circumstances—such as a child custody proceeding, or proceedings where your emotional condition has been determined to be an important element—a judge may require my testimony if he or she determines that the resolution of such issues demands it.

There are some situations in which I am legally required to take action to protect others from harm, even though this action may reveal some information about a client's treatment.

1. If I believe that a child, an elderly person, or a disabled person is being abused, I must file a report with the appropriate state agency.

2. If I believe a client is threatening serious bodily harm to another, I am required to take protective actions, which may include notifying the potential victim, notifying the police, or seeking appropriate hospitalization.

3. If a client threatens to harm him- or herself, I may be required to seek hospitalization for the client or to contact family members or significant others who can help provide protection.

These first three situations have rarely arisen in my practice. However, should such a situation occur, I will make every effort to fully discuss it with you before taking any action.

4. I occasionally find it helpful to consult about a case with other professionals. In these consultations, although I make every effort to avoid revealing the identity of my patient, this cannot be guaranteed. Also, the consultant is legally bound to keep all information confidential. Unless you object, I will not tell you about these consultations unless I feel it is important in our work together.

Although this written summary of exceptions to confidentiality should prove helpful in informing you about potential problems, it is important that we discuss any questions or concerns you may have at our next meeting. As you might suspect, the laws governing these issues are quite complex, and I am not an attorney. While I am happy to discuss these issues, a formal consultation with an attorney may be desirable if you feel you need specific legal advice.

Your signature below indicates that you have read the information in this document and agree to abide by its terms during our professional relationship.

_____     _____
Signature                                                                              Date

_____     _____
Psychotherapist's Name                                                          Date

**FIGURE 2.2.**  *(page 4 of 4)*

Once the treatment process begins, the relationship progresses most smoothly when both parties are conscientious about punctuality and follow through on agreed-upon assignments. This serves to provide a reassuring and secure foundation for the intensive work of psychotherapy, and at the same time conveys that all parties have made a mutual and earnest commitment. The frequency of appointments is agreed upon, based on the psychological and practical needs of the patients. As goals are met, increased spacing of appointments (e.g., from weekly to twice monthly to once monthly) assists in preparing for the termination process and eases patients into new routines.

## Timing and Pacing of Feedback

Patients often feel a sense of emotional vulnerability and fragility after acquired brain injury. Many if not most of their suppositions and aspirations in life are shattered. Therefore, introducing feedback to improve a patient's awareness, acceptance, and realism requires careful timing and pacing. It is imperative that the psychotherapist be judicious about how much, when, how, and in what context the psychoeducation process unfolds. This often necessitates picking one's battles, chunking the feedback into digestible subcomponents, and engaging the patient in dialogue about his or her emotional state. In general, new information can be perceived as troubling or even shocking, particularly in the context of organic unawareness. It should first be shared within a private session with the patient, rather than in a more public forum, such as a group setting. The psychotherapist should also try to avoid introducing emotionally laden and potentially disturbing topics on Fridays; otherwise, patients' rigidity, perseveration, and depression will tend to erupt over weekends. It is best to introduce unsettling material when a patient is emotionally calm and most logical— in other words, "striking when the iron is cold" (Yalom, 2002, p. 121).

## Collateral Data and the "Advisory Board"

Giving patients collateral data in the form of feedback from family members, patient peers, successful "graduates" from the psychotherapy process, employers, coworkers, and friends provides powerful elucidation and reinforcement of treatment principles (Klonoff et al., 2008; Klonoff, Lamb, Henderson, Reichert, et al., 2000). Telling stories about other patients with similar challenges or treatment impasses is also highly effective (Prigatano & Klonoff, 1988).

Often a psychotherapist can encourage a patient to develop a personal "advisory board," made up of trustworthy confidants who will share honest and constructive feedback. This becomes especially necessary during life episodes (both within and outside of treatment) in regard to which the patient questions or discounts therapeutic input. Ideally, as the working alliance builds, the patient begins to consider the psychotherapist as a valued member of his or her advisory board.

## Psychoeducation and Directiveness

Because of patients' deficits in executive functions, attention, concentration, and memory, psychotherapists generally must take a more directive and information-dispensing approach in their interventions (Klonoff, 1997; Prigatano & Klonoff, 1988; Whitehouse, 1994). This provides the structure, forethought, and guidance necessary for patients to plan and execute goals, including plotting their psychological course of action. However, a psychotherapist's role is to assist patients, not to dictate to them or usurp their right to personal choice and self-determination. Generally, a therapist supplies useful exercises and facilitates dialogue to assist a patient with conceptualization, problem solving, goal setting, and execution. The psychotherapist must then closely monitor the patient's progress toward achieving goals and adapt the therapeutic approach to meet the patient's evolving needs or tribulations.

## Note Taking and Journal Keeping

Note taking is integral to the psychotherapeutic process after brain injury (Klonoff, 1997; Kortte, Hill-Briggs, & Wegener, 2005; Whitehouse, 1994). A patient arriving for a session without a notebook is like a marathon runner arriving for a race without running shoes; it is possible to run long distances in bare feet, but not desirable or effectual. Some psychotherapists may argue that note taking detracts from the dialogue process; however, in my clinical experience, note taking is vital for these patients. It helps them acquire the ability to summarize, synthesize, and eventually integrate the content of discussions.

Note taking should occur at intervals during a session when it appears appropriate to stop and summarize a discussion, or alternatively at the end of the session. Deciding how and when a patient should take notes requires clinical acumen, flexibility, and practicality. In general, the more severe the patient's cognitive deficits are, the more frequent the breaks to take notes should be, and the more assistance the patient will require to formulate and record the salient points. Often patients need help determining where and how to take notes, and what notes to take. For example, patients with aphasia or higher-level abstract reasoning difficulties often have difficulty deducing main ideas and/or formulating them into coherent, concise, and cohesive bullet points. Therefore, the psychotherapist may need to dictate some notes to serve as examples. Patients with executive function deficits may need cueing as to where in their notebooks to place the notes, as well as how to keep notes in chronological order. In cases where a patient is unable to write because of motor or vision deficits, the psychotherapist needs to take the notes him- or herself (often on a computer, to facilitate their readability).

At the beginning of sessions, time should often be taken to revisit previous discussions by reviewing notes, even if the therapist has to read them to the patient (Klonoff, 1997; Langenbahn et al., 1999; Whitehouse, 1994). This is especially important for patients with severe memory problems, who have discontinuous, fragmented, confabulated, or no recollection of prior events. The written record also allows a patient to review previous discussions outside of formal sessions, providing a permanent source for reconstruction of previous dialogue. Asking the patient to look over notes at the outset of sessions and summarize the main points also provides a useful cognitive exercise and practice with abstraction and deductive thinking. A patient who is comfortable with doing so can be encouraged to share psychotherapy notes with relevant family members, to help them gain insight into their loved one's postinjury psychological constructs and challenges. This enhances the support system's capacity to empathically relate to the patient. Often patients share that they have later gone back and reviewed their notes during troubling periods, and have found solace and guidance in doing so.

Yalom (2002) describes the process of "cyclotherapy," wherein themes in psychotherapy are continually revisited in order to deepen the process of exploration and revelation. Therefore, patients who are experiencing intense emotional distress or resistance also benefit greatly from note taking, as it allows a healthy "breather" in the discussion and provides the opportunity to write down major concepts and insights that can later be further digested and explored. For patients who have a tendency to distort or misinterpret feedback, structured note taking also serves as a useful therapeutic tool to keep the discussion on track, neutral, and clarified.

A patient who is capable of keeping a journal can be encouraged to use this tool between appointments. It provides a wealth of information to the psychotherapist regarding the patient's experiences, thoughts, and feelings, especially in the context of forgetfulness. Stream-of-consciousness journal entries also enhance self-reflection and an unhindered flow of ideas, which might be censored within the therapy room (Kerner & Fitzpatrick, 2007).

### "Rehab Lingo"

"Rehab lingo," or user-friendly language, can greatly enhance the acceptability of feedback to patients. For example, when describing problems with irritability or agitation, I might use the expression "snarky"; this is less jarring and confrontative, and preserves the working alliance. Similarly, instead of using a sterile neuropsychological term such as "mental flexibility," it is better to say "going with the flow" or "shifting gears." Patients and families are more inclined to appreciate the positive intent of feedback when it is more colloquial and "softer" in its presentation. Using terminology that is germane to the patient's personal lifestyle and lexicon helps make the process more tolerable and "speaks" to the patient. For example, a piano player with impulse control problems was encouraged to "set a slower speed" on his "internal metronome" to better gauge his reactions.

### Slogans and Mantras

Slogans or catchy phrases assist patients in priming their psychological energies (Sherer, Oden, Bergloff, Levin, & High, 1998). These tag phrases handily cue patients in a more engaging manner. For example, "Just do it" reminds patients of the need for initiative, ingenuity, and task execution.

Mantras are useful tools to maintain patients' focus on their treatment priorities and goals. A mantra usually consists of a word or phrase symbolizing pertinent challenges and aspirations. Mantras also encapsulate main guiding principles for patients' day-to-day happiness and stability. Daily mantras are particularly helpful for patients with severe memory problems, who benefit from brief and frequent therapeutic reminders. Examples include "I think I can, I think I can" (Piper, 1986) in instances where patients display self-doubt, and "Silence is golden" for difficulties with hyperverbality. The mantra should be written and placed in an accessible location for patients to refer to as often as possible (e.g., in the front of the datebook, or posted at home on a mirror or refrigerator door). The wording and concepts contained in mantras should be tailored to the particular patient and based on his or her interests, culture, and lifestyle. They are most often discovered through psychotherapeutic dialogue, and implemented conjointly and enthusiastically by the psychotherapist and the patient. They can also serve as comfortable and empowering cueing devices for family members.

## Metaphors

Metaphors are other potent mechanisms for illustrating principles on a symbolic and figurative level. They also provide practice for patients in less concrete, more abstract thinking (Sherer et al., 1998). Like mantras, metaphors should be meaningful to each individual patient and based on his or her unique background, preferences, and circumstances. For example, when a patient who was a wood craftsman terminated treatment and moved to a different state to attend a university, he was presented with a "new tool kit" of principles and coping mechanisms from the psychotherapy sessions that he could access and apply to his new life.

## Diagrams and Drawings

Diagrams and drawings are personal favorites of mine for illustrating and elucidating principles and issues that arise during the psychotherapy process. Like many other techniques described above, they are instrumental for patients with deficits in executive functions (e.g., abstraction and seeing the "big picture") and memory. Diagrams and drawings provide concrete and accessible ways to conceptualize and synthesize issues (Kortte et al., 2005; Langenbahn et al., 1999; Prigatano & Klonoff, 1988). For example, Figure 2.3 is a beautiful visual depiction of the power of the working alliance and collaborative process; it can remind patients in times of turmoil and disillusionment that their therapists and support networks are partners in their journey of recovery. Or a staircase diagram can help remind patients that the recovery process is gradual and stepwise. Like mantras and metaphors, diagrams and drawings need to be customized to each patient.

## Additional Psychotherapy Exercises and Complementary Media

Additional psychotherapy exercises can include constructing lists of pros and cons or pie charts to help with decision making, and writing essays to expand, reinforce, and integrate psychotherapeutic constructs. Such exercises are powerful vehicles for dialogue and help guide a patient's self-reflection and adaptation. They can be conducted in either individual or group psychotherapy. Complementary media, including books, journal articles, movies, art, and music, are all core tools. Further examples are given in later chapters.

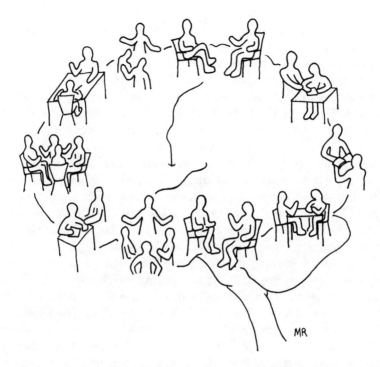

**FIGURE 2.3.** A drawing depicting the power of the working alliance and collaborative process for patients with brain injury.

## COORDINATION OF CARE

Given the variety of injury sequelae, patients with brain injury typically benefit from a team approach that coordinates care and treats the patients holistically. This approach can also benefit a psychotherapist, as it introduces the expertise of multiple specialists and thus lessens the therapist's burden of responsibilities. For example, a speech–language pathologist or occupational therapist can provide "nuts-and-bolts" training for a patient in using a datebook system in the home and school or work environments, enabling the psychotherapist to focus some of his or her energies on increasing the patient's psychological acceptance of the tool.

In addition, cotreatment and close coordination of services should result in the reinforcement of primary therapeutic principles by multiple specialists, which will provide validation and support for the psychotherapist's efforts. Naturally, such coordination will require the formation of liaisons with the referring rehabilitation physician, neurologist, psychiatrist, and so forth. It is important to remember that the patients' motivation and willingness to pursue their psychotherapy and broader rehabilitation goals will depend to a great extent upon the purposeful and collegial interaction of all therapists and physicians involved in the treatment process. When the professionals function synergetically, pooling their knowledge and working collaboratively toward the recovery of each patient as a whole individual, the treatment process is generally most efficacious (Klonoff et al., 2003).

Patients' outcomes can only be as good as the energies, harmony, vision, and ideals of the professionals who are guiding the process.

The psychotherapist sometimes functions as a team leader and may carry unique responsibilities and wear multiple "hats": those of an administrator; a personnel manager; a cognitive therapist; the "psychotherapist at near distance" for the patients he or she treats directly; and a "psychotherapist at far distance" for those he or she consults for. Core skills include empathy, open-mindedness, flexibility, hope, vision, and optimism—all expressed not only in work with the patients and families, but also in interactions with team members. These qualities, of course, must be tempered by a realistic and pragmatic "game plan," with an orientation toward the development of achievable goals. At the same time, the team leader should have a "cosmic view," with the internal capacity to envision and be appropriately decisive about the best course of action. He or she must then galvanize and support the team, patients, and families to accomplish goals in a stepwise manner, minimizing unwarranted misdirection. Moreover, the team leader's ability to understand and explain the underlying psychodynamics between the patients and therapists, in conjunction with how these play out within the team dynamics (Hartman, 1971), will help to integrate the team. The team leader can bolster the therapists' commitment and energy reserves through demonstrating a strong sense of loyalty toward and advocacy for the team. His or her guidance and insights are instrumental when the team is considering complex psychological and compliance issues, which can be particularly stressful and unnerving. Finally, when the psychotherapist conducts regular staff meetings, time should be allocated for introspective dialogue and replenishment of the team's emotional resources; doing so will increase the collective momentum and promote effective goal setting for the patients.

## THE REIMBURSEMENT PROCESS

Depending on the country, region, or state where they reside, patients being referred for psychotherapy may need a physician's prescription for such therapy to ensure reimbursement. Reimbursement for psychotherapy after brain injury either can be embedded in overall payment for a program of outpatient therapies, or can be paid directly to a psychotherapist as part of a private practice. In situations where the psychotherapist is functioning as part of a treatment team, it is preferable to include services for psychotherapy as part of the full complement of services within overall contractual arrangements; psychotherapy services are typically billed as part of mental health benefits using the neurological diagnosis. When it is feasible to do so, delegating this time-consuming and sometimes laborious job to a specific individual with expertise in these duties (e.g., an insurance verifier) frees the psychotherapist to devote his or her specialized skills toward the instrumental goal of patient care.

In general, most private third-party insurance companies in the United States will pay for a specified number of yearly psychotherapy sessions. In more favorable situations, there may be unlimited visits; however, reimbursement for these is usually based on medical necessity and/or medical review. Obtaining preauthorization and benefit information before the start of psychotherapy is required, so that the patient and therapist are fully aware of reimbursement factors and limitations. From an ethical standpoint, this is also critical, so that all parties are aware of the allocated number of visits; this will enable the setting and accomplishment of realistic goals within feasible parameters, and will prevent problems with premature termination or abandonment of care. In some situations (e.g., workers' compensation), there is more latitude in the time frame for therapy, although all parties should be attentive to attaining subgoals and not exploiting precious resources. Funding agencies also appreciate adherence to these accountability principles, so that valuable resources are not squandered when patients (and/or families) are not making the requisite commitment and effort essential to maximize their recovery and rehabilitation potential.

Sometimes state agencies are viable funding sources. Examples include state department of economic security (DES) independent living rehabilitation services (ILRS), which allocate funds to improve patients' level of independence in the home and community, or DES vocational rehabilitation services (VRS), whose fundamental mission is to return patients with neurological injuries to gainful employment. Usually, however, these agencies require that a patient has no other comparable insurance benefits.

Whenever possible, it is extremely helpful for a patient's family to request assistance from an insurance case manager who can individualize the convoluted maze of insurance benefits. It can also behoove the psychotherapist to develop and maintain strong working relationships with counselors within the state agencies, and with case managers within private third-party companies and workers' compensation. For example, the therapist can hold monthly meetings with a VRS counselor, a patient, a family member, and (when appropriate) other treating therapists to provide an update on the patient's progress and goals. This facilitates a deeper understanding of, and greater professional investment in, the intricacies of the psychotherapy and neurorehabilitation process. Regular and clear documentation is also helpful in procuring further financial support for psychotherapy. When problems arise, direct dialogue with insurance plans' medical directors is sometimes beneficial in the education process. Buttressing the clinical principles with peer-reviewed research demonstrating the efficacy of psychotherapy specifically, and neurorehabilitation in general, is also recommended to legitimize the treatment process (e.g., Klonoff et al., 2006, 2007).

## CASE STUDY

Dr. Smith was a 48-year-old dental surgeon who had suffered a cerebral infarct due to a spontaneous right internal carotid artery dissection. This resulted in left-sided hemiparesis. Dr. Smith was referred from an outside medical setting and initiated psychotherapy approximately 6 months after his stroke. Although Dr. Smith had suffered a serious right-hemisphere stroke, he had made a remarkable recovery within the first 6–8 weeks afterward. His social history indicated that he was extremely bright and a gifted surgeon, suggesting the advantage of cognitive reserve capacity (Satz, 1993). He was also very personable, and his background history indicated that he was happy and well adjusted.

Dr. Smith had partial awareness of his stroke-related deficits, in that he iden-tified primarily physical sequelae, including gait disturbance, hemiparesis of the left arm and hand, and left-sided visual neglect. He also had a rudimentary appre-ciation of cognitive changes, as he acknowledged that it took him longer to review paperwork. When asked about other possible intellectual changes, Dr. Smith was contemplative but noncommittal. He hypothesized that he was unable to return to work in his present condition. Dr. Smith developed excellent beginning rapport with the psychotherapist during the initial consultation, and expressed a genuine interest in continuing treatment in order to master the full ramifications of his stroke, so as to reattain his prior work status.

After confirmation of his health benefits, Dr. Smith agreed to undergo a neuropsychological assessment. He also enrolled in an outpatient setting, where the therapists coordinated their efforts to treat patients holistically. He agreed to undergo multidisciplinary assessments to delineate his overall neurological sta-tus.

After the initial assessment is conducted and a working alliance has begun to form, the psychotherapist must begin to increase the patient's awareness of his or her situation. This is the topic of the next chapter.

# CHAPTER 3

# Increasing Patients' Self-Awareness

## SELF-AWARENESS AND ORGANIC UNAWARENESS

"Self-awareness" is a complex, multimodal construct that has been defined as the "capacity to perceive the 'self' in relatively 'objective' terms while maintaining a sense of subjectivity" (Prigatano & Schacter, 1991, p. 13). It involves a continual interaction of thoughts and feelings, and reflects the highest level of organization and integration of brain structures (Prigatano & Schacter, 1991). Self-awareness requires self-reflection, incorporating judgment and insight (Sohlberg, 2000). Researchers have struggled with how best to quantify this elusive construct, as well as its functional implications, including realistic goal setting (Fleming, Strong, & Ashton, 1996; Pagulayan, Temkin, Machamer, & Dikmen, 2007).

Much has been written regarding the theoretical, anatomical, physiological, and neuropsychological correlates of "organic unawareness" (or "anosognosia") related to hemiplegia, hemianopia, linguistic deficits, traumatic brain injury, dementia, and memory disorders (Flashman, Amador, & McAllister, 2005; Prigatano & Schacter, 1991). Cheng and Man (2006) have identified three common elements of unawareness: (1) lack of objective knowledge, due to cognitive impairment and/or nonprovision of relevant information; (2) difficulty in applying objective information or self-knowledge of deficits to daily life (i.e., the functional applications); and (3) impaired neuropsychological functions (e.g., goal setting, self-prediction, and self-monitoring of psychological factors).

Within the field of neurorehabilitation, and specifically during psychotherapy after brain injury, the remediation of deficits in awareness requires an appreciation of its complexity, dimensions, diversity, and fluidity (Coetzer, 2006; Langer, 1994).

In this context, a useful working definition of *self-awareness* is the understanding and acknowledgment of postinjury neurological strengths and difficulties, as well as their functional implications (Klonoff, 1997; for a recent review, see Ownsworth et al., 2007).

Improvements in self-awareness and self-insight are prerequisites for a patient's active personal investment, progress, and recovery after brain injury (Anson & Ponsford, 2006a; Hartman-Maeir, Soroker, Oman, & Katz, 2003; Klonoff, 1997; Prigatano, 2008b; for a review, see Toglia & Kirk, 2000). Importantly, poor self-knowledge is associated with reduced independence and productivity, weaker interpersonal skills, and poorer psychosocial outcome (Ownsworth et al., 2007).

Certain anatomical correlates and constructs are particularly relevant in impaired self-awareness, including diffuse and multifocal lesions after traumatic brain injury (Flashman et al., 2005; Prigatano, 2005a). Perhaps most importantly, frontal system dysfunction has been linked to impaired self-awareness (Fleming & Ownsworth, 2006; Hoofien, Gilboa, Vakil, & Barak, 2004; for a review, see Stuss, 1991). This can manifest itself in a variety of ways, including indifference or a deficient critical attitude toward problem areas; detachment; absence of introspection; dissociation between knowing and doing; and disturbances in self-continuity, self-regulation, and metacognition (Cicerone et al., 2006; Stuss, 1991). Stuss (1991) has also postulated that frontal system disorders of self-awareness will vary, depending on the particular damaged areas. Impaired executive functions, such as judgment, selectivity, initiation, flexibility, problem solving, decision making, and self-monitoring, will greatly affect self-awareness (Bivona et al., 2008; Noé et al., 2005; Stuss, 1991). More recently, self-awareness has been subdivided into "metacognition," or knowledge from the past and present in conjunction with planning for the future; and "online awareness," which encompasses self-monitoring and self-regulation (Noé et al., 2005; Toglia & Kirk, 2000).

Right-hemisphere damage has also been linked to impaired awareness, specifically hemispace/hemi-inattention, hemiplegia, and hemianopia (Bisiach & Geminiani, 1991; Fleming & Ownsworth, 2006; Goldberg & Barr, 1991; Klonoff, Sheperd, O'Brien, Chiapello, & Hodak, 1990; McGlynn & Schacter, 1989). Clinical manifestations include patients' underestimating their overall limitations, including the severity of their neuropsychological sequelae (e.g., left-sided neglect and impulsivity) and their difficulties in appreciating the "big picture" (Hartman-Maeir et al., 2003; Klonoff et al., 1990). In addition, although there may be recognition of discrete neurocognitive impairments, the impact of these on daily functioning is often substantially minimized (Klonoff et al., 1990). This translates into patients' "biting off more than they can chew" in the realms of financial management and work.

## A BASELINE DETERMINATION OF AWARENESS

Before initiating the psychoeducation process, the psychotherapist needs to gauge the patient's degree of awareness of his or her injury-related deficits and preserved strengths. A preliminary determination of this is made during the consultation and early sessions (see Chapter 2). However, as the treatment process evolves, the psychotherapist can use a working model of the relative contributions (both organic and nonorganic) to the patient's clinical presentation of unawareness. Model parameters include the nature of the brain injury; preinjury emotional status and adjustment; current affect and demeanor; the degree and domains of awareness; and the patient's capacity for generalization. This will help the psychotherapist understand the root causes of the patient's belief systems, utterances, and behavior. Once the psychotherapist ascertains approximately where the patient is on the spectrum of awareness (high, medium, or low), he or she will know how to intervene most effectively. Table 3.1 summarizes these parameters and the diagnostic techniques that are useful in this conceptualization process, as well as a patient's attributes that function as either facilitators or impediments to his or her baseline degree of awareness.

## Nature, Location, and Acuteness of the Brain Injury

Key variables associated with organicity are the nature, location, and acuteness or chronicity of the brain injury. The more profound the level of organicity, the greater the impact on the patient's capacity for self-insight and behavioral change within the therapeutic relationship, as well as in community settings. As stated above, impaired self-awareness is often correlated with diffuse, frontal, and right-hemisphere damage.

**TABLE 3.1. Baseline Determination of Patients' Awareness**

| Parameters | Diagnostic techniques | Awareness impediments | Awareness facilitators |
|---|---|---|---|
| Nature, location, and acuteness of the brain injury | Medical history; neuropsychological assessments; collateral assessments | Frontal lobe and right-hemisphere damage; diffuse injury | Positive trajectory of recovery; chronic injuries with real-life input |
| Preinjury emotional status and adjustment | Psychosocial history; clinical interview; objective evidence | Unhealthy and/or pervasive defense strategies | Healthy emotional makeup and ego resources |
| Affect and demeanor | Astute clinical observation; collateral input | Agitated, brittle, or argumentative | Bewildered, nonplussed, surprised |
| Degree and domains | Questionnaires; clinical interview; Deficit Rating Scale (see Chapter 2, Figure 2.1); collateral input; clinical observation | Limited and constricted perspective; discordance with collateral input | Broad and deep perspective; concordance with collateral input |
| Capacity for generalization | Clinical interview; adjunct postinjury objective data | Poor concordance between self-perception and objective data | Preliminary appreciation of functional implications |

Techniques to assess organicity and injury localization include a thorough review of the medical history, including acute neurosurgical and neurological information. The qualitative and quantitative results of recent and historical neuropsychological assessments provide an additional pertinent context, as well as a time line on which to evaluate the patient's current degree of awareness. Reports from affiliated specialists (e.g., physical and occupational therapists and speech–language pathologists) are also necessary for an appraisal of the patient's neurological status. Quantitative and qualitative observations are invaluable for formulating the patient's degree of awareness. From the nature and degree of deficits and the estimated trajectory of recovery, the psychotherapist can better predict the patient's likely predisposition for awareness training; less severe injuries with more rapid neurological improvements lay a better foundation for inculcation of awareness. Patients with chronic (vs. acute) injuries may have been forced to develop better self-insight, secondary to the unavoidable bombardment of real-world feedback, experiences, and often failures.

### Preinjury Emotional Status and Adjustment

Additional considerations are the patient's preinjury emotions, coping, and adjustment, as these impinge significantly on the expression and remediation of organic unawareness (Ownsworth, McFarland, & Young, 2002). As depicted in Chapter 2, medical records, a thorough history, personality testing (e.g., with the MMPI-2 [Butcher, 2005; Graham, 2006] and the MCMI-III [Millon, 2005]), and objective indicators of life accomplishments (e.g., preinjury academic and work accomplishments) unearth major clues to the patient's preinjury adjustment. Premorbid psychological health and resiliency bode well for tolerating the often stark realizations patients will confront as part of awareness training. Likewise, problematic preexisting coping strategies, including minimization, avoidance, or entrenched denial, may hinder the awareness development process.

### Affect and Demeanor

In determining the patient's degree of awareness, the psychotherapist should observe the patient's demeanor and affect, as well as solicit collateral feedback from family members and others. Astute clinical observation and empathic responsiveness are crucial elements in ascertaining the patient's mood and disposition. Patients with "pure" organic unawareness, who have the potential for self-awareness, most often react as nonplussed, surprised, or bewildered when deficit areas are shared by the psychotherapist. Patients who are highly agitated, psychologically brittle, or argumentative during inquiry about injury-related deficits are more likely to struggle during awareness training.

### Degree and Domains of Awareness

There are various forms of unawareness, including a patient's propensity for partial/implicit knowledge of deficits, even though the patient explicitly denies the existence of deficits (Prigatano & Schacter, 1991). For example, after traumatic brain injury patients most often accurately perceive and focus their energies on physical disabilities, but significantly underestimate their emotional, behavioral, interpersonal, and cognitive deficits (Fischer, Trexler, & Gauggel, 2004; Hart, Sherer, Whyte, Polansky, & Novack, 2004; Hoofien et al., 2004; Trahan, Pepin, & Hopps, 2006).

The patient's span and depth of insight into deficit areas can be assessed via structured interviews, questionnaires, and/or clinical observations (Flashman et al., 2005; Fleming et al., 1996). The Patient Competency Rating Scale (Prigatano et al., 1986) is a useful clinical tool in ascertaining the patient's self-perception of potential areas of challenge, as it provides self-assessment in multiple domains (e.g., memory, activities of daily living, and mood); these are rated on a 5-point spectrum, ranging from "can do with ease" to "can't do." In general, endorsements of problem areas are suggestive of at least budding awareness, especially if there is some agreement between these endorsements and collateral input.

## Capacity for Generalization

In addition to assessing the patient's awareness of deficits, the psychotherapist must assess his or her awareness of the consequences of these deficits. This is best accomplished by asking the patient about how his or her injury has affected functional activities, such as staying alone in the home, driving, and/or work. It is also helpful to have access to supplemental objective postinjury data, including school grades and (when possible) performance evaluations from work. Poor concordance between postinjury factual information and the patient's self-perception is indicative of limited self-awareness.

Assessment of these variables will indicate the extent to which the patient is aware of his or her deficits, can describe them, and (ideally) can relate them to functionality. This is the point of entry into deeper discussions of, and interventions for improving, awareness; it represents the crucial bridge between contemplation and action (Fleming et al., 1996).

The process of increasing a patient's self-awareness after brain injury can be depicted as a continuum: The patient moves from relative unawareness to burgeoning awareness. As this process proceeds, the patient will experience catastrophic reactions from time to time, and most often will grapple with some degree of depression. In fact, there is an inverse relationship between the degree of unawareness and the concomitant degree of emotional distress; decreasing patients' unawareness is difficult if not impossible to do without increasing their emotional distress. Awareness training and treatment for catastrophic reactions and depression are best conducted in a treatment context that offers multiple forms of intervention. The balance of this chapter describes specific techniques for raising patients' self-awareness and addressing the emotional aftermath, through individual psychotherapy, adjunct therapies, cognitive retraining, a psychoeducation group, and group psychotherapy. The case of Dr. Smith, introduced at the end of Chapter 2, is used to illustrate points throughout this discussion.

## INDIVIDUAL PSYCHOTHERAPY INTERVENTIONS

### Awareness Training

Awareness training is predicated on a trusting and sound working alliance between the psychotherapist and the patient; otherwise, the patient will retreat into a defensive stance (Flashman et al., 2005; Schönberger, Humle, & Teasdale, 2006b). In addition, the psychotherapist must be skilled and sensitive about the timing and pacing of any feedback, so as not to overwhelm, unduly discourage, or demean the patient. Sometimes in the attempt to convince or "prove a point" to the patient, the therapist can become confrontative and convey too much information; most often this will backfire and alienate the patient.

During awareness training, patients tend to narrow their perceptions and focus on discrete and obvious aspects of functioning (e.g., "my walking," "my talking"). Therefore, both psychoeducation and treatment should encompass the full, multifaceted range of each patient's deficit set (e.g., executive functions and safety awareness). Both more subtle deficits and broader deficits may be ignored by the patient, but both can have a substantial impact on outcome, including productive work (Hoofien et al., 2004; Klonoff et al., 2007; Shames, Treger, Ring, & Giaquinto, 2007; Sherer et al., 2003). Patients are educated to widen their focus in order to optimize their recovery. Awareness training techniques include sharing the assessment results; counterbalancing information ("new news") with affective release; and making use of metaphors, mantras, and diagrams for "new news."

### Sharing Assessment Results

As stated above, assessment findings in one or more areas (e.g., neuropsychology, speech–language therapy, occupational therapy, and physical therapy) provide a springboard for the awareness dialogue. However, exposure to written documentation with quantification of specific deficit areas (complete with percentile and grade equivalent scores) often propels a patient from relative unawareness and "blissful ignorance" to distress, fright, or even panic. Therefore, in order to avoid a possibly counterproductive inundation of information, the sharing of findings often needs to be organized and prioritized for the patient. One technique is to summarize the "top" (most salient) three to four problem areas, and to introduce other associated deficits gradually in future sessions. When the psychotherapist is describing the size of each deficit, it is more sensitive to employ terms such as "small," "medium," and "large," rather than clinical jargon (e.g., "mild," "moderate," and "severe"). Depending on the patient's psychological readiness, review of a normal probability curve relative to his or her test performance is another helpful visual aid. Interpretation of neuropsychological and other evaluation findings should also take into account the patient's preexisting abilities, so as to provide comparison standards that are genuinely representative of the individual (Lezak et al., 2004). Relating specific deficits to the damaged anatomical areas is an additional integral aspect of the psychoeducation process. It is often advisable to employ models and pictures of the brain to help validate the discussion. When patients are ready, review of their CT and MRI scans in relationship to acquired deficits also bolsters their knowledge base.

Given how upsetting this feedback can be, it is very important for the therapist to counterbalance news of deficits with relative strengths and the "rescue" role of compensatory strategies. This helps prevent a patient from becoming overwhelmed, disillusioned, hopeless, or angry. Recording the evaluation findings in the patient's notebook will help him or her to remember, consolidate, and come to terms with the information. The following illustrates the process of sharing assessment results by continuing with the case of Dr. Smith.

### CASE STUDY

Soon after the initial interview, Dr. Smith began individual psychotherapy in conjunction with his multidisciplinary evaluations. More extensive inquiry during the first few sessions indicated that his baseline level of awareness was rudimentary. He had suffered a significant right-hemisphere stroke fairly recently and was unaware of the nature and extent of his cognitive limitations. However, his affability and positive preinjury adjustment gave him the foundation to undertake awareness training. He recognized that he was unable to drive or work yet, indicating the capacity to generalize his current discrete impairments to the real world.

Dr. Smith had not had a comprehensive neurorehabilitation workup since the early postacute period, and had not undergone any form of neuropsychological testing. This was in part by his own choice, as he was reluctant to be exposed to his possible shortcomings. An evaluation encompassing all disciplines was completed, and the results of each segment were reviewed with him orally by the evaluator from each therapy domain. The psychotherapist then provided Dr. Smith with a report summary—orally at first—of his retained strengths and deficit areas.

The results of Dr. Smith's evaluation were sobering: "Medium" deficits were identified in the areas of left upper-extremity function (motor control, tone normalization, sensation, strength, and dexterity), bilateral gross motor coordination, and visuoperceptual skills. His demeanor became crestfallen. However, the neuropsychological testing also revealed a number of well-preserved and even outstanding skills, which the psychotherapist enumerated with Dr. Smith. These included his vocabulary and overall language skills, as well as his verbal learning and recall. Self-relative deficits were then postulated, including "medium" deficits in his speed of information processing, attention, visual recall, visuoperceptual and visuospatial skills, and executive functions (including new concept formation, impulse control, planning, problem solving, organization, and strategy generation). All of these findings had profound implications for his reintegration to work. As part of the dialogue, Dr. Smith's CT and MRI findings were reviewed; deficit areas were related to damaged anatomical areas, with the aid of brain diagrams and a brain model. As an emotional buffer, the therapist split feedback about these deficit areas over two sessions, and only then gave the results to Dr. Smith in detailed written form.

The psychotherapist recommended a 6-month course of psychotherapy. Dr. Smith was initially perplexed by the length of the recommended course, assuming that he would progress more quickly. Understandably, he also described feeling overwhelmed and discouraged by the enormity of his challenges, while at the same time relieved to know that he was in "good hands." He felt that the treating therapists (including his psychotherapist) were dedicated to providing the necessary therapies for as long as necessary to ameliorate his various deficits.

## Counterbalancing "New News" with Affective Release

After the patient is exposed to the overview of his or her neurological strengths and difficulties, follow-up sessions should buttress and expand this knowledge base, while at the same time facilitating understandable affective catharsis. The psychotherapist can accomplish this through open-ended questions that encourage patients to reflect and elaborate on what they have learned, as well as on how they feel about the information. Examples include "How would you summarize where you are at in your recovery right now?" or "How did you feel about our last session when we reviewed your test results?" Follow-up discussions should allow the patient to meander between the intellectual (i.e., "brain") responses and the emotional (i.e., "heart") reactions, without constraining the process by imposing a rigid therapeutic agenda. The therapist can be most helpful in gently encouraging the patient to give ample energies to both the cerebral and affective levels.

## Mantras, Metaphors, and Diagrams for "New News"

The use of mantras, metaphors, and diagrams can assist in psychoeducation and the process of increasing awareness. The following are some useful examples.

### "PATIENCE, TRUST, AND COLLABORATION"

Very often patients are tempted to abandon the treatment process, secondary to their bewilderment or exasperation with the psychoeducation process. The mantra "Patience, trust, and collaboration" represents the three pillars of an early working alliance. It provides a simple yet effective rubric to calm the patient and guide him or her through the awareness maze.

### "THE VOLUME IS TURNED UP"

Sometimes patients will contradict and dispute feedback about their problem areas, commonly postulating that their supposed neurological difficulties were evident preinjury. In this situation, it can be very helpful to explain that brain injury can exaggerate an individual's preexisting personality and/or behavioral characteristics (Prigatano, 1999). This aspect of brain injury can be explained by comparing it to a stereo or other sound system: It can "turn up the volume" on preinjury problems (Prigatano, 1999). This metaphor respects the patient's preinjury personality makeup, yet gently incorporates the contribution of the injury, thereby furthering the awareness process.

### ACTIONS–CONSEQUENCES

Due to executive system dysfunction, patients often do not see the connections— or draw inaccurate connections—between their thoughts or actions and the possible consequences of or responses to these. The education process often must focus on these connections. For example, a patient may verbalize that he or she has significant problems with new learning, but will follow up with the intention to cram for an upcoming test. Politely identifying the inherent contradiction between the identified problems and the proposed response, and the potential hazards of this course of action, will assist the patient in drawing more accurate inferences about the implications of his or her choices.

## DIAGRAMS: "CONNECT THE DOTS" AND "PUZZLE PIECES"

Diagrams can be quite versatile in helping patients "connect the dots" or assemble the "puzzle pieces" of their injury-related sequelae. That is, they can help patients place details within the "big picture." For example, a diagram of puzzle pieces is helpful in defining the main elements of executive functions; each piece can be labeled (as judgment, decision making, impulse control, etc.). Connecting the dots is useful in plotting a strategic plan or course of action. It helps the patient identify and sequence the necessary steps to accomplish a goal. For example, two steps needed to achieve the goal of driving are improving distractibility and multitasking.

## "THE HONEYMOON IS OVER"

Some patients experience a sense of relief and reassurance upon initiating the psychotherapeutic relationship and embarking upon the information-gathering expedition. With dawning awareness, they feel empowered and inspired to work diligently to overcome their shortcomings. However, for some patients, this phase can be short-lived; the more they learn about their new predicament, the less invigorated they feel. A helpful metaphor for this reaction is "The honeymoon is over," as it validates the understandable transition from initial zest to "the long road ahead."

## "DON'T KILL THE MESSENGER"

Induction of awareness creates understandable and predictable emotional distress in patients. Often patients will unleash their anger or distrust on the person who is conveying disturbing feedback. Asking such patients not to "kill the messenger" helps them recognize that the therapist is merely the conduit, not the reason for the effects of the damage. This can reduce the intensity of patients' reactions and help them separate the message from those who convey it.

## A "HEART-TO-HEART" DISCUSSION

Sometimes the psychotherapist feels the need to have a "heart-to-heart" discussion with a patient, as a way to help him or her take seriously the importance of "facing facts." It is usually employed when the degree of unawareness is very pervasive and resistant to other interventions, and/or when the psychotherapist is genuinely concerned that detrimental or even dangerous conclusions and plans are being implemented, due to markedly deficient awareness. This can be an effective way to capture a patient's attention; however, as all more direct, straightforward interventions must be, it needs to be couched in an atmosphere of sincere concern and a sturdy working alliance.

Sometimes the initial education process about injury-related deficits precipitates many hard-to-answer questions from the patient. These often fall into the category of wanting (or pressuring) the psychotherapist to answer specific long-range questions, such as "Will all of these problems go away?" or "Will I make a 100% recovery, and how long will it take?" It is advisable for the psychotherapist to tread gently, encouraging a "wait-and-see" attitude for long-term answers. In the meantime, it is best to encourage patients to focus on short-range goals (ones that can be accomplished in 1–2 months), and to emphasize active retraining and compensations. This avoids quashing the patients' motivation and hope, and instead empowers them to work diligently to overcome their limitations.

## Alleviating Emotional Distress

### Catastrophic Reactions

Catastrophic reactions are almost inevitable external manifestations of improved self-awareness. Goldstein (1952) was the first to describe the behavioral state that occurs when a patient struggles and fails to perform tasks after brain injury that were completed with ease before the injury. Goldstein (1952) stated that the patient "may appear dazed, become agitated, change color, start to fumble, become unfriendly, evasive, and even aggressive" (p. 255). He also identified anxiety as the underlying reason for catastrophic reactions, related to the "threat of self-realization" over not being able to accomplish a task. Catastrophic reactions take multiple forms, all of which relate to intolerance for one's acquired imperfections (Klonoff et al., 1993). These include the more classic manifestations of anger, frustration, sadness, tearfulness, and anxiety. The most common and pervasive one is feeling overwhelmed. Less obvious but equally serious reactions include avoidance, shutting down, minimization, disavowal, and concealment (Klonoff et al., 1993; Riley, Brennan, & Powell, 2004). Often patients refer to catastrophic reactions as "meltdowns" or "hitting the wall." Overall, they reflect a patient's self-realization of ineptitude, which assaults his or her sense of psychological well-being.

The psychotherapist should educate patients so that they know what catastrophic reactions are and can recognize them. This starts with a basic definition of a "catastrophic reaction" (i.e., a strong emotional reaction to current difficulties in accomplishing tasks that were easy before the injury). In "rehab lingo," catastrophic reactions are referred to as "CRs." This normalizes and humanizes them. An effective treatment technique to address catastrophic reactions is "empathic responsiveness" (Schwaber, 1979). That is, the psychotherapist enters the patient's subjective reality and listens attentively to the patient's description of these experiences. The psychotherapist is like a detective, helping to perceive and illuminate with patients their "triggers" (the specific catalysts for the reactions), as well as what coping techniques are effective at diminishing the reactions' frequency and intensity.

Practically speaking, empathic responsiveness involves asking the patient to walk the therapist through the specifics of a recent upsetting event, with particular attention to the antecedent circumstances that precipitated the catastrophic reaction. This process assists the patient in understanding the connection between inner feelings of pain and overt behaviors; it also legitimizes his or her frustrations (Klonoff et al., 1993). This type of inquiry is useful in acquiring an appreciation of the patient's idiosyncratic activators and expressions of catastrophic reactions.

Once the psychotherapist and the patient have acquired insight into the specific sources and forms of the patient's catastrophic reactions, practical steps can be taken to reduce their occurrence. Recommendations include the modification of the environment to reduce or eliminate conditions that overwhelm the patient. These can include developing and implementing personalized compensatory strategies, and finding "best-fit" community environments where the patient feels that he or she can succeed and flourish (Klonoff et al., 1993). Education for family members and support for the patient's social network are also vital, so that they do not inadvertently precipitate or escalate catastrophic reactions (Klonoff et al., 1993).

## Depression

Organic unawareness, by definition, precludes intense emotionality over losses. Therefore, enhanced self-insight is a double-edged sword. It is positive as an antecedent for the patient's eventual improved adjustment and better quality of life, including the assimilation of a more representative and reality-based self-perception of injury-related assets and challenges. However, it can also precipitate a patient into depression (Fleminger, Oliver, Williams, & Evans, 2003; Gouick & Gentleman, 2004; Malec, Testa, Rush, Brown, & Moessner, 2007; Schönberger, Humle, & Teasdale, 2006a). Depression can also be the consequence of frequent and intense catastrophic reactions; in fact, a decline into a depressed state can be considered the pervasive counterpart to periodic catastrophic reactions. To complicate matters, depression can be caused by pathophysiological factors, such as moderate or severe brain injury involving the frontal, subcortical, and limbic areas (Ghaffar & Feinstein, 2008; Gouick & Gentleman, 2004; Pies, 2008; see Rogers & Read, 2007, for a review).

Common symptoms associated with depression include vegetative signs (e.g., insomnia or excessive fatigue, low energy, reduced libido, and weight loss); psychological symptoms (e.g., low self-esteem, self-depreciation, apathy, and anhedonia); behavioral accompaniments (e.g., social withdrawal and crying); and cognitive factors (e.g., hopelessness, worthlessness, and guilt) (Fleminger et al., 2003; Ghaffar & Feinstein, 2008; House, 2003; Kant, Duffy, & Pivovarnik, 1998). With intensified awareness and appreciation of their losses, patients may also capitulate to feelings of sorrow, gloominess, despair, disillusionment, emptiness, shame, worthlessness, hostility, self-hatred, violent rage attacks, and self-destructive behavior (Gans, 1983; Klonoff et al., 1993). Other associated manifestations include anger, fear, anxiety, suffering, grief, and mourning, culminating in a profound sense of loss (Langer, 1994, 1999; O'Callaghan, Powell, & Oyebode, 2006). As described in Chapter 4, the postinjury existence can become so unbearable that a patient may become vulnerable to suicidal outcry (Klonoff & Lage, 1991, 1995).

During awareness training, the psychotherapist must be vigilant about the emergence of depressive symptomatology in the patient. This requires frequent "checking in" regarding the patient's mood, as well as careful observation of the patient's affect, level of engagement in the therapeutic process, and involvement in pleasurable community activities, (e.g., family life, hobbies). A useful technique is to have the patient keep a mood log in his or her datebook—that is, to have the patient rate his or her mood each day, on a scale from 1 (very depressed) to 10 (very happy). It is often helpful to review the specific symptomatology associated with dysthymia and depression (see, e.g., American Psychiatric Association, 2000) as part of the psychoeducational process. The psychotherapist should recommend exercise as an effective adjunctive treatment for depression (Fann et al., 2009). Collateral input from significant others is also essential, to be sure that the psychotherapist has an accurate perception of the patient's mood and adjustment in community settings.

### Anxiety

Another common consequence of awareness training is increased anxiety. Initially, this can be associated with catastrophic reactions; the patient realizes that he or she cannot perform tasks competently, and becomes anxious and self-conscious about his or her ineptness. This can then spread to more global worries about broader issues of functionality (e.g., "Will I work again? Will I drive again? How will I care for my family?"). In addition, anxiety can be associated with lesion locations, including the right hemisphere and the temporolimbic areas (Williams, Evans, & Fleminger, 2003). Other manifestations of anxiety can include fearfulness, rumination, indecision, self-doubt, avoidance, or somatic manifestations. Empathic listening and supportive reassurance are integral treatment techniques to help allay patients' fears and worries (Hiott & Labbate, 2002). Education about the optimal balance of anxiety and productive output, using a version of the Yerkes–Dodson diagram (Eysenck, 2006), helps patients recognize the deleterious effects of excessive worry. Similarly, the well-known Serenity Prayer is a helpful mantra to redirect patients' energies toward productive and proactive thinking. Skill building and relaxation training are other effective techniques to ameliorate patients' anxieties (Williams et al., 2003).

### The Role of Psychiatric Intervention and Psychotropic Medication

Psychiatric intervention is invaluable in the psychotherapy process, especially with intensification of emotional distress. In my setting, the psychiatrist works on a consultation/liaison basis; she and a psychotherapist meet conjointly with a patient usually once or twice per month until the patient's mood is stabilized, at which time the frequency of visits is reduced. Family members attend part or all of the sessions, depending on the patient's level of cognitive impairment, as well as his or her level of comfort with family attendance. The psychiatrist's more intermittent contact with the patient affords a more objective point of view, which is often very beneficial to both the patient and the psychotherapist. In addition, the presence of another empathic expert on the psychiatric sequelae of brain injury often clarifies and enriches the understanding of the emotional turmoil the patient is experiencing.

Psychotropic medications are often indispensable tools in the "tool kit" for improving a patient's foundational coping skills as well as emotional control. They can help reduce the frequency and magnitude of catastrophic reactions, and can ameliorate depression. Patients can then cope better with their life-altering and often grievous circumstances, and this improved coping allows the psychotherapeutic process to blossom. A number of medications are helpful in this regard, including SSRIs (e.g., sertraline; G. A. Lage & P. Bollam, personal communication, n.d.; Vaishnavi et al., 2009). The "rule of thumb" is to consider using medications when the patient's catastrophic reactions, anxiety, depression, or other emotional disturbances are interfering with his or her capacity to obtain maximum benefit from psychotherapy (and/or other rehabilitation activities) and are adversely affecting functional goal attainment (G. A. Lage & P. Bollam, personal communication, n.d.).

A close liaison and a collaborative relationship with a psychiatrist are mandatory for the provision of integrated care. This includes an appreciation for the possible development of "therapeutic triangles"; these are transference reactions involving the psychotherapist, the treating psychiatrist, and the patient (Bradley & Bentley, 2003). For example, many patients after brain injury react negatively to the recommendation of psychotropic medication; most often they view the introduction of medication as a sign of weakness. They want to "get over it" without a "crutch." This often results in a negative transference reaction to the prescribing psychiatrist. Alternatively, when patients experience rapid symptom relief, they may view the treating psychotherapist as inadequate in meeting their psychological needs, instead preferring an "instant cure" from the psychiatrist. Dialogue, mutual respect, education, and an appreciation of the dynamics of two professionals collaborating in patient care will enhance the overall treatment for the patient.

## CASE STUDY

After the initial sharing of assessment results with Dr. Smith, the next several weekly individual psychotherapy sessions were devoted to continued dialogue and education about his injury-related sequelae. In the initial follow-up session, Dr. Smith described the "new news" as an "awakening." Dr. Smith said that he had anticipated some areas of difficulty on an "intellectual level," but he felt "blindsided psychologically" by their breadth, their magnitude, and their implications for his returning to the practice of dental surgery. He was particularly shaken by the severity of the cognitive results, because he felt that his professional aspirations had evaporated. On the one hand, his basic understanding of brain–behavior relationships had enabled him to predict logically that his cognitive skills would be affected; on the other hand, he quickly resorted to "killing the messenger" by challenging the validity of the testing process, and adamantly insisting that some of his deficits (e.g., in organizational skills) were preexisting. The therapist introduced the metaphor of the brain injury's "turning up the volume" on possible preexisting weaknesses. This acknowledged Dr. Smith's historical self-view, with an overlay of new, stroke-related changes.

In subsequent sessions, Dr. Smith was overcome by emotion, shedding many tears and lamenting over how he had toiled so diligently to achieve professional stature, a solid community reputation, and a professorship at an acclaimed dental school. He described feeling "devalued," with his life "out of control." By his report, this behavior was new; he described his preinjury behavior as stoic, with a tendency to "bottle up emotions." His psychotherapist reframed this affective release as a sign of his growing awareness and a testament to his courage and openness in facing his new reality. In addition, Dr. Smith was complimented on his (unexpected) superior ability to contemplate his deficits so readily in the context of right-hemisphere damage. This was even more impressive, given his ability to grasp the implications of his deficits for his work functions.

Dr. Smith's dawning awareness advanced to an increasingly lucid self-perception of incapacities. This precipitated a cascade of catastrophic reactions, when he felt exceedingly overwhelmed, anxious, and frustrated with his inabilities. His left-sided physical problems affected basic skills (e.g., tying his shoelaces and buttoning his shirts); how then would he ever perform oral surgery? This soon gave way to depressive periods, characterized by despair and feelings of worthlessness, because of his perceived incompetence.

Dr. Smith initiated consultations with a psychiatrist within the first 3 weeks of initiating psychotherapy. He himself recognized that he was overwhelmed and dysphoric, with insomnia and other depressive symptoms. His psychotherapist attended this first consultation and all follow-up visits. Dr. Smith expressed appreciation for this attendance, as he felt that it coordinated his psychological care more effectively and efficiently. He had been prescribed an antidepressant by another psychiatrist during the acute phase of recovery; however, it was the opinion of the new psychiatrist that another medication would be more effective, given the persistence of his mood disorder and catastrophic reactions. Dr. Smith willingly switched medications to sertraline. Dr. Smith continued to see the psychiatrist on a monthly basis over the next 5 months, and when necessary the dosage of medication was increased to accommodate new challenges and pressures, especially once Dr. Smith returned to work.

During the turmoil of Dr. Smith's dawning awareness, the frequency of individual psychotherapy sessions was increased to twice weekly. To fortify the psychoeducation process, capitalize on his verbal strengths, and contextualize his personal circumstances, Dr. Smith was given a series of published articles on catastrophic reactions, memory remediation, and sequelae of right-hemisphere stroke. Dr. Smith loved to read, and he voraciously studied the articles; he then proceeded to research his neurological condition further, stating that "knowledge is power." He would bring germane articles to sessions, which were reviewed conjointly. He expressed appreciation for the format and content of this imparting of knowledge, as it bolstered his spirits to operate on the "scientist" level and within an "academic" context.

Dr. Smith's psychotherapy also took a pragmatic approach to help with awareness training. His cognitive strengths and difficulties were written in columns, with an associated diagrammed "game plan" of how to attack the problems in individual psychotherapy and in his other therapies. He felt empowered by this "broad-band approach" to his multiple sequelae. This included homework exercises and games on the computer to address his specific deficit areas (e.g., attention, visual memory, and executive functions such as abstract reasoning). Dr. Smith had always been determined and goal-oriented; these therapeutic activities helped to anchor him emotionally, and thus helped him to plot a practical and workable therapeutic course.

Before his stroke, Dr. Smith had lived alone; however, given his social isolation from his work colleagues, he became lonely and melancholy. Therefore, his psychotherapist recommended that his parents—who were retired, and with whom he had an excellent relationship—come to live with him for a period of time, to provide emotional sustenance and assist with practical daily activities (e.g., driving, financial decision making). Given Dr. Smith's motivation, it was also decided to increase the frequency of his other rehabilitation therapies from 4 to 5 days per week; this heartened him, and he eagerly tackled his deficits. His psychotherapist also collaborated with his physical therapist to institute an appropriate home exercise program. These practical solutions reduced the intensity and frequency of his catastrophic reactions and improved his mood and outlook.

As part of individual psychotherapy, and to assist Dr. Smith in embracing and expressing his personal feelings of loss, he was encouraged to watch the movie *The Doctor* (Feldman, Glick, Ziskin, & Haines, 1991) as a depiction of catastrophic reactions and depression in another health care professional. In this movie, a heart surgeon practices medicine in a detached and unemotional manner; he even counsels young physician residents not to become emotionally involved with their patients, so as not to compromise their clinical judgment. This attitude is transformed radically when he is diagnosed unexpectedly with throat cancer. Now "the shoe is on the other foot," and he is faced with the stark personal confrontation of his own human frailties. The doctor is ensnared by fear, loneliness, and vulnerability, and his feelings of invincibility are shattered. His wife and a patient with terminal brain cancer help the doctor cope and become emotionally present with others. Watching this movie and discussing it in psychotherapy proved extremely validating for Dr. Smith. It facilitated deeper introspection and communication about his personal feelings and reactions. It also intensified his personal resolve to return to the humanistic practice of healing patients.

## ADJUNCT THERAPIES FOR GENERALIZING AWARENESS TRAINING

"Self-awareness" has also been defined as "the position of the self within the social milieu" (Stuss & Benson, 1986, p. 246). Remediation of the multiple components of awareness requires techniques that are both broad and deep. The process of self-awareness and realization needs to be generalized from personal knowledge ("I have this problem") to individual and group interactions in the clinic environment ("My deficits affect me this way"), and ultimately to the outside community ("My deficits will translate this way in the real world").

Multiple sources of input, therefore, are important in the awareness process; patients are less likely to deflect, minimize, or reject feedback when they hear it from many people both inside and outside the psychotherapeutic setting (Brown, Lyons, & Rose, 2006; O'Callaghan et al., 2006). A number of structured therapeutic techniques can also facilitate the process of patients' generalizing their self-awareness (Fleming & Ownsworth, 2006). These include holistic treatment, compensatory and facilitatory approaches, structured experiences, direct feedback, video-recorded feedback, confrontational techniques, cognitive therapy, group therapy, game formats, and behavioral interventions (Ben-Yishay et al., 1985; Flashman et al., 2005; Fleming & Ownsworth, 2006; Mateer et al., 2005; Prigatano, 2005b; Sherer et al., 1998). These multiple interventions enhance patients' self-awareness.

Collaborative evidentiary techniques in the form of specific, jointly determined therapeutic challenges and modalities are therefore pivotal as part of the psychotherapeutic process, in order to enlighten the patient about his or her postinjury capabilities and limitations. For a psychotherapist working in a team setting, collateral information from clinic-based activities (including cognitive retraining scores, language exercises, physical measurements, and homework), as well as datebook use and Home Independence Checklist scores, are fundamental tools for assisting the patient in developing an accurate self-appraisal of his or her postinjury strengths and obstacles. Clinical observations gleaned by the psychotherapist during unstructured clinic activities (e.g., breaks, lunch hour, or community outings) provide rich supplemental information, as these activities more closely simulate real-world settings and involve fewer constraints. Another helpful method is video-recording the patient's speech and physical capacities, once the patient has the psychological fortitude and willingness to embrace this technique. Written behavioral logs delineating target areas for self-monitoring, in conjunction with hourly ratings by cotherapists (see Chapter 8), are other beneficial tools for the awareness development process. These collaborative evidentiary techniques afford a consummate multidimensional perspective using objective and concrete evidence of performance, which can be more difficult for the patient to ignore or dispute.

Feedback from family members and friends, school grades, and work observations greatly enhance the meaningfulness and relevance of these new insights. In addition, input from fellow patients is not only a powerful source of awareness training, but can be more palatable than other types of feedback, as it is considered to emanate from an unbiased place of personal resonance. This can take the form of clinic-based patient group discussions. Alternatively, the psychotherapist can arrange one or more conjoint appointments with two patients who have similar backgrounds and aspirations, but who are at different places in the recovery and rehabilitation process (one more of a novice, and the other more seasoned). This enables a peer mentorship relationship to evolve. Moreover, when here-and-now clinical observations of the patient's behaviors (Yalom, 2002) are processed close to the time of their occurrence, the patient is assisted in appreciating his or her injury effects and their impact on the environment.

## COGNITIVE RETRAINING

The inclusion of cognitive retraining exercises in the psychotherapist's repertoire represents one of the best applications of the collaborative evidentiary process. It is a powerful mechanism to unearth patients' strengths and weaknesses, because it provides concrete data in the form of scores and learning style. "Cognitive retraining" is a specific form of cognitive remediation that employs both restorative and compensatory approaches in order to remediate neurocognitive and neurobehavioral deficits, and to promote functional competence in a broad array of everyday life situations (Ben-Yishay & Diller, 1993; Klonoff et al., 2007; Prigatano et al., 1986). Patients participate in these sessions at least a couple of times per week if this is feasible, to allow for sufficient practice and inculcation of the awareness process. At the outset of each session, the overall purposes of cognitive retraining are reviewed. These are to improve patients' thinking skills; to improve their awareness of their strengths and difficulties; and to help them learn compensations that will assist them in the home, school, and work environments (Klonoff, O'Brien, Prigatano, Chiapello, & Cunningham, 1989; Klonoff et al., 1997).

### Session Procedures

As long as a patient has the cognitive capability to handle distractions, it is actually helpful to have background sounds during cognitive retraining, thereby simulating community environments (e.g., home, school, and work) where ambient noise and distractions are expected (Klonoff et al., 2007). If the treatment setting permits, two patients can work at the same time with the therapist. Although I use a specific set of cognitive activities during cognitive retraining, there is no "magic" associated with these tasks; any thinking or language task can be integrated into a constructive treatment experience. It is most efficacious to include 8–15 short tasks that draw upon a broad range of abilities, including speed of information processing, sustained attention, working memory, new learning, visual scanning, visuoconstruction skills, language skills (e.g., oral reading, vocabulary, and spelling), impulse control, mental flexibility, and attention to detail. Sample tasks include word search puzzles; an activity resembling the word game Boggle; data matching; scanning tasks for target letters, numbers, and symbols; and design construction using colored blocks (see Klonoff et al., 1997, 2007, for other examples). A personal favorite of mine is having patients write the first (or last) letter of 10 sentences that relate to the awareness process (e.g., "Compensations make all of the difference"). All tasks are timed, and should vary with respect to the mode of response (oral vs. written), stimulus (verbal vs. visual), and degree of therapist involvement (interactive vs. more independent) (Klonoff et al., 1989).

Each task should have a purpose sheet that is reviewed before the start of the task. The sheet includes the cognitive skills addressed, functional examples, and space for the patient to note his or her individualized compensatory strategies. General functional examples are described for each task, so as to relate the fundamental cognitive skills (e.g., visual scanning, attention, and concentration) to everyday abilities (e.g., driving). As patients proceed in their recovery, specific applications of the task skills to their work/school endeavors are identified. Ideally, with time and practice, patients' awareness improves and they can construct their own lists of functional applications. This calls for them to take a metacognitive perspective on the effects of their brain injuries, and to think of ways to generalize the use of their new skills to other settings (Ben-Yishay & Diller, 1993; Worthington & Waller, 2009). This counteracts a tendency to interpret the activities on a concrete and artificial basis.

### How Cognitive Retraining Aids Self-Awareness

The principal benefits of cognitive retraining sessions are the learning process regarding retained skills and awareness of difficulties; the creative development and implementation of useful compensatory techniques for difficulties; and an appreciation of how postinjury strengths, difficulties, and compensations will affect functional status (Klonoff et al., 2007). These then become part of the patient's armamentarium of effective coping tools.

Through cognitive retraining exercises, patients develop "emergent awareness," or recognition of a problem when it occurs (Barco, Crosson, Bolesta, Werts, & Stout, 1991). However, a higher-order form of awareness—one that is necessary for generalization of skills into community settings—is "anticipatory awareness," or the recognition that a deficit-related problem will arise before it takes place (Barco et al., 1991). For this reason, meaningful quantitative data are derived from and applied in cognitive retraining sessions (Klonoff et al., 1989). For example, in my setting, all tasks are standardized in their administration by treating therapists, and data have been collected on 327 prior patients. From these, percentile scores have been developed for each task, also stratified according to age. Patients identify "expected scores," based on their perception of the percentile level at which they should be performing. They also set personal "attainable goals," which may be lower than the expected scores, depending on the nature and extent of their deficits. These two sets of scores are also noted by the patients on the task purpose sheets. This augments the awareness development process and prepares patients psychologically for expected challenges in community environments. The process of creating a data set of expected scores based on prior patients' task performance can be replicated in any setting, as long as tasks are administered and scored consistently.

Patients are responsible for detailed scoring, mathematical calculations, and record-keeping protocols (Klonoff et al., 1989, 1997). These responsibilities enable both assessment and retraining of procedural memory—an important underlying skill for community functioning (Klonoff et al., 2007). Depending on patients' procedural memory and overall cognitive skills, it is advisable to develop and choose from three levels of procedural checklists (Klonoff et al., 2007): (1) a prefabricated detailed, step-by-step procedure checklist of how to perform and score the task, which patients complete by marking off each step sequentially; (2) patient-generated detailed step-by-step procedures, which they devise and create in typewritten form; or (3) limited and relevant notations of only those protocol steps that they would otherwise confuse or omit. Patients can memorize the setup, execution, and scoring protocols whenever possible. Development and utilization of procedural checklists provide invaluable information about a patient's procedural memory, learning capacity, organization skills, and sequential thinking. Of course, not all patients follow the progression from extensive checklists to no checklists and the extent to which they can (or cannot) becomes vital information to analyze and discuss as part of the awareness development process.

The psychotherapist should always conduct "error analyses" with each patient as needed. These consist of analyzing the underlying reasons for poor scores (distractibility, catastrophic reactions, memory problems, mental fatigue, impulsivity, etc.). Such analyses are crucial to patients' developing a sophisticated understanding of their deficit areas. Patients should also have the opportunity to graph their scores as a cognitive exercise; this allows them to visualize and appraise their individual challenges and progress. This procedure also addresses visuospatial skills, planning, and organization.

Cognitive retraining provides an abundance of useful qualitative data on patients' behavior, motivations, interpersonal skills, and coping styles (Klonoff et al., 1989, 2007). These are partially derived from observation of the patient–patient interactions when two patients are working together, including their mutual reactions to relative areas of strengths and difficulties, punctuality, pragmatic communication abilities (e.g., turn taking), organizational skills, and distractibility. Patient–therapist interactions simulate student–teacher and employee–employer relations, including patients' reactions to directions and constructive feedback, as well as frustration tolerance.

## Compensatory Strategies

Central to the effectiveness of cognitive retraining exercises are the development and implementation of compensatory strategies. Collaborating with and educating patients about the necessity, utility, and generalization of these strategies is critical to the awareness development process. Patients initially perform all tasks without compensations, therefore providing a baseline (Klonoff et al., 1997). After one to three trials, specific and personalized strategies to improve performance are introduced, in order to demonstrate their power. Common cognitive examples include using a ruler for visual scanning, double-checking one's work for error reduction, and self-monitoring impulsivity problems. Typical behavioral compensations include focusing on receptivity to feedback if a patient is resistant or "snarky," and adjusting expectations for catastrophic reactions. A sign that a patient is successfully developing awareness (and acceptance) is the patient's ability to independently invent and apply practical strategies to new tasks.

To address and enhance the awareness process, all patients develop lists of their strengths, difficulties, and compensations (Klonoff et al., 2007). Patients type these lists, both to help consolidate this knowledge and to enhance their bimanual dexterity. These lists are reviewed at the outset of every cognitive retraining session and are updated commensurate with their progress and new challenges during the course of the patients' recovery. Therapists must guide patients in recognizing and describing their relative areas of strengths and difficulties. These include not only their cognitive and physical strengths and difficulties, but the patients' emotional reactions to their perceived deficits and coping strategies. The therapist must also be creative in developing beneficial and applicable compensations, and in relating the overall psychoeducation and compensation training process to home, work, and school environments.

### Psychological Issues and Cognitive Retraining

Cognitive retraining sessions are a ripe setting for catastrophic reactions. Patients are regularly confronted not only by their deficits, but by the discrepancies between their perceptions of their skill sets and the realities of their scores. The external manifestations of feelings and coping styles are rich sources of information about each patient. The psychotherapist can follow up on these emerging psychological issues with patients. This can be accomplished either as part of the cognitive retraining sessions or in individual psychotherapy sessions, which afford more privacy. Psychotherapy sessions are also very useful for addressing issues of organic unawareness, denial, or disavowal (see Chapter 5). For example, if a patient is minimizing difficulties, the therapist can gently present data on the expected and the actual performance of tasks. This helps educate the patient about his or her relative strengths and difficulties. The pace and timing of such feedback are based on the patient's receptivity and on the therapist's thorough understanding of the patient's neuropsychological strengths and deficits, as well as their impact on day-to-day functioning. More often than not, the success of the awareness development process in cognitive retraining is predicated on the therapist's level of sophistication and clinical sensitivity in educating the patient and interpreting the clinical observations and data (Klonoff et al., 1997).

Several other typical behavioral challenges to self-awareness can be processed in individual psychotherapy, including cognitive rigidity and difficulty in seeing the "big picture." For example, patients may have difficulty appreciating the applicability of cognitive retraining patterns to the real world. The therapist should use specific examples to help patients recognize how the quantitative scores and behaviors (e.g., alertness, interpersonal interactions) apply to the patients' community-based responsibilities and aspirations. Resistance to the use of compensatory strategies constitutes a major "red flag" for adaptation in community environments, and should be discussed in this context. Cognitive retraining sessions are also an excellent setting in which to evaluate and monitor patients' level of motivation and concerted effort. Typical pathognomonic patterns of suboptimal effort include inexplicable and wide fluctuations in scores, as well as a highly passive approach to task protocols and completion, without the usual associated emotional distress.

**CASE STUDY**

In the third week of his therapies, Dr. Smith began cognitive retraining with his psychotherapist, participating in about four sessions per week. Emphasis was placed on addressing all the neurocognitive, behavioral, and upper-extremity sequelae of his right-hemisphere stroke: left-sided hemiparesis; visual neglect and problems with visual scanning; distractibility; procedural learning difficulties and memory interference effects; problems with visuospatial skills and attention to visual details; organizational difficulties; and impulsivity. Figure 3.1 is Dr. Smith's list of his strengths, difficulties, and compensations. The pertinence of cognitive retraining tasks to the real-world work environment was emphasized from the inception of the sessions. For example, when Dr, Smith was completing an analogue of the Word Fluency Test (Strauss et al., 2006), the relevance to lectures and conference presentations was pointed out. The importance of the balance between

| Strengths | Mantras/metaphors |
|---|---|
| Good vocabulary | "Master strategist" |
| Good spelling | "Patience/patients" |
| Open to feedback | |
| Open to compensations | |
| "Quick study" | |

| Difficulties | Compensations |
|---|---|
| 1. Left-sided motor weakness | 1. Use clipboard and left hand to stabilize paper |
| 2. Left-sided neglect | 2. Colored margin on the left |
| 3. Impulsive | 3. Slow down and focus on accuracy; "stop, look, and listen" |
| 4. Attention to visual detail | 4. Slow down, use ruler, and triple-check; use "checks and balances" |
| 5. New procedural learning | 5. Develop procedure checklists; be vigilant and study in advance |
| 6. Scribbling/poor legibility | 6. Write legibly; slow down |
| 7. "Big picture," prioritization, judgment, and time management | 7. Stand back and be mindful; self-monitor; learn to delegate; focus on content (vs. form) |
| 8. Not organized | 8. Become organized and use strategies systematically |
| 9. "Mini" catastrophic reactions | 9. Acknowledge and discuss them in individual psychotherapy |
| 10. "Flight into health!!!" | 10. Adhere consistently to the compensations in and outside of therapy |

**FIGURE 3.1.** Dr. Smith's cognitive retraining list of strengths, difficulties, and compensations.

speed and accuracy was related to possible written inaccuracies in manuscripts or patient records.

Dr. Smith recognized his propensity for catastrophic reactions when he encountered unexpected and unwanted failures on tasks. The slogan "Patience/ patients" was adopted and revisited during each session, to help remind him to allow sufficient time for his healing process and to affirm his hope of returning to the healing of patients. This phrase was a sustaining thought during times of duress and disheartenment.

The metacognitive aspects of cognitive retraining were essential preparation for Dr. Smith's return to work as a practicing oral surgeon and professor. He was assisted in recognizing the "big picture" of how the cognitive retraining tasks and his level of performance corresponded to his work duties and potential. For example, Dr. Smith was trained to be vigilant about time management by focusing on being punctual to sessions. As an exercise in multitasking, he was expected to watch the amount of available time per session (e.g., 40 minutes) and to monitor his task completion in the context of ending on time, without being rushed or truncating the thorough execution of a task. This was designed to simulate managing his time effectively when seeing patients in a clinic or lecturing students. Initially, prefabricated procedural checklists for task completion were provided; with time, Dr. Smith was expected to generate his own procedural checklists, as a precursor to developing a systematic and error-free approach to his work duties. He and his therapist also engaged in error analyses. Gradually, when performing new tasks, he was given the responsibility of inventing appropriate compensations, based on the task components and his areas of relative strength and difficulty. This not only empowered him in the treatment process, but provided him invaluable training in becoming a "master strategist" to avoid potential problems related to his residual deficits.

Dr. Smith's psychotherapist helped him apply his insights from cognitive retraining to other work activities. For example, before his return to work, Dr. Smith prepared lectures for his dental students. His specific list of strengths, difficulties, and compensations (see Figure 3.1) was incorporated in this process. Specifically, Dr. Smith was counseled to double- and triple-check his work; to use a 6-inch ruler to assist with reading for details; to incorporate "checks and balances" when reviewing data analyses; and to "stop, look, and listen" when requesting input and feedback from colleagues.

## PSYCHOEDUCATION GROUP

In addition to individual psychotherapy and cognitive retraining, patients can participate in a psychoeducation group. This group is designed to improve the patients' understanding and insight about their own injuries (Klonoff, Lamb, Henderson, Reichert, et al., 2000). One possible format is to have 8–12 patients meet four times per week for 45-minute sessions. A psychoeducation group is ideally facilitated by a neuropsychologist/psychotherapist and a speech–language pathologist. Information is best provided in the form of PowerPoint slides and handouts. In my setting, this type of group has four modules: the PEM (see Chapter 1, Figure

1.2); neuroanatomy; memory; and strengths and difficulties. Each module lasts about 6 weeks. There are didactic lectures and group exercises, as well as videos to supplement the psychoeducational process (Klonoff, Lamb, Henderson, Reichert, et al., 2000).

Because the group is conducted in a classroom format, it provides an opportunity for students to practice essential school reentry skills, including note taking, auditory comprehension, speed of information processing, multitasking, and social interaction skills. With the exception of the strengths-and-difficulties module, there is a quiz at the completion of each module; the quiz tests the patients' understanding and retention of the material. There are two versions of the end-of-module tests. The first version is relatively general and is administered in an open-book format. It is given to nonstudents and severely impaired patients. The second version, which is more detailed and comprehensive, is given to students and patients returning to gainful employment. This second version is first completed from memory, after which patients use their notes to add missing answers, in order to reinforce the acquisition of knowledge. Two scores are computed: one with and another without notes. The following is a brief description of each module.

## The PEM

A primary teaching tool in psychoeducation group is the PEM (again, see Chapter 1, Figure 1.2). The group spends approximately 6 weeks reviewing the model and studying the terminology. Following that, patients place themselves in the model by rating their phase and "color" (coping status) for the physical, cognitive, and social/emotional domains. As part of an awareness exercise, each patient then receives input from the other group members, as well as from the therapist(s) facilitating the discussion. Review of this model emphasizes for patients the perils of the crisis ("red") or warning ("yellow") zones. At the same time, it provides a roadmap for a brighter, productive, and meaningful future ("green" zone).

## Neuroanatomy

In the second module, patients study basic neuroanatomy. They first review the module's purposes, which are to help them (1) understand how the brain works; (2) learn how injuries affect the brain and the ability to function; and (3) become their "own best experts." Information pertinent to general principles of recovery are reviewed, as are various types of brain injuries (e.g., traumatic brain injury, aneurysm, anoxia, brain tumor). The parts and functions of the brainstem, cerebellum, hemispheres, and lobes of the brain, as well as other subcortical structures, are reviewed. PowerPoint slides of parts of the brain are used to illustrate the content. The symptomatology associated with damage to each area is emphasized, followed by discussion of patients' perceptions of their own specific deficits. After studying the coursework, patients also review their MRI and CT scans in the group to personalize the education and awareness process. This boosts each patient's knowledge about the anatomy and pathophysiology of his or her injury.

## Memory

In the third module, patients learn about the specific neuroanatomy and substrates of memory. They are introduced to different types of memory systems (e.g., procedural memory and prospective memory), as well as the different stages of memory (e.g., sensory memory, short-term memory, and long-term memory). The module also reviews common types of memory failures, with an emphasis on helpful compensations or learning strategies (e.g., mnemonics and associations). As a memory exercise, patients memorize a "roll call" list; this includes each patient's first and last name, type of injury, and birthplace, as well as personal preferences (such as favorite food, type of car, and color). Patients take turns trying to recall this information for the entire group. This provides an opportunity to practice helpful mnemonic strategies and introduces a "fun" component to the group discussion. Patients also decide on daily memory assignments, and patients and therapists then bring in various objects and mementos to the group (e.g., pictures from a vacation). This also facilitates practice with their datebooks. Consistent follow-through by all participants for several sessions is rewarded by a pizza party.

## Strengths and Difficulties

In the strengths-and-difficulties module, a list is compiled with each patient. This is separate from cognitive retraining's list of strengths, difficulties, and compensations, described earlier. The list for this module is compiled first with the patient's input, and then with contributions from the group members and the therapists. Three domains are addressed: the physical, the cognitive, and the social/emotional. Often patients are assisted by their individual psychotherapists in developing their lists before a group discussion, to reduce their level of anxiety or frustration. The therapists also construct their own lists with group input, which normalizes the process. The contributions of group members are structured according to the "sandwich technique": Input begins with a positive statement, which is followed by the constructive feedback, and concludes with another positive statement. This increases each individual's receptivity to and comfort with the process.

### CASE STUDY

Dr. Smith attended a psychoeducation group and completed all four modules. Figure 3.2 is his list of strengths and difficulties. His test scores at the end of the PEM module were 97% without notes and 100% with notes, indicating good assimilation and recall of the material. Approximately 10 weeks after his admission, Dr. Smith provided self-ratings of his placement in the PEM. He indicated that he was in Phase 4 of the "green" (adaptive coping) zone on the physical, cognitive, and social/emotional dimensions. Peer input and therapists' ratings placed him in Phase 5 of the "green" zone. Dr. Smith's self-view was that his less advanced Phase 4 rating related to his periodic catastrophic reactions about his deficits and his perceived slow pace of recovery. He also felt that he was still learning more about the consequences of his stroke, especially in relationship to his projected functional status at work. This discussion helped the therapists better appreciate

|  | Strengths | Difficulties |
|---|---|---|
| Physical | Improving gait pattern<br>Functionally independent | Decreased left-sided strength<br>Increased left-sided tone<br>Decreased balance<br>Decreased endurance |
| Cognitive | Verbal expression<br>Reading comprehension<br>Vocabulary<br>Spelling<br>Quick learner | Deductive reasoning<br>Organization and problem solving<br>Attention to details<br>Impulsivity<br>Seeing the "big picture"<br>Time management |
| Social/<br>emotional | Open to feedback<br>Interactive<br>Helpful, kind, friendly, polite<br>Encouraging to others and supportive<br>Good sense of humor<br>Resilient<br>Family support | Some impatience<br>Mild depression<br>Catastrophic reactions<br>Unrealistic expectations of self |

**FIGURE 3.2.** Dr. Smith's psychoeducation group list of strengths and difficulties.

Dr. Smith's internalized emotional distress, which was followed up in individual psychotherapy sessions with his psychotherapist.

Dr. Smith also gave a mock lecture in the psychoeducation group prior to his transition to the university teaching environment. This was considered part of his treatment process, and during the preparation phase, Dr. Smith received therapeutic assistance and input from his psychotherapist and speech–language pathologist. This task provided invaluable practice with executive functions, including prioritizing and organizing his program in the context of his other multiple responsibilities, as well as judgment and decision making regarding the amount and type of content to include, based on the audience. The lecture was designed to be appropriate for dental students, and he was expected to develop a PowerPoint presentation. After the lecture, Dr. Smith received input from his peers in the group. The lecture was also video-recorded and was subsequently reviewed with him in individual speech and psychotherapy sessions for content, delivery style, time management, and quality of slides. Feedback included that he was fluent, well organized, thorough, relaxed, engaging of the audience, and able to juggle the content demands effectively within the time constraints. This "in-house" practice was instrumental in rebuilding Dr. Smith's confidence in his teaching and lectureship skills.

## GROUP PSYCHOTHERAPY

A critical therapeutic venue for the awareness development process is group psychotherapy (Delmonico et al., 1998; Klonoff, 1997). This provides a much-needed interpersonal forum for learning from group members, based on their similar experiences and vantage points (Delmonico et al., 1998; Prigatano et al., 1986).

One possible format for group psychotherapy is four sessions per week, each for 40 minutes; it may be facilitated by one (or two) clinical neuropsychologist(s) or psychotherapist(s), with 6–10 patients participating. The decisions about whether and when to integrate a patient into the group are made primarily by the individual psychotherapist treating the patient (with possible input from the other therapists), the patient, and his or her family. Participants must be emotionally ready for peer interaction and guided self-reflection about topics related to their injury knowledge, coping techniques, and realistic decision making for the future. Other criteria include sufficient cognitive and language recovery to benefit from the group discussion, and sufficient impulse and temper control to discuss sensitive topics without becoming irate or insulting toward others (Klonoff, 1997; Klonoff, Lamb, Henderson, Reichert, et al., 2000; Prigatano et al., 1986). The group is open-entry/open-exit, and patient participants vary considerably with respect to their age, etiology, injury acuteness, and amount of treatment they have received (Klonoff, 1997).

When patients begin the group, they are given a handout that summarizes the purpose and etiquette of the group (see Figure 3.3). From the patients' point of view, group psychotherapy provides the opportunity to share feelings and "gripes"; to obtain opinions and support from peers who "walk in their shoes"; problem solve about common challenges and concerns (e.g., change in driving status, catastrophic reactions); and to enjoy a sense of camaraderie. Some have described it as a "fraternity" with the toughest initiation imaginable. The group's exchanges and interrelationships instill perspective, scope, and hope to the group members.

Group psychotherapy has some structure to assist patients with memory problems. Each session reviews the name and purpose of the group, as well as the previous session's discussion (Prigatano, 1999). The group facilitators take notes on an easel pad to keep track of salient information, which patients copy into their notebooks (Klonoff, 1997). In addition, summaries of meaningful topic areas are provided in handout form so that patients will have accessible and permanent records of the discussions, especially when they have difficulties with divided attention, writing, and/or spelling.

Both the form and content of group sessions vary, as shown in Figure 3.3. They include free discussion; didactics; guided exercises; review of journal articles, readings, and movies; patients' self-disclosures; viewpoints at the time of therapy termination; and visits by therapy "graduates." Participants are always encouraged to raise topics of personal interest or relevance to the awareness process.

There is considerable fluidity and flexibility in what is discussed in the group and how, based on the needs and preferences of the group members. The topics for free discussion listed on Figure 3.3 are those frequently raised by group members. Open discussions allow the patients to "vent" or "decompress" about their frustrations and hassles. Once feelings are "off their chests," patients are more psychologically primed for psychoeducation. Given the sensitive nature of the topics and the understandable emotional angst that patients may experience, the group psychotherapists need to be proactive in guiding the group discussion. It is often helpful to approach patients in individual psychotherapy first to ascertain their comfort with particular topics or self-disclosure; this will ensure that they do not feel "ambushed" or unnecessarily disturbed by the group discussion.

## Group Psychotherapy Introduction

Q: Name of the group?    A: Group psychotherapy.
Q: Purpose?    A: To discuss feelings.
Q: Why is this important?    A: How you feel determines how you act; how you act determines how others react to you.

## General Rules and Etiquette

1. Respect others' opinions and provide feedback in a sensitive manner.
2. Discussions are confidential.
3. Group members should take notes summarizing the key points.
4. Any topic that relates to feelings about the recovery and rehabilitation process can be raised for discussion in the group.

## Form and Content of Awareness Topics

1. *Free discussion of topics raised by group members*
   a. Why are people telling me I'm unaware?
   b. Why do I need a datebook?
   c. Why can't I drive?
   d. Why do I have to be in all of these therapies (e.g., community outings, communication pragmatics group, current events)?
   e. Why are psychotropic medications being recommended?

2. *Guided didactics and discussions introduced by group leaders*
   a. Role of working alliance and trust in outcome.
   b. Awareness challenges in "new" versus "old" injuries.
   c. Subcomponents of executive functions.
   d. Catastrophic reactions ("CRs").
   e. Postinjury personality changes.
   f. What is depression?

3. *Guided exercises*
   a. Autobiographies: Who was I before my injury?
   b. Self-ratings (0 = none, 1 = small, 10 = big) of executive function deficits.
   c. Personal examples of "CRs," associated emotions, and coping strategies.
   d. Self-ratings of readiness to drive.
   e. Creating my own ideal program schedule.
   f. Self-ratings of the benefits of each therapy.
   g. Self-identified goals and projected length of treatment.

4. *Handouts and movies*
   a. *The Karate Kid* (Weintraub, Louis, Smith, & Avildsen, 1984).
   b. *Failure to Launch* (Rudin & Dey, 2006).
   c. *Good Will Hunting* (Armstrong et al., 1997).

**FIGURE 3.3.** Handout for group psychotherapy. (Introduction from Prigatano et al., 1986).

The guided didactics and discussions also provide a forum for psychotherapists to tackle areas that can pose barriers to patients' progress in their rehabilitation, as well as to help the patient appreciate the commonality of their emotional conditions and functional predicaments.

Guided exercises are an interactive modality for exploring patients' level of awareness. In general, patients provide self-ratings from 0 to 10 (0 = no problem, 1 = small problem, 10 = big problem); they then receive input from their peers and group facilitators. This enables dialogue regarding each patient's self-perception relative to the perceptions of others—a central component of the group interchange process. It is also a powerful way to work on developing awareness. Construction of brief autobiographies is an engaging technique for patients to become better acquainted with each other beyond the context of their injuries. It also helps to "open the door" for meaningful dialogue about how their existence has been altered by their injuries. The discussion of movies sometimes occurs in conjunction with community outings (see Chapter 8); patients and therapists will watch a movie together and answer specific questions afterward. The patients' answers and reactions are then explored in group psychotherapy to enhance the introspective process. For example, the movie *The Karate Kid* (Weintraub, Louis, Smith, & Avildsen, 1984) is used in this manner: Patients are encouraged to apply various messages in the movie to their recovery process, with the aid of the sample discussion questions in Figure 3.4. Such exercises can enhance patients' appreciation and application of formal therapeutic activities to an assortment of functional daily tasks.

Other benefits of group psychotherapy include the opportunity for current patients to witness the achievements and therapy terminations of their peers. In my experience, patient "graduates" have visited groups months and even years after their discharge, to discuss their candid feelings and reflections about the recovery and rehabilitation process in light of their lives in the real world. This can provide education, balance, and optimism for the current patients, who are often experiencing periods of disillusionment about the slow pace of their recovery and/or the tedium of rehabilitation. Dynamic discussion with peer input is often more readily acceptable to patients and can reinforce awareness constructs raised by treating therapists. Group exchange also alleviates postinjury loneliness and alienation, and normalizes the often painful realization process. The group forum facilitates empathic responsiveness toward others, with more senior group members helping to mentor and encourage newer ones. It is empowering to patients to become the "helpers" instead of the "helped."

## CASE STUDY

Dr. Smith began group psychotherapy in conjunction with starting his cognitive retraining and psychoeducation group. Awareness topics and exercises included his autobiography; a self-rating of the benefits of the psychoeducation group (which he rated highly); factors related to successful return to driving (including relevant therapies and his own performance levels in cognitive retraining); the definition and management of catastrophic reactions; the sources and treatment of depression; and expectations of his capacity for returning to work as an oral

(Short answers: 2–3 sentences for each question. Use a separate sheet of paper.)

1. When Mr. Miyagi talks to Daniel about learning karate, he refers to a "Yes–No" versus a "Guess so" attitude. What does this mean? How does it relate to your rehabilitation?

2. Name three techniques Mr. Miyagi uses to help Daniel learn karate.

3. How does Mr. Miyagi's approach (e.g., "Wax on—right hand/Wax off—left hand") relate to your rehabilitation?

4. What do you think about the relationship between Mr. Miyagi and Daniel?

5. What are two main messages of the movie?

6. Relate the following statements by Mr. Miyagi to your neurological recovery and rehabilitation:

    a. "Not everything is as it seems."
    b. "Trust the quality of what you know, not the quantity."
    c. "Come back tomorrow."
    d. "First stand, then fly."

7. Describe three practical activities/chores you do, and explain why they relate to your neurological recovery.

8. Use three words to describe the main character and what he learns.

9. What is Mr. Miyagi's real name?

10. How many times do they say "Wax on . . . /Wax off . . . "?

11. Did you like the movie? Yes ____ No ____

    Why or why not?

**FIGURE 3.4.** Psychotherapy questions for *The Karate Kid*.

surgeon. Dr. Smith used the group effectively to discuss his personal precipitants and manifestations of catastrophic reactions, including becoming frustrated and despairing about his stroke-related cognitive difficulties (e.g., inattention to detail, visuospatial skills) and physical problems (e.g., left-sided hemiparesis), as well as their impact on his daily functioning and work potential.

One month after starting the group, Dr. Smith participated in the group exercise of devising his own schedule, which was highly concordant with that recommended by his treating therapists. This suggested a good appreciation of the type of the treatment he was receiving and its benefits. Two months later, he participated in a group self-awareness exercise where patients shared their perception of areas of neurological recovery. He reported self-perceived changes in his gait, left-hand functionality, organization, and prioritization skills. At that time, he estimated that he would require an additional 3 months of therapy in order to return successfully to work as an oral surgeon, compared with the 6-month estimate proposed by the group facilitators. This suggested an underestimation of the complexity of the recovery and work reintegration process, related to remnants of organic unawareness. The group discussion assisted Dr. Smith in recalibrating his time projection.

Dr. Smith watched *The Karate Kid* (Weintraub et al., 1984) and responded to the questions in Figure 3.4. Relevant themes included the role of strong mentorship, with kindness, compassion, and strict discipline. Dr. Smith had a long-time mentor who was a "beacon of hope" during his dental career and his neurological recovery. Dr. Smith valued the clinic-developed procedural checklists, and utilized a similar protocol when developing new lecture plans. The "First stand, then fly" metaphor was a helpful guidepost when he was discussing his gradual reintegration into his work and teaching environments.

During Dr. Smith's group participation, a former patient came to speak. He had undergone rehabilitation and subsequently returned successfully to his pre-injury occupation as a pilot. There were a number of parallels between Dr. Smith and this patient: Both had sustained strokes, were highly educated and ambitious before their injuries, and had highly technical and complex jobs that affected others' safety and well-being. Both had grappled with the possibility of being unemployable, and both required substantial retesting and reevaluation to be cleared to work again in their chosen professions. Both individuals admitted to feelings of "hating to fail," and both struggled with worry and chagrin related to the profound uncertainty about their futures. Both upheld the intrinsic value of compensatory strategies and earnestly incorporated the guidance and constructs of their neurorehabilitation. This particular speaker was highly informative and inspiring to Dr. Smith, as through the eyes of this other patient he could envision his own return to his vocational calling in some form.

This chapter has described the complex process of increasing self-awareness of injury-related deficits and retained strengths in the recovery process. As patients' awareness evolves, issues of sense of self and identity emerge. Patients begin to wonder who they are after their injuries. The next chapter discusses the handling of these challenges in psychotherapy.

# CHAPTER 4

# Sense of Self and Identity

*with* Stephen M. Myles

$A$s Chapter 3 has described, the development of awareness is accompanied by inevitable distress, including fear, anxiety, grief, and emptiness (O'Callaghan et al., 2006). Furthermore, the burgeoning awareness precipitates dilemmas and yearnings over the loss of purpose and identity (the "old me"), compounded by disdain for the "new me" (O'Callaghan et al., 2006).

Inherent in the conceptualization of identity and the self are stable and enduring qualities, in part drawn from life experiences. However, brain injury often devastates an individual's core internal state. Memory loss affects the continuous integration of events, which threatens the integrity of the self and the core identity (Brown et al., 2006; Piolino et al., 2007). Loss of self after brain injury is also associated with (1) loss of clear self-knowledge; (2) loss of self by comparison (i.e., alterations in self-image from the past to the present); and (3) loss of self in the eyes of others (i.e., the mostly negative perceptions of brain injury and brain-injured persons by others in society) (Nochi, 1998). Others have conceptualized changes in sense of self as a "crisis of the conceptualized self," in which a patient recognizes that he or she is not the same person (Myles, 2004) and experiences feelings of insecurity, vulnerability, and uncertainty (Howes, Benton, & Edwards, 2005).

We propose a working definition of *self* based on the Kohutian definition. That is, self emanates from the "interplay of inherited and environmental fac-

---

**Stephen M. Myles, DClinPsy,** is a Clinical Neuropsychologist at the Center for Transitional NeuroRehabilitation, Barrow Neurological Institute, St. Joseph's Hospital and Medical Center, Phoenix, Arizona.

tors" (Wolf, 1988, p. 182) and can be characterized as the "essence of one's being," or as the foundational personality attributes and sense of who one is (Lewis & Rosenberg, 1990). A subcomponent of the self consists of *values*, defined as the individual's core beliefs that endure over the lifespan. Other manifestations of the self include *identity*, defined as the person's subjective characterization of his or her individuality in the social context; and *social roles*, or the individual's societal position and responsibilities as perceived and defined by both the person him- or herself and members of the social network. Identity and social roles have a fluid interrelationship, and are influenced by family history and culture.

Although elements of the core self, values, identity, and social roles are retained after brain injury, the injury's consequences often result in their major alteration and/or evolution. Some authors have focused on the grief and loss associated with changes in sense of self (Chamberlain, 2006; Persinger, 1993). Others have emphasized positive aspects, such as "posttraumatic growth," which includes positive changes in self-perceptions and an emerging philosophy of life (McGrath & Linley, 2006; Vickery, Gontkovsky, Wallace, & Caroselli, 2006).

This chapter explores helping patients as they grapple with a disrupted sense of self. Grief and mourning are discussed first as the overarching processes of alteration in the patients' being. As patients become aware of the impact of their injuries on their sense of self, identity, values, and social roles, psychotherapy can assist them in self-discovery, redefinition, and self-determination.

## GRIEF AND MOURNING

"Grief" has been defined as distress, suffering, or other affective reactions to a loss (Genevro, Marshall, & Miller, 2004; Middleton, Raphael, Martinek, & Misso, 1993; Wilkinson, 2000). After brain injury, patients are exposed both to subjective indices of loss (i.e., their self-perceptions of their acquired deficiencies) and to objective evidence (e.g., changes in employment status, income, and driving). Grief is an often unavoidable product of increased awareness of the brain injury's consequences. It is generally manifested as shock, sorrow, fear, anger, self-reproach, and/or anxiety (Coetzer, 2006; Hinkebein & Stucky, 2007; Langer, 1994; O'Callaghan et al., 2006). In its more severe forms, it can create feelings of hopelessness, helplessness, and despair, especially when the losses are perceived as catastrophic or permanent (Langer, 1994). Some have depicted this state as "partial death" (Tadir & Stern, 1985). Irreconcilable grief may escalate to suicidality. Particularly salient for patients with brain injury is the interaction among multiple variables, including the pathophysiology of the injury, its impact on emotional expression, the patient's neuropsychological status, and personal grief reactions (Coetzer, 2006). The individual's gender, social context, religion, and culture also influence the nature and expression of grief, which can be cyclical (Chamberlain, 2006; Matthews & Marwit, 2006; Niemeier, Kennedy, McKinley, & Cifu, 2004; Paletti, 2008; Stroebe & Schut, 1999). May (1977) described the effect of disability on the individual's sense of self as "dissolution of self."

If "grief" is conceptualized as a process of self-dissolution, into a deep emotional well, "mourning" can be viewed as the metamorphosis of raw affect into a reconstitution process. Mourning can also be viewed as the assimilation of new feelings into an altered worldview, or as the capacity to redefine oneself and reintegrate into life (Balk, 2004); this capacity can include including transcendence (Chen, 1997), self-transformation (Paletti, 2008), or reconstruction of meaning (Matthews & Marwit, 2006). Following brain injury, therefore, grief and mourning reactions, play specific parts in the patient's evolving sense of self, identity, values, and social roles.

## SENSE OF SELF

After brain injury, patients' internal sense of self may change in part because of organically based personality changes. For example, research has implicated prefrontal brain damage in a poorly integrated postinjury self (Mathiesen & Weinryb, 2004; Ylvisaker & Feeney, 2000). However, brain injury can have diverse effects on personality, and there is inherent variability in the preinjury self. Complicating the process is the view that one's "essence of being" (the sense of "I" or "me") is actually constructed from multiple selves (Heller, Levin, Mukherjee, & Reis, 2006). Redefining and integrating a patient's sense of self are predicated on enhancing awareness, so that the patient can "find the bits of the puzzle" (Brown et al., 2006, p. 940).

In individual psychotherapy, the psychotherapist sets out upon a joint venture with the patient to discover the new essence of this multidimensional self, in juxtaposition with (and eventual merging with) aspects of the prior multifaceted self. Treatment works best when the patient is comfortable with "storytelling" about the self—that is, describing and reflecting on his or her core personality attributes and their manifestation in the patient's preinjury versus postinjury lifestyle. In this process, the psychotherapist should first encourage the patient to explore the preinjury self, because often there are foundational remnants that the patient clings to. Judicious listening with open-ended questions by the psychotherapist will assist the patient in articulating perceptions of his or her core personality attributes before the injury. These include questions such as "What were you like as a person prior to this injury?" and "Who in your family do you most take after, and why?" Other helpful techniques include looking at photo albums, discussing salient life events through autobiographical essays, and discussing sources of inspiration (influential books, movies, music, etc.). Personality testing (e.g., with the MMPI-2 or MCMI-III) is a helpful supplemental tool to explore preinjury attributes: Was the individual sociable, impulsive, independent, and so on?

The patient is next encouraged to document in list form his or her postinjury qualities, and then to compare and contrast these with preinjury features. Open-ended questions also facilitate this process—for example, "How are you different as a person now, and why?" The psychotherapist should be patient and nurturing in this process, because superimposed upon the familiar (and sometimes lost) attributes are newly emerging and often foreign characteristics, which can be troubling and frightening to the patient.

Another effective treatment tool for exploring a patient's sense of self is a sentence completion task. In the task we use, the patient finishes 36 half-completed

*Instructions:* Please complete the following sentences any way you want.

1. Since the injury, my sense of who I am . . .
2. Since the injury, my physical abilities . . .
3. Since the injury, I feel . . .
4. Since the injury, the way I see myself . . .
5. Since the injury, my thinking abilities . . .
6. Since the injury, my sense of connection with other people . . .
7. Since the injury, when I think of myself . . .
8. Since the injury, when I think about my body . . .
9. Since the injury, when I think about the future, I feel . . .
10. Since the injury, my feelings about myself . . .
11. Since the injury, when I think about my role in my family . . .
12. When I think about life before the injury, I feel . . .
13. Since the injury, what matters to me . . .
14. Since the injury, when I think about work . . .
15. Compared to before the injury, my emotions . . .
16. Since the injury, my role in life . . .
17. Since the injury, my self-esteem . . .
18. Compared to before the injury, my level of stress . . .
19. Since the injury, my place in the world . . .
20. Since the injury, my confidence . . .
21. Compared to before the injury, I get upset . . .
22. Since the injury, my sense of purpose . . .
23. Since the injury, when I compare myself to other people . . .
24. Compared to before the injury, I feel sad . . .
25. Since the injury, the things that are important to me . . .
26. When I compare myself to how I was before the injury . . .
27. Compared to before the injury, I worry . . .
28. Since the injury, I am . . .
29. Since the injury, my relationships with the people close to me . . .
30. Compared to before the injury, I feel anxious . . .
31. Since the injury, my life is . . .
32. Since the injury, my ability to deal with problems . . .
33. Compared to before the injury, I get frustrated . . .
34. Since the injury, when I think about my life . . .
35. Since the injury, my ability to cope with stress . . .
36. Compared to before the injury, I feel angry . . .

**FIGURE 4.1.** Sense of self following brain injury: Sentence completion task.

sentence stems that compare postinjury to preinjury life (Myles, 2007) (see Figure 4.1). This tool can qualitatively elucidate the patient's perceptions of changes in cognitive, emotional, behavioral, and physical aspects of the self. This self-appraisal may be positive (i.e., the patient is acquiring an improved sense of being in various domains); neutral (i.e., there are no significant changes); or negative (i.e., the patient feels miserable about his or her postinjury sense of self). Discussion of the individual's answers can serve as a springboard for self-reflection on current values, in the context of historical core beliefs.

Deciphering a new sense of self should take into account the effects of neurological sequelae on personality style, in combination with the emergent attributes based on the brain injury as a major life-altering event. To this end, the psychotherapist can guide the patient in understanding the relative contribution of these factors by correlating neurological with behavioral symptoms (e.g., temporal lobe injury can produce increased distrust; frontal lobe injury can facilitate greater openness).

Collateral input can also be helpful in patients' redefinition of self. For example, emotional strengths are identified and listed as part of the strengths-and-difficulties module in the psychoeducation group (see Chapter 3). The patient's family and significant social network can add unique historical perspectives. Often, too, the psychotherapist can assist patients in witnessing the evolution of their sense of self through here-and-now (Yalom, 2002) observations of personality style. Frequently there is an amplification of certain desirable characteristics (e.g., sensitivity, empathy), which are imbued by his or her personal experience and loss. These old and new attributes then coalesce into a new sense of self.

## CASE STUDY

At the age of 47, Dr. Derksen, a physician, was diagnosed with a low-grade ependymoma of the fourth ventricle. In fact, he diagnosed the tumor himself by recognizing the symptoms and by reviewing his own brain scan. However, he was horrified to discover his own postoperative deficits, including dysarthria and problems with swallowing, balance, gait, stamina, vision, hand dexterity, and coordination. Initially Dr. Derksen was very reluctant to consider psychotherapy, preferring to focus his energies on other treatment disciplines to improve his functional status. He hesitantly agreed to begin the psychotherapy process 2 weeks after starting his other therapies in an interdisciplinary treatment setting. Approximately 4 weeks after that, he began attending group psychotherapy.

It was apparent to his psychotherapist that Dr. Derksen was experiencing considerable turmoil about the uninvited and devastating transformations in his sense of self. His medical predicament had abruptly and irrevocably catapulted his sense of self from the "diagnostician/observer of illness" to the "personally afflicted." Within the newfound safe haven of the psychotherapeutic relationship, he tentatively explored, articulated, and eventually integrated his prior self with aspects of his newly discovered, foreign self. Now, in his role as a patient, he was forced to evaluate life from the vantage point of both a healer and an ill person. With guidance, Dr. Derksen came to recognize that his essence of being was in fact composed of multiple selves, all embodying the commonalities of a competent, nurturing, loving, and empathic human being.

One prominent self that he tended to downplay was his vibrancy within the family unit, mainly because of the guilt he was feeling about placing such a burden on his wife and young children. Early in treatment and periodically thereafter, Dr. Derksen was encouraged to use his psychotherapy sessions to vent his deep disquiet and sorrow about the impact of his illness. The psychotherapist alternated her listening perspective with reminders and illustrations about his many forms of involvement with his children and his loving relationship with his wife. Over time, through the grief and mourning process, he was helped to accept and cherish the fact that he was still a devoted husband and father.

Dr. Derksen also wrestled in sessions with the real and frightening possibility of tumor regrowth, which persisted in the shadowy background and constituted an ominous threat to his life expectancy. This represented his "vulnerable" self. During one session he wept, convinced he was "living on borrowed time." To help him delve further into this theme, the psychotherapist recommended the movie *Life as a House* (Cowan & Winkler, 2001). Dr. Derksen was inspired by the main character's (George's) resolve in the face of his own mortality to be an "architect" of new and vibrant house/life energies, characterized by love, physicality, and heartfelt communication with those he treasured most in life. As George says, "Something bad forces something good."

Other dimensions of Dr. Derksen's postoperative sense of self that were cultivated in psychotherapy were new roles as a communicator and advocate for persons with brain injury. Initially, Dr. Derksen was shy, noncommunicative, and opposed to sharing his feelings candidly in group psychotherapy; this reluctance was also related to his self-consciousness about his dysarthria. However, he soon came to recognize the commonality of the torturous life journey he and his fellow patients were traversing. Through the relational climate, his psychotherapist helped him feel comfortable with sharing his own perspectives, as well as with soliciting frank impressions from his patient peers. As an example, by carefully weighing his colleagues' input from their vantage point as health care consumers, he became a stronger advocate for the brain-injured population through community outreach projects. Gradually, through the combination of dialogue and self-reflection, Dr. Derksen transformed his feelings of anguish, helplessness, and disillusionment into meaningful actions.

Two months after the initiation of psychotherapy, Dr. Derksen voiced an interest in writing, particularly poetry. His psychotherapist urged him to pursue this endeavor. This represented the emergence of his "creative" self; he described this as a process of "reconciling." Gradually, the discussion of his poetry became his personal battlefield for his struggles. Through the sharing and analytical process—first with his psychotherapist, and later with his loved ones—he reinvigorated his core being.

Another self that his psychotherapist highlighted consisted of Dr. Derksen's considerable expertise and accomplishments in the field of medicine. This self was exemplified not only in his own keen recognition of his neurological changes, but importantly in the widespread community respect for his reputation as a

> With battered visage and bludgeoned brain
> To tilt the head just so . . .
>       There, the vision is still for the moment.
>       I can see the world as it was
>       But not the same ever again
> Much is lost
>       And cloaked grief hovers close,
>       Sucking the air soundlessly.
> There is a deeper stillness
> An awesome, silent strength
> That bears me on a soaring wing
> Beating steadily as my heart
> Powerful, sure, and constant.
>
>                                    —Timothy Derksen

**FIGURE 4.2.** An untitled poem by Dr. Derksen. From Klonoff (2005). Copyright 2005 by Catherine Derksen. Reprinted by permission of Mrs. Derksen and the Barrow Neurological Institute.

knowledgeable yet caring practitioner. Through the psychotherapeutic process, he grieved over his current inabilities to perform surgical procedures; he tended to minimize his other true talents outside of his technical know-how. With further collaboration and contemplation, however, he reconfigured the "successful" physician as compassionate and dedicated.

Dr. Derksen derived encouragement for returning to the practice of medicine from individual and group psychotherapy. He was reconstituting his "doctor" self. His psychotherapist took a leadership role in advocacy and liaisons with the necessary professionals to facilitate this process. His wife also remained staunchly supportive. Approximately 9 months after his initial diagnosis, Dr. Derksen gradually returned to the practice of medicine. Ultimately, through the psychotherapy process, Dr. Derksen emerged to redefine the essence of his being as "counting my blessings, proclaiming my rarity, going the extra mile, using the power of choice, and doing all things in love."

Figures 4.2 and 4.3 are samples of Dr. Derksen's poetry. In the first poem, he reflects on his damaged self, referring to his "battered visage," "bludgeoned brain," and double vision. He laments his losses, proclaiming that "Much is lost/ And cloaked grief hovers close." His new sense of self is fighting to find hope and meaning, through "An awesome, silent strength . . . Powerful, sure, and constant." Dr. Derksen's second poem, "Vespers," captures his deepened sense of self as a healer, as he juxtaposes his personal imperfections with those of his ill patient, resonating with deeply shared intuitive knowledge and empathy on the fragility of health and life.

At the conclusion of his rehabilitation and psychotherapy, Dr. Derksen delivered a good-bye speech to his family, his peers, their families, and his treating therapists, including his psychotherapist. He said:

Today, out of habit, I mimic a radio voice,
pedantic love-to-hear-myself sales pitch,
but the slick words trip over my sluggish tongue
and trail, quieted by a quick cerebral flush.

For a moment I can hear grief's whispers again
behind the curtain, reminding me how he hovers
persistent and sexless as a faucet drip, sick
seduction to engage in that bottomless dialogue.

But I focus then to visit a woman twice my age,
plagued by her own fading spells, and wonder
at the uncharted waters we both sail, rudderless
and peering through mists at jumbled constellations.

She with the dry cataracts and pruned gyri and
I stumbling with concealed radiant brand, attempt
a dance of normalcy and longing to the music
of measured sighs and syncopating hearts.

—Timothy Derksen

**FIGURE 4.3.** Dr. Derksen's poem "Vespers." From Klonoff (2005). Copyright 2005 by Catherine Derksen. Reprinted by permission of Mrs. Derksen and the Barrow Neurological Institute.

"I only want to remark on one aspect of this wondrous process as it has impacted my life. And that lies in the conviction that this has all been a gift to me. . . . The sense I have is one of gratitude. To be sure, that gratitude was preceded by other sentiments—in fact, some of these not so seemly sentiments still rise up from time to time. There has been anger and frustration, sadness and, at times, a deep sense of loss that all but blocks out the sun. . . . There are all too many people adrift around us who have never had the availability of such resources when confronted with the tragedy of brain injury. And somehow even that realization feeds my gratitude. Because now, more than ever, I can truly recognize and intervene more effectively with these conditions in my patients who come to my office. . . . Thank you all for your part in restoring fullness and hopefulness in my life. Let us not forget one another."

## NARCISSISTIC RAGE

Within this journey, the patient will encounter the "stormy seas" of life experience, once he or she is exposed to assaults on his or her self-esteem. The resulting narcissistic rage can be directed either toward oneself, toward the external objects perceived to the causes of the narcissistic insults, or both (Baker & Baker, 1987; Kohut, 1972). Such rage is the reaction of the self when it experiences helplessness, shame, and loss of integrity; this "disintegration anxiety" represents the sense of loss of self, humanness, and wholeness (Kohut, 1984b). There is fragmentation of the self, characterized by feelings of emptiness, depression, worthlessness, or hopelessness. Narcissistic rage can be differentiated from catastrophic reactions: The former represents an explosive reaction to a destroyed sense of "me" and the global disintegration of the sense of self, whereas the latter are intense but short-lived emotional reactions to specific stimuli.

It is essential to address narcissistic rage in remediating dissolution of the sense of self. This is accomplished by first providing a working definition: *Narcissistic rage* is rage engendered by an assault (by the effects of the injury) on the patient's sense of inner being, resulting in a shattering of his or her core essence and self-defining capabilities. Following this, the patient is encouraged to express the understandably intense feelings of fury and self-hatred associated with this assault, so as to expel these emotions in a healthy and protected setting. Coupled with this process is helping the patient identify the specific deficits that are precipitating such strong visceral reactions; this self-insight helps to insulate the patient from future intense rage reactions. The psychotherapist should assist the patient in understanding and integrating the realities of the injury's effects (Klonoff & Lage, 1991). This is accomplished by acknowledging the problem areas that undermine the sense of efficacy and competency, while devoting equal attention to residual talents and skill sets (Klonoff & Lage, 1991). This helps the patient to reconstitute him- or herself psychologically. Given the intensity of the emotional turmoil, the psychotherapist must be creative in psychotherapeutic interventions, using whatever "tools in the tool kit" to best and broadly assist the patient; these may include dialogue, dream analysis, journal keeping, and/or art or music therapy. Psychotropic medications are also often instrumental in helping with mood regulation and ameliorating intense and pervasive bouts of depression and hopelessness.

### CASE STUDY

Linda, a 31-year-old woman, experienced the onset of complex partial seizures. She was diagnosed with a grade 2 oligodendroglioma in the left temporal lobe. During the next 5 years, she underwent two brain surgeries, chemotherapy, and radiation treatments, including gamma knife treatment. Prior to her diagnosis, she had been a successful mechanical engineer and an avid outdoorswoman, enjoying hang gliding, hiking, and running.

Linda received comprehensive therapies, including psychotherapy. Her significant neuropsychological deficits included problems with attention and concentration, memory (new learning and retention), initiation, multitasking, auditory processing, higher-level language comprehension, and abstraction. Her growing awareness of these changes created emotional chaos and profound despair. She felt panicky and distraught over her growing realization of lost capabilities and fractured hopes for work, marriage, motherhood, and even independent living. She suffered episodes of narcissistic rage over these glaring and impending losses.

Linda was seen weekly in psychotherapy for 2 years, and was also followed bimonthly by a psychiatrist for psychotropic medications. Mirroring Linda's interests and talents, the psychotherapeutic interventions utilized a variety of approaches: talk therapy, psychopharmacology, dream analysis, journal keeping, and art therapy. With guidance, her artwork created a powerful therapeutic bond in psychotherapy and was a cathartic outlet for her misery and feelings of loss. In this way, she was able to objectify her feelings about her brain tumor and its disruption of her life dreams. Figure 4.4 is a drawing Linda did soon after the initial diagnosis of the tumor. The left side of the diagram denotes her pretumor lifestyle, characterized by joy, fulfillment, and exhilaration, including hang gliding. She graphically depicts her transposition to the barren landscape associated with the destructiveness of the tumor, including her feelings of emptiness and anguish. The two eyes confront the terrifying collision of her two realities, with a transformation to the chained existence of a terminal illness.

Figure 4.5 also eloquently depicts Linda's narcissistic injury and sense of profound loss. The left side of the drawing represents the turbulence, bleakness, desolation, and despair associated with her tumor diagnosis. Linda's journey through the rehabilitation program (the "ADHNR" bridge) shows her transition from feelings of worthlessness and purposelessness to a renewed sense of redefinition, vitality, and meaning, as illustrated by her new path to fresh life and beauty on the right side of the drawing.

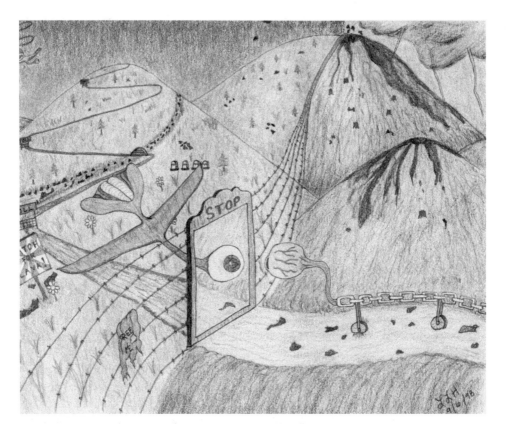

**FIGURE 4.4.** The contrast between Linda's pre- and postillness lifestyles. From Klonoff (2005). Copyright 2005 by James Afinowich. Reprinted by permission of Mr. Afinowich and the Barrow Neurological Institute.

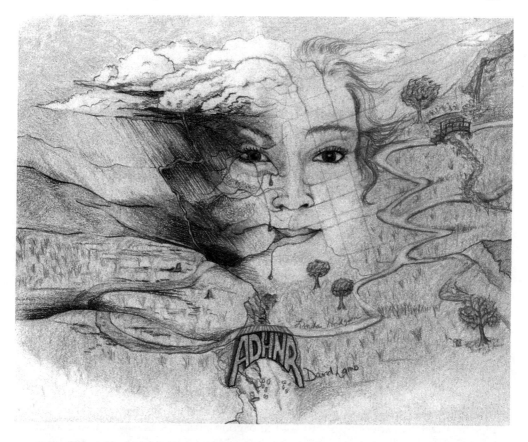

**FIGURE 4.5.** Linda's and her therapist's drawing of her journey through the rehabilitation program (across the "ADHNR" bridge). From Klonoff (2005). Copyright 2005 by James Afinowich. Reprinted by permission of Mr. Afinowich, David Lamb, PhD, and the Barrow Neurological Institute.

Linda's almost daily journal entries chronicled her experiences, aspirations, disappointments, and ultimately the complex interplay of her emotions. Her entries became her voice when she could no longer easily gather and articulately speak her thoughts; she shared all of her writings with her psychotherapist. This, in combination with talk therapy, helped her recognize the catalysts and manifestations of her narcissistic rage. The catalysts included her chagrin with ongoing hallucinations, seizures, and severe aftereffects of chemotherapy, radiation, and gamma knife treatment. At times the challenges were so seemingly insurmountable that she descended into feelings of self-indignation, hopelessness, and despondency. Her sense of "me" was so eradicated by illness that she struggled to find purpose to her life. Her journal keeping became a way to reconstitute herself and consolidate her connections to her loved ones.

A goal of the psychotherapy was to provide Linda with new ways of enhancing her quality of life, including alternative forms of self-expression and connection with nature (an integral part of her pretumor lifestyle). Although she could no longer go hang gliding, she was encouraged to continue hiking. She often wanted to hike alone as an outlet for self-reflection. Often she took her drawing pad and colored pencils, capturing the beauty of her surroundings while contemplating her life circumstances. Despite her intermittent seizures, her psychotherapist advocated for this freedom with her treating physicians, emphasizing the "dignity of risk" (M. Pepping, personal communication, n.d.) and the importance of her continued self-sufficiency and autonomy. She wrote in one journal entry:

> "It was beautiful walking on the sand this evening. God had gotten tired of the footprints and the boring texture and color. He brought on the rains. His painting is beautiful. He took the paintbrush and caressed it over the ground as if directing soft and mesmerizing music. With each step you could see where the gentle flows intertwined and, at times, imagine the percussion of stone against stone."

Although Linda recognized that her health precluded motherhood, she desperately yearned for a connection with children. Her psychotherapist therefore arranged a volunteer work experience doing art activities with youngsters waiting for clinic appointments in a hospital. Linda relished this opportunity; she wrote: "Two teachers who had babies as patients loved my turkey puppet design and asked if they could have them to use for their school classes."

Linda's primary relationships remained central to her emotional well-being and greatly helped to counterbalance her narcissistic rage and feelings of emptiness because of her profound losses. Her psychotherapist recommended that she continue to go on trips with her hang-gliding buddies, so as to enjoy nature and the socialization experience with "old and good" friends. She was also encouraged to travel whenever possible to see friends and family; she often combined this travel with ventures into the wilderness or other beautiful locales. In another journal entry, she wrote:

> "Her catching the big fish was the highlight, of course, but the hilarious part came when it got off the hook and it flipped and flopped and jumped towards the water. I was not going to let it get away. I was losing my shoes on the rocks as my hands tried to grab the fish, and I tripped onto my knees as he slid into the water. I turned around to see how my best friend was taking it; she burst into laughter. Then we both ended up bent over laughing so hard we couldn't breathe. You'd think we were silently crying."

Her psychotherapist also persuaded Linda to find other outlets for artistic expression, including community college classes in the fields of art and computer graphics. At first she was terrified of these classes; she would become overwhelmed with the intensity of the workload and hovering deadlines. She would then actively avoid working on her projects, which contributed further to her feelings of worthlessness and incompetency—or, as she described it, her "damaged and defective self." As a pragmatist, her psychotherapist wrote letters to her professors explaining her neurological condition, and also served as her advocate with the college's resources program for disabled students; she thus received the necessary accommodations to enable her to benefit from and enjoy her art classes, unhindered by academic and time constraints. Other pursuits her therapist suggested she undertake included developing a logo for a business operated by a relative, and overseeing the formatting and construction of a yearly newsletter for her neurorehabilitation program. All of these projects helped rebuild her self-esteem and provided meaningful improvement in her quality of life; she described them as providing "mental equilibrium."

Months later, as Linda boldly faced her trepidation about the uncertainty of her life, she wrote:

> "I look up at what I wrote. . . . If someone were to just look at the words on the paper, they would see anger. But [my psychotherapist] knows me better. She knows that I had tears in my eyes . . . my fears come out as heat, trying to fight the cause and chase it away. I have a lot of fighting left within me. I'm pissed at this tumor. As it gets bigger, I get angrier. And the anger reflects my fears. I have doors up around me, but these doors are different than they were prior to (my psychotherapy). . . . She's helped me redesign them. We've added holes where she feels they're necessary. . . . They're lighter and faster, but stronger in the healthy, necessary areas."

Linda also chronicled that her sessions with her psychiatrist and medications also helped her "not retreat, and not give up." She wrote that "he usually has one of two looks . . . smiling or supportive; he's got the sweetest way of tapping into my brain." Their empathic attunement seemed to quell her despair and hopelessness.

Ultimately, Linda grappled with the existential significance of her condition—her grief and mourning over her losses, and the meaning of her suffering. When, together with her psychotherapist, she read excerpts from Viktor Frankl's *Man's Search for Meaning* (1984), she commented: "It doesn't bring me down; just brings me back." She also wrote:

> "Jenny [my friend] and I were talking last night and somehow got on the subject of health versus happiness. She surprised me by saying she would take her health. She said she respects my preference for happiness; when I was 'quote' healthy before, I was so unhappy. And now that I have 'cancer,' I feel like I'm the happiest I've been my whole life. Not due to the tumor of course, but to the changes that have been brought about."

## SUICIDALITY

Patients surviving brain injuries are at risk for suicide (Fleminger et al., 2003; Leon-Carrion et al., 2001; Simpson & Tate, 2007). Contributory factors include intense and abrupt changes in these individuals' life situations (e.g., failed relationships, social alienation, compromised health, and/or faltering careers). Patients feel stripped of their identity, autonomy, and aspirations, and suicide becomes the ultimate expression of self-destructive behavior due to narcissistic injury (Klonoff & Lage, 1991; see Klonoff & Lage, 1995, for a review). Patients' postinjury personality attributes of impulsivity and cognitive rigidity may also predispose them to desperate acts (Klonoff & Lage, 1995). High-risk patients are also likely to have a preinjury history of depression, suicidal ideation, intent, or attempts, including injury-related covert or overt self-destructiveness (e.g., single high-speed motor vehicle accidents). Recent research has identified increased injury severity, male gender, older age, unemployment, pre- and postinjury comorbid psychiatric and alcohol use disorders, and pre- and postinjury suicidal ideation/attempts as correlates of suicide after traumatic brain injury (Mainio et al., 2007; Simpson & Tate, 2007).

The psychotherapist must be alert to potential warning signs of self-harm and knowledgeable about suicide prevention (Ghaffar & Feinstein, 2008; Simpson, Winstanley, & Bertapelle, 2003). Figure 4.6 summarizes suicide prevention techniques after brain injury. Regular proactive screening for feelings of hopelessness, and a structured risk assessment interview when necessary, are valuable tools (Kuipers & Lancaster, 2000; Simpson & Tate, 2007). Treatment interventions include creating an ambience of empathic attunement and nurturance, in combination with providing assistance in practical problem solving. This approach combats the patient's cognitive distortions (especially rigid and concrete thinking), while generating viable alternatives and implementing solutions (Klonoff & Lage, 1995; Kuipers & Lancaster, 2000; Leon-Carrion et al., 2001; Simpson & Tate, 2007). Close liaison and cotreatment with a psychiatrist are crucial, for both his or her expertise and capability to expedite hospitalization if needed. Antidepressant medications (e.g., sertraline and paroxetine) are often essential adjuncts to psychotherapy (Klonoff & Lage, 1995; Simpson & Tate, 2007). Some clinicians employ contracts that are completed with suicidal patients as tangible records of their commitment not to resort to self-harm, and of constructive alternatives for safety and coping (Kuipers & Lancaster, 2000).

A psychotherapist should closely monitor a suicidal patient's access to potentially lethal tools (Klonoff & Lage, 1995; Simpson & Tate, 2007), given the problems with judgment and impulsivity in this population. Such monitoring includes

- Alertness to warning signs
- Regular proactive screening
- Empathic ambience
- Collaborative problem solving
- Liaison and cotreatment with a psychiatrist
- Psychotropic medications
- No-self-harm contracts
- Monitoring of access to lethal tools, including medications
- Long-term psychotherapeutic supports
- Provision of emergency contact information and resources
- Assistance in finding renewed meaning in life

**FIGURE 4.6.** Techniques for suicide prevention after brain injury.

recommending family control of medication, with access to only 1-month sup-plies, to counteract medication hoarding. In addition, firearms should be removed from the home to maximize the patient's safety (Klonoff & Lage, 1995). Long-term psychotherapeutic supports are often necessary, in the form of support groups, social networks, and intensification or reinitiation of psychotherapy during crisis periods (Klonoff & Lage, 1995; Kuipers & Lancaster, 2000). Each patient should be provided with an emergency contact card listing crisis contacts (Simpson & Tate, 2007), and family members should be apprised of life-preserving options (e.g., calling 911 or taking the patient to the emergency room), as well as of other available agencies and professionals (Kuipers & Lancaster, 2000). Assisting the patient in finding renewed meaning or "self-reinvention" (Jourard, 1971) is one of the most potent antidotes for suicidal risk, as the patient becomes reinvested in a new identity, different forms of productivity, and a new life meaning (Klonoff & Lage, 1995).

## VALUES

After brain injury, patients often engage in a desperate quest for meaning in life (Prigatano, 1999). They experience profound feelings of ennui and purposeless-ness once they recognize their losses. Their executive function deficits affect goal setting, planning, and flexible thinking, and they feel baffled, directionless, and unable to fathom the abstract notion of a meaningful existence. However, life val-ues motivate human existence (Jemmer, 2006), and thus can provide consoling guideposts on this journey to redefinition. As such, work on values in psychother-apy shifts a patient's preoccupation from a "loss perspective" to both an "assets perspective" and a "restorative orientation," which are adaptive and hopeful (Ben-Yishay & Daniels-Zide, 2000; Stroebe & Schut, 1999).

One approach to values work comes from "acceptance and commitment ther-apy" (ACT; Hayes, Strosahl, & Wilson, 1999), which has recently been adapted for the brain-injured population (Myles, 2007). The four-step ACT process begins with patients' exploring their values in a wide variety of life domains (i.e., work, leisure, community, family, friendships, intimate relations, parenting, spiritual-ity, education/learning, and health/exercise). Patients generate statements about what is important to them in key life domains (e.g., "It is important to me to be a caring, supportive, and honest friend to others"). Emphasis is placed on the pro-cess of living, as opposed to the outcomes of actions. Using a 10-point scale (1 = least important, 10 = most important), patients then rate the relative importance of the different life domains in which they have generated values statements.

In the second step of the ACT process, patients rate how consistent their recent behavior (e.g., over the past 2 weeks) has been with their expressed values (1 = not at all consistent, 10 = very consistent). In the third step, patients are assisted in identifying goals, the achievement of which will increase the consistency between their behaviors and expressed values. Finally, the patients are guided to select and follow through with specific tasks aimed at achieving these goals. ACT is effi-cacious in directing the psychological healing process toward personally valued "metagoals."

John, a 26-year-old computer software programmer for a video game company, sustained a severe traumatic brain injury in a rollover motor vehicle accident. Postinjury physical sequelae included significant double vision, balance problems, gait disturbance, right-side (dominant-side) hemiparesis, and overall slowed motor responses. A comprehensive neuropsychological evaluation indicated severe deficits in speed of information processing, attention, executive systems, and verbal memory, with a tendency to confabulate. During the assessment, John was "snarky," with low frustration tolerance.

John began individual psychotherapy 6 weeks postinjury, as a vital element of his neurorehabilitation program. During the course of the initial interview, it became clear that John's career was very important to him. For the most part, his affect was blunted and he seemed dysphoric; however, when he was describing his vocation, John's mood brightened and he became notably more talkative and expressive. He identified returning to work as his "number one goal" and was mortified about how his absence from work would affect the progress of current projects. Another area of life that was clearly of consequence to John was his relationship with his parents. He complained that it was alien and disconcerting to be living with his parents again, as he had moved out when he was 17 years of age, and the relationship since then had been distant. He expressed regret about this and said he wanted to be a "better son" to his parents now. His psychotherapist made a mental "note to self" to explore further the role of work and family in John's life at a later date.

Initial sessions were spent in gathering additional background information about his relevant personal history and current psychological functioning. John described how, as a teenager, he had struggled academically; he had little interest in the core high school curriculum and was a C student. However, he had developed an interest in computers early in life, and he taught himself basic programming skills. He actively pursued his interest in programming throughout his adolescent years. Then he was hired at age 17 by the owner of a software company, whom he met at a computer games conference. Initially, his job duties involved simple office "gofer" tasks, but as his knowledge and skills developed, he became a programmer and eventually worked his way up to a supervisory position. To him, work signified competence, success, and respect—all of which had eluded him in high school.

Before his accident, John was also active outside of work, in both healthy and unhealthy ways. He had a strong interest in "extreme" sports, including skateboarding, snowboarding, and riding all-terrain vehicles (ATVs), which he said fulfilled his need for "action and excitement." He also acknowledged regular recreational use of street drugs and an excessive number of casual dating relationships. He described himself as very money-oriented and proud of his salary, most of which was spent funding his self-proclaimed "high intensity" lifestyle.

John was seen twice per week in psychotherapy. His initial awareness of his deficits was limited, secondary to the severity of his frontal lobe injury. It was felt that this organic unawareness protected his identity during the early stage of the recovery process. Simply put, he was too unaware of the consequences of the injury for his sense of self to be threatened by them.

As his awareness grew, John became fraught with narcissistic rage. He was educated about this, as it became clear that his identity was under assault. He wondered whether his accident was somehow "punishment" for his past life. Meanwhile, tensions had erupted in John's relationship with his parents. Fiercely independent before his injury, he felt demoralized at having to return to live in the family home. He felt as if he were "living under a microscope"—as if his every move and mood were being analyzed. From his parents' perspective, John was uncooperative and reckless. His mother bemoaned that it felt like "having him as a teenager all over again." Through cognitive retraining exercises, John's cognitive deficits became overwhelmingly apparent to him. This reawakened the feelings of aggravation and ineptitude that he had experienced in school; he grieved that all his hard work and achievements had been for nothing.

As a part of exploring how John's injury had affected his sense of self, his psychotherapist proposed the sentence completion task (Myles, 2007; see Figure 4.1) as a therapeutic tool 3 weeks after initiating psychotherapy. Overall, John's responses (see Figure 4.7 for some examples) indicated considerable existential angst about his identity and place in the world. However, interwoven with his feelings of loss and pain were threads of desire and hope for positive life changes and a new sense of self.

The psychotherapy process explored John's key life values—that is, his core beliefs and "guiding lights" for a meaningful existence (Hayes et al., 1999). Three domains—work, family relationships, and health/exercise—were indispensable in the reconstitution of John's postinjury sense of self.

In the realm of work, John identified his values as follows: "to work to my potential, to always be open to improving and learning new skills, and to treat my coworkers respectfully." John rated the consistency of his recent behavior with these core values as 4/10 (1 = not all consistent, 10 = very consistent). He confessed that his resistance to recommendations for cognitive compensations (e.g., consistently using his datebook) and his "snarkiness" toward others were inconsistent with his stated values. To increase the consistency of his behavior with his expressed values in this domain, he set himself the goals of self-monitoring his irritable behavior and increasing his acceptance of feedback. He used the lyrics to "Respect" as sung by Aretha Franklin (Redding, 1965/1967) as a mantra to remind him of his goals. As steps toward achieving these goals, he planned to inquire about beneficial compensations for cognitive difficulties, and to record and apologize for any incidents of "snarkiness."

In the sphere of family relationships, John's values included being "a caring, considerate, and appreciative son" to his parents. Initially, he rated the consistency of his recent behavior with his values as being only 2/10. He identified the frequent verbal tantrums and quarrels with his parents as contradictory to his values. With further introspection, he recognized that many of these arguments arose from his dismissal of their suggestions and apprehensions about his safety. For example, despite his severe diplopia and balance problems, he was adamant about taking long walks in the dark without his leg brace. To increase the consistency of his behavior with his expressed values in this domain, John set himself the goals of being amenable to safety ideas and regularly expressing his appreciation to his parents for their devotion. As steps toward these goals, he planned to schedule a weekly "milieu meeting" with his parents to brainstorm about fun but safe sports

| Sentence stem | Response |
|---|---|
| 1. Since the injury, my sense of who I am . . . | " . . . is lost. I don't know who I am or where I'm going." |
| 3. Since the injury, I feel . . . | " . . . useless, broken, no good to anyone." |
| 5. Since my injury, my thinking abilities . . . | " . . . are like a child—I feel slow and stupid." |
| 9. Since the injury, when I think about the future, I feel . . . | " . . . confused, afraid, like I'm lost." |
| 11. Since the injury, when I think about my role in my family . . . | " . . . I feel like a burden—I can't do anything for myself." |
| 13. Since the injury, what matters to me . . . | " . . . has changed. I want to get on the right path again." |
| 14. Since the injury, when I think about work . . . | " . . . I get scared that I will never get back to it." |
| 15. Compared to before the injury, my emotions . . . | " . . . are close to the surface and harder to control." |
| 16. Since the injury, my role in life . . . | " . . . is unclear, but I know I don't want to make the same mistakes as before." |
| 17. Since the injury, my self esteem . . . | " . . . is up and down, like I'm on a roller coaster." |
| 20. Since the injury, my confidence . . . | " . . . is shot. I used to be sure of myself, and now I'm not." |
| 22. Since the injury, my sense of purpose . . . | " . . . is more clear to me—I didn't care about God, and now I know that he saved me for a purpose." |
| 29. Since the injury, my relationships with the people close to me . . . | " . . . are better and mean more to me." |

**FIGURE 4.7.** Examples of John's answers to the sentence completion task (see Figure 4.1).

and family excursions. He also set himself a daily assignment in his datebook: to complete a simple household chore to reduce his parents' burdens.

In the domain of health/exercise, John explored his fascination with "extreme" sports. It became evident that it was the "rush" he experienced while flying through space, whether on a skateboard, a snowboard, or an ATV, that enthralled him. However, further inquiry led to the realization that he also derived huge satisfaction from his athleticism, including the ability to control his body lithely and perform feats of physical prowess without injury. This realization enabled him to express his values in this area as follows: "It's important to me to do things to optimize my health (eating, sleeping, and exercising). It's also important to learn more about what my body is capable of and to maximize my physical potential." He rated the consistency of his recent behavior with these values as being 5/10, recognizing that he was pushing himself too hard in his physical workouts (e.g., overexerting himself at the gym by using excessive weights and repetitions). John and the therapist agreed that his first goal in this area would be to improve his diet—he tended to eat "junk food" and had gained a significant amount of weight.

A second goal was for him to identify and pursue a form of exercise that would give him a sense of triumph from testing his limits and maximizing his potential, but in a harmless way. Specific tasks he set included meeting with a dietician to explore, plan, and follow through with healthy eating options, and participating in a therapeutic yoga class to improve his knowledge and control of his physical capabilities.

In weekly sessions, John and his psychotherapist reviewed his progress in following through with his specific tasks in quest of his greater goals. Thus he discovered harmony between his actions and his expressed values. Individual psychotherapy also assisted John in embracing that, unlike specific tasks and goals, personal values are about the *process* of living rather than the *outcomes* of actions. In other words, values are never fully and finally achieved; they serve as sustaining and inspiring life principles.

As part of group psychotherapy, John also participated in a powerful values-related activity—the "tombstone" exercise (Hayes et al., 1999, pp. 215–218). Patients are guided to contemplate what they envision carved on their tombstones at the end of a long life by those people who knew them best. In John's group, patients were also asked to imagine what others would say about how they lived their life principles (as opposed to their material achievements—income, awards, etc.) from the present time forward. John shared that he would like to be remembered by others as "a dedicated worker," a "true friend," and "a loving and kind son." He also watched the movie *The Ultimate Gift* (Eldridge et al., 2006) with his patient peers, and then participated in a group exercise in which he personalized his own 12 life gifts. For example, for the gifts of gratitude and family, he vowed to appreciate and admire his family members for their love and commitment. For the gift of friends, he pledged to focus more on "two-way street" relationships. From his endeavors in individual psychotherapy, John was able to provide concrete examples of his new behaviors in these areas, which served to reinforce his commitment to his values.

Overall, values work in the form of structured and guided exercises helped John to redefine his postinjury sense of self. He now perceived himself to be competent, successful, and respected at work, through giving his ultimate commitment and energies, without preoccupation with financial reward. Values work also shifted his focus away from feelings of self-hatred and regret about his preinjury mistakes and unhealthy hedonistic choices, and toward his present values, choices, and consequential actions. In a later psychotherapy session, he spontaneously remarked: "I believe now that this accident happened for a reason. I'm a better person, and I like the new me so much more."

## IDENTITY AND SOCIAL ROLES

"Identity," as defined earlier, is a person's subjective characterization of individuality within the social context. Related to this is "self-esteem," which can be defined as one's worth as a person with a particular identity; it is the valuation of oneself by oneself (Tafarodi & Ho, 2006). An important subcomponent of self-esteem is body image, which can also be substantially and adversely affected after brain injury (Howes, Edwards, & Benton, 2005a, 2005b). Therefore, brain injuries may have a profound impact on patients' identity and self-valuation (McGrath, 2004); most often there is a resultant shattering of identity, at least temporarily. Overall, patients' ultimate attainment of an optimal and stable outcome is predicated on the successful reformation of their ego identity, including self-acceptance, acquiescence to their fate, and peace of mind (Ben-Yishay & Lakin, 1989; Ben-Yishay et al., 1985).

Important subcomponents of identity are "social roles," which are self-designated and/or assigned positions and responsibilities within the immediate family, community, and society. Both general and specific factors that contribute to social roles can be radically altered postinjury (Hallett, Zasler, Maurer, & Cash, 1994). General factors include internal qualities and characteristics that promote joy, satisfaction, and meaning in one's role definition. For example, recent research indicates that postinjury marital stability may be better when the preinjury relationship has been of lengthier duration and greater maturity (Kreutzer, Marwitz, Hsu, Williams, & Riddick, 2007). Relationship satisfaction is also maximized when the patient shows empathic responsiveness (Burridge, Huw Williams, Yates, Harris, & Ward, 2007).

A specific factor that influences and defines social roles is gender. Male social roles that may be affected by brain injury include husband, boyfriend, father, and son; the affected female roles include wife, girlfriend, mother, and daughter (Gutman, 1999; Mukherjee, Reis, & Heller, 2003; Schopp, Good, Barker, Mazurek, & Hathaway, 2006). Disruptions in gender roles can affect the patient's self-esteem, body image, intimate relationships, life expectations, and rites of passage (e.g., creation of families) (Gutman & Napier-Klemic, 1996). The psychotherapist needs to ascertain his or her patients' gender-specific aspirations and, to the extent possible, support them in their quest for personal fulfillment. It is worth noting that brain injury sometimes serves as an impetus for reprioritization of patients' life goals; indeed, they often invest more energy and commitment in their relationship roles after injury than before, when their efforts have often been more materialistic and acquisition-driven.

Due to the social context, effective psychotherapeutic interventions for assessing and addressing identity and social roles usually necessitate a combination of individual treatment and conjoint treatment with those parties who actively participate in a patient's daily life. It is usually incumbent upon the psychotherapist to rely on pertinent assessment data to help the patient understand the role of various neurological sequelae in his or her subjective impressions of identity and social role formation. As detailed in Chapter 3, the patient must have a keen appreciation of specific strengths and deficits and their implications for community-based functions.

With complex dilemmas (e.g., a patient's capacity for parenting), it is recommended that the psychotherapist not become dogmatic or dictatorial in his or her recommendations, but instead help the patient make use of meaningful tools with which to reach his or her own conclusions. These can include pros-and-cons lists, journal entries, essays or other homework assignments on applicable topics, or diagram formats (e.g., a steppingstone depiction of necessary steps to accomplish subgoals). Other treating professionals (e.g., a rehabilitation physician, neurologist, and psychiatrist) can also help to share the burden of such a weighty decision, although it ultimately rests on the shoulders of the patient (and his or her social network). Importantly, family participation and devotion (or lack thereof) are vital contributors to reacquisition of social roles, as the family's division of labor, emotional support, and functional aid, usually set the ultimate bar (or barrier) for social role attainment within the family system. Therefore, conjoint treatment sessions are essential in helping all parties recognize the realities of, constraints on, and opportunities for family life (marriage, parenting, etc.).

The psychotherapist should also take a pragmatic approach to helping patients fulfill their social roles optimally. This includes discussing educational materials for parenting skills in sessions; training patients in datebook use to track important home responsibilities; and developing job-specific checklists (e.g., for supervising young children's homework).

The psychotherapist's empathic listening stance is critical when patients are grieving over physical changes and body image concerns. One tactic is to remind patients of their values (e.g., inner beauty vs. external manifestations), to help them focus on salient and meaningful elements of their core being. The psychotherapist can also help patients access extra treatment to maximize their comfort with their appearance (e.g., working with a dietician, physical therapist, or physical trainer). Small-group work with same-gender patients is a very beneficial forum for sharing and collaboration.

## CASE STUDY

Anne was age 19 when she sustained a traumatic brain injury as a bicyclist. CT and MRI scans indicated a left frontotemporal subdural hematoma, and left-to-right shift consistent with edema. She was unconscious for 1 week, with a Glasgow Coma Scale score of 10; she received traditional outpatient therapies for 4 months. She then completed an associate's degree in communications, taking an extra year to complete her coursework and utilizing resources for disabled students. She obtained a job working in a senior center as an assistant to the activities director. Despite the effects of her traumatic brain injury, she was very well liked because of her sensitivity and empathy toward her elderly clients. Her performance evaluations lauded her compassion, ingenuity, common-sense approach, and optimism.

Five years after her injury, Anne married her childhood sweetheart, Mark. He was extraordinarily loving toward her and awestruck by her emotional resiliency and courage in rebuilding her life. Despite her work and marital successes, Anne was miserable, often secluding herself at home and rejecting the affections of her husband. After 3 months of intermittent and severe depression, she was referred by her rehabilitation physician for psychotherapy. A neuropsychological evaluation was performed to help with diagnostic formulation. Anne's strengths included basic language comprehension, sustained attention, alternating attention, planning, problem solving, and academics (including reading comprehension and vocabulary). She showed mild to moderate deficits in the areas of speed of information processing, verbal learning and recall, and selected executive functions (including flexible thinking and multitasking).

Early psychotherapy sessions revealed that Anne suffered from considerable self-doubt and a very poor self-image. As a child and teenager, she had been a dancer; after the injury, she had right-leg weakness, necessitating the use of an ankle–foot orthosis. Her body image was damaged; she considered herself unattractive and unfeminine. During the third session, Anne began to sob and revealed that she felt "empty" as a woman, because she felt she was a burden to her husband. She also dreamed of having a baby, but was desperately afraid that because of her brain injury, she could never be the mother she wanted to be. She had very fond memories of her own childhood, with a close and loving relationship with her own mother. She feared that her physical and cognitive disabilities would prevent her from being a capable parent.

Anne was seen weekly for 2 months to specifically address her qualms as a wife. Marital sessions were also held, in which Mark highlighted her talents and tried to reassure her about his enduring passion and commitment. Although she "heard" his feedback during the sessions, her insecurities and recrimination about subjecting him to her disabilities would reemerge between sessions, and her emotions would spiral downward to renewed misery and self-contempt. With her psychotherapist, she developed and utilized the metaphor of "emotional avalanches" to help her recognize this cyclical and self-defeating pattern in her behavior. For example, after a session where she experienced a catastrophic reaction about her memory failures, Anne was given a homework assignment. To help expand her perception of her identity, she was asked to rework a journal entry, taking into account her attractive traits. The original entry grumbled about her deficiencies at a work party sponsored by her husband's employer.

### Original Entry

"It upsets me because this is what he ended up with. He deserves better and I don't know why he even wants to take me. I feel like an ass crying about it now, but I can't help it. . . . It bothers me because I forget so easily."

### Reworked Entry

"Last week I went to a potluck with Mark. Although I have a memory problem, it was good that I was there with my husband, because I'm a nice person and I think most people like me. I'm a patient person, and I'm stronger emotionally because of everything I've been through in my life. I'm even more compassionate because I understand how it feels to have challenges or setbacks in life. When people meet me, I come across as sensible, honest, and down to earth. Because I'm physically able, I can walk around and get my food and visit with people. If I tell people 'my story about my story,' they will see how determined and hard-working I am. It's good I went to the party to be with Mark, and I have a lot of things to offer."

These discussions and written exercises helped Anne appreciate her inner fortitude and bolstered her self-esteem. Eventually, at the suggestion of her psychotherapist, Mark also wrote Anne a letter proclaiming his confidence and faith in her:

"I just wanted to write you a letter letting you know how wonderful you are. You bring just as much to our marriage as I do. We are both decision makers in this marriage. You are not an added responsibility in my life; you are a blessing, and I am thankful for every day spent with you. We help each other because we love each other. You are beautiful, smart, kind, and strong. I love you, and I hope that one day you believe in yourself as much as I believe in you."

This letter was a turning point in the psychotherapy and in Anne's perception of their relationship. It provided a concrete representation and constant reminder of his commitment to their marriage.

The emphasis in the therapy then shifted to her dilemma about motherhood. Anne felt that bringing a child into the world with a "disabled" parent would be "selfish." She perseverated on her slower thinking and residual memory problems, convincing herself that she did not have the "intellect" to be a good mother. She expressed guilt and shame that her husband would have a double burden: her disabilities and a helpless infant. Together, Anne and the psychotherapist constructed a mantra based on her capacity to be nurturing and supportive of others in her environment (e.g., her husband and her work colleagues and clients). She placed it at the front of her datebook:

"Follow my own advice → look at the positives in myself; don't fret; don't 'what if'; having good self-esteem will help my child have self-esteem."

Gradually, she became more proficient at inhibiting negative thoughts and proclamations, with a more balanced and even complimentary self-image.

Anne's definition of parenting also appeared to be predominantly preoccupied with concrete factors—that is, what she could or could not *do* versus who she *was* as a person. This concrete thinking seemed to be related to her frontal lobe injury. The tactic taken in psychotherapy was to help her become more open-minded and view parenting on a more abstract and humanistic level. Anne's neuropsychological test findings reflecting adequate attentional, planning, problem-solving, and academic/intellectual skills, as well as her prior work accomplishments, helped to convince her that she in fact possessed these fundamental skills.

Sessions also focused on the cognitive-behavioral approach of defining the attributes and the meaning of a truly "good" mother. Together, Anne and the psychotherapist compiled a list of the "essences of parenthood." These included the capacity to experience and display love, devotion, patience, nurturance, and protection toward her infant; the ability to discriminate and teach right from wrong; and reasoning, judgment, and common sense. To help reinforce her new belief that she had the enduring core characteristics indispensable for motherhood, Anne devised a list of preinjury versus postinjury personality attributes to help give her a visual representation of the totality of her contributions as a wife and mother (Figure 4.8). Through this exercise, she was better able to embrace the uniqueness of her maturation and her courage in tackling life's adversities.

Anne utilized group psychotherapy sessions to further explore her feelings about social role strivings. The psychotherapists facilitated a discussion about per-

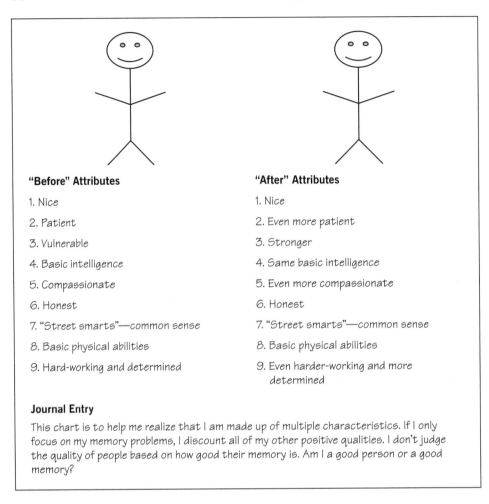

**"Before" Attributes**

1. Nice

2. Patient

3. Vulnerable

4. Basic intelligence

5. Compassionate

6. Honest

7. "Street smarts"—common sense

8. Basic physical abilities

9. Hard-working and determined

**"After" Attributes**

1. Nice

2. Even more patient

3. Stronger

4. Same basic intelligence

5. Even more compassionate

6. Honest

7. "Street smarts"—common sense

8. Basic physical abilities

9. Even harder-working and more determined

**Journal Entry**

This chart is to help me realize that I am made up of multiple characteristics. If I only focus on my memory problems, I discount all of my other positive qualities. I don't judge the quality of people based on how good their memory is. Am I a good person or a good memory?

**FIGURE 4.8.** Anne's pre- and postinjury personality attributes.

sonal aspirations and by asking these questions: "What are your life goals?" and "What's your legacy; how do you wish to be remembered?" Anne confided to the group her misgivings about parenthood. Then, for a music therapy exercise, Anne chose the theme song from the movie *Rocky* (Conti, Connors, & Robbins, 1976) and related Rocky's personal quest to her elusive dream of motherhood. Verbalizing her dream helped to demystify the process, and her peers provided resounding support and encouragement. This helped to validate Anne's hope for a joyful and fulfilled future.

Anne had substantial devotion from her parents, who lived nearby and expressed an eagerness to provide whatever practical assistance she needed; they were delighted about the idea of a grandchild. Her psychotherapist recommended to Anne that she be flexible and receptive in her parenting approach. Several family sessions were held, involving and educating all parties, to help reassure Anne of their loyalty and confidence in her as a potential mother.

Anne and Mark were also encouraged to watch the movie *The Wizard of Oz* (LeRoy & Fleming, 1939), to illustrate that she indeed had the requisite decision-making ability and could surmount her trepidation. Soon after, she became pregnant. Her mood oscillated from ecstasy to panic as the pregnancy progressed. She was seen twice per month during her pregnancy to help prepare her psychologically for her new role, including educational materials. At the psychotherapist's advice, Anne and Mark produced a videographic record of the pregnancy to create a permanent chronicle of events. At the monthly patient aftercare group (see Chapter 9), Anne was honored by her peers with a "Baby Blessings" cake, prior to the delivery.

After the birth of her daughter, Claire, Anne experienced some episodes of feeling melancholic, overwhelmed, and inadequate in her new role. To help with the acclimation process, the psychotherapist solicited the assistance of an occupational therapist. Both therapists worked collaboratively to help Anne reconstruct her datebook and Home Independence Checklist (see Chapter 6), and to create a "parent notebook" tailored to the needs and responsibilities of being a new mother. This included sections for doctors' appointments; feeding, bathing, and sleeping records; developmental milestones; and age-appropriate play activities. She even created a checklist for packing the diaper bag! Anne was ritualistic about using her datebook to log all of the wonderful events. She also kept a daily journal, so as to have a point of reference for Claire's growth and development. Her psychotherapist encouraged Anne to join a moms' group through her church as another outlet for socialization and education.

During this adaptation phase, the psychotherapist suggested that Anne and Mark watch the movie *Stepmom* (Barnathan & Columbus, 1998); this movie's plot mirrored Anne's transition from a parental position predominated by insecurities and blunders, to one of thoughtfulness and competency.

After termination of her therapy, Anne wrote her psychotherapist a thank-you card stating:

"11:20 P.M. I'm sitting here now on my couch in my house with my husband and my baby. What a blessing! I'm a much stronger, confident, independent woman now, and I'm proud of that. I will continue to compensate for my disability—because I'm not done yet ☺."

The process of helping a patient regain a sense of self, values, identity, and social roles is intertwined with helping the patient better accept his or her postinjury predicament. This acceptance process is elaborated upon in the next chapter.

# CHAPTER 5

# Increasing Acceptance

## THE NATURE AND DETERMINANTS OF ACCEPTANCE

Patients' acceptance of their life circumstances after brain injury is a crucial part of the adjustment process. *Acceptance* means patients' ability and willingness to cope with their new reality and identity. Patients need to have sufficient residual skills to appreciate and cope with their injury-related changes, including requisite executive functions, such as flexible problem solving and "big-picture" thinking.

Given that brain injury often causes radical, profound, and enduring life changes, the process of acceptance is painful, arduous, complex, and prolonged. In fact, some authors have proposed that the brain injury creates a "transcrisis state," in which there is a precarious homeostasis with often inadequate resolution of situational crises, due to chronic and long-term sequelae (Davis, Gemeinhardt, Gan, Anstey, & Gargaro, 2003; Gilliand & James, 1988). Generally, there is no endpoint to the acceptance process, but instead an evolving maturation of new practicalities and ideals.

As articulated in Phase 5 of the PEM (see Chapter 1, Figure 1.2), patients manifest acceptance through embracing and using compensatory strategies (Klonoff, 1997; Prigatano et al., 1986). Such compensations are tools and techniques that assist patients in "getting around" their problem areas, and thereby improving their functioning (Klonoff, Lamb, Henderson, Reichert, et al., 2000; Klonoff et al., 2007; Prigatano et al., 1986). At first, compensations are generally recommended by treating therapists. As patients' acceptance grows, they often develop their own workable tools to maximize their performance. Figure 5.1 shows how use of compensations becomes its own reward as functioning improves. When functioning improves, a patient's mood improves, and compensatory strategies become part of the learned repertoire.

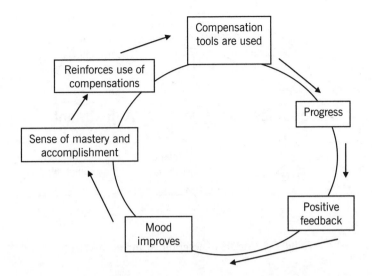

**FIGURE 5.1.** Compensation process.

Resiliency and coping capacity are key determinants of acceptance. After brain injury, patients who demonstrate residual resiliency and adaptive coping skills fare better overall with respect to self-esteem, social reintegration, work outcome, and quality of life (Anson & Ponsford, 2006c; Dumont, Gervais, Fougeyrollas, & Bertrand, 2004; Schutz, 2007; Tomberg, Toomela, Pulver, & Tikk, 2005; see Dawson & Winocur, 2008, for a review). Conversely, after brain injury, a coping style characterized by worry, wishful thinking, self-blame, ignoring the problem, and withdrawal has been associated with elevated levels of anxiety and depression, greater psychosocial dysfunction, and lower self-esteem (Anson & Ponsford, 2006b; Curran, Ponsford, & Crowe, 2000). Maladaptive coping behaviors (e.g., escape/avoidance) have a negative impact on patients' overall postinjury health, work/school status, and marital adjustment (Blais & Boisvert, 2007; Dawson, Schwartz, Winocur, & Stuss, 2007; Tomberg, Toomela, Ennok, & Tikk, 2007; again, see Dawson & Winocur, 2008, for a review).

Researchers have also identified empowerment as an important tool. Through improving their knowledge base and support, patients with acquired brain injury can optimize their coping capacity and future planning (Man, 2001). Enhanced acceptance and a positive attitude toward disability are associated with better quality of life (Snead & Davis, 2002).

## ADJUSTMENT = ADAPTATION + ASSIMILATION

The acceptance process gradually undergoes a metamorphosis into adjustment (see Figure 5.2). Postinjury *adjustment* can be defined as the interplay between patients' external adaptation to the physical environment and an internal process of assimilation, in which preexisting plans, expectations, and hopes are reformulated into a meaningful existence. It must be emphasized that the process of first

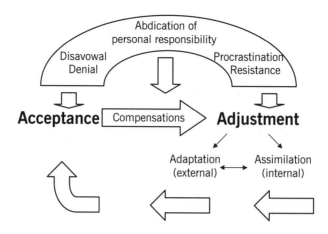

**FIGURE 5.2.** Model of acceptance and adjustment.

acceptance and then adjustment is both cyclical and evolving; with additional insights, patients are further challenged to accept, assimilate, and adapt. As a patient faces adversity, the *assimilation* process integrates the "old self" into a "new me," including his or her identity, inner being, and life philosophy. This redefinition and self-transformation process (Balk, 2004; Paletti, 2008) is fluid and often includes periods of inner strife, contrasted with personal growth and fulfillment. *Adaptation* is the patient's reintegration into the mainstream of his or her family, societal, and cultural milieus, including specific activities of daily living, productive work or school, and hobbies. Chapter 9 discusses adjustment, adaptation, and assimilation in greater detail.

Chen (1997) has suggested that crisis reminds individuals of their spiritual needs. Both spirituality and religious faith can help a patient cope with his or her limitations through recreating a meaningful life and relationship with the world (McColl et al., 2000a). Religious faith operationalizes spirituality into institutionalized beliefs and practices. These can become a powerful source of sustenance by providing a rubric for the transformative experience (Dalai Lama & Cutler, 1998; McColl et al., 2000a), and thus enabling a patient to make sense of apparently nonsensical losses.

Spirituality themes that contribute to the acceptance and adjustment process after brain injury include the patient's feeling closer to his or her family, identifying "true friends," developing increased trust in others, realizing life's purpose, and acknowledging personal vulnerabilities (McColl et al., 2000a, 2000b). Postinjury spiritual well-being can also facilitate hope and "awe or reverence" (e.g., patients' noticing and appreciating the world around them; see McColl et al., 2000a, for a review).

## CONSIDERATIONS IN THE ACCEPTANCE PROCESS

Certain behaviors and beliefs can interface and/or interfere with the complicated process of acceptance. This section reviews denial, disavowal, resistance, procrastination, and abdication of personal responsibility as potential considerations (and sometimes obstacles) to the acceptance process.

## Denial

"Denial" has been defined as "difficulty recognizing and/or accepting the existence, nature, degree, and/or impact of one's condition" (Kortte & Wegener, 2004, p. 187). Some authors have differentiated between neurogenic unawareness (anosognosia) and psychogenic unawareness (denial) (O'Callaghan et al., 2006), although sometimes the two coexist (Cicerone, 1989; Kortte, Wegener, & Chwalisz, 2003). A working definition of *denial* is the patient's persistent psychological disbelief in his or her disability, in the face of objective evidence to the contrary.

The adaptive benefit of denial is controversial. Historically, it was considered a premorbid personality style, involving a protective defense mechanism against painful thoughts (Langer, 1994; Lewis, 1991; for reviews, see Weinstein, 1991; Prigatano & Klonoff, 1998; Ownsworth et al., 2002; Kortte & Wegener, 2004). Others see denial as a necessary steppingstone in the acceptance process; it is viewed as providing a temporary reprieve that enables the patient to feel better about his or her losses and circumstances (Cicerone, 1989; Kortte & Wegener, 2004; Langer, 1994; see O'Callaghan et al., 2006, for a review). It should also be noted that there are various forms of denial, and that these are not mutually exclusive (Weinstein, 1991). Often patients deny selected aspects of their disabilities; which aspects they deny may be related to how psychologically threatening the reality is and/or how noticeable the problems are (Cicerone, 1989). As such, denial can be considered psychological "blind spots" or the inability to recognize injury-related perturbations. Manifestations of denial after acquired brain injury include excuses, rationalizations, resistance (see below), defensiveness, minimization, and avoidance (Kortte et al., 2003; O'Callaghan et al., 2006; Prigatano & Klonoff, 1998).

## Disavowal

If denial sounds like "Problem? What problem?", disavowal sounds like "It's a problem; no, it isn't a problem." *Disavowal* is intermittent acknowledgment of a problem. Reduction of postinjury denial and disavowal is a fluid and evolving psychological process, and must be addressed delicately and empathically during individual psychotherapy. The process of awareness training, as discussed in Chapter 3, addresses organic unawareness and gently eases patients into conscious appreciation of painful elements of their condition (Lewis, 1991). This can be considered "adaptive disavowal," whereby patients gradually acknowledge their injury-related sequelae.

## Resistance

Embedded in the process of psychotherapy is the phenomenon of *resistance*, or the "curious observation that some painfully distressed patients seeking assistance from expensive and highly trained professionals reject their therapists' best advice, fail to act in their own best interest, and do not respond to the most effective interventions that can be mustered on their behalf" (Beutler, Moleiro, & Talebi, 2002, p. 207). Resistance encompasses both a dispositional trait and in-therapy behaviors of opposition, anger, irritation, and suspiciousness (see Beutler et al., 2002, for a review; see also Ownsworth & McFarland, 2004). In psychodynamic approaches, resistance is customary and automatic; it is a way of avoiding and yet communicating unacceptable drives, feelings, fantasies, and behaviors (Messer, 2002). Resistance has also been conceptualized as having an adaptive function of enabling a patient to feel assertive, autonomous, and separate from others, as well as to communicate distress and cope (Messer, 2002). Resistance and defiance of the acceptance process can be intensified for patients with a preinjury history of narcissistic problems, as these patients have an especially poor tolerance for imperfections and failure (Klonoff & Lage, 1991). The feeling of being "damaged goods" can erupt into narcissistic rage (see Chapter 4).

In interpersonal psychotherapy, resistance constitutes moments during sessions whereby a patient's interpersonal behavior sabotages the intervention process (Van Denburg & Kiesler, 2002). After brain injury, affective and mood alterations (e.g., irritability, poor self-regulation) can impede the flow of exchanges. Resistance has also been described as the tendency to resist modifying behavior outside of the therapy session (Messer, 2002). This can be a result of underlying psychodynamics, or it can be another by-product of the brain injury, secondary to difficulties with memory and/or executive functions.

Common manifestations of resistance, also applicable to the effects of brain injury, include refusal to follow through on homework assignments; repeated decisions and actions that contradict agreed-upon recommendations in treatment; intense expression of emotions; in-session avoidance (e.g., silences, "don't know" responses, diversions away from salient subject matter); and "gratuitous debates" (Newman, 2002). Patients may also minimize or hide the effects of their injuries, and/or may refuse to disclose relevant personal information to appropriate parties (Klonoff, 1997). These represent "yellow" warning behaviors in Phase 5 of the PEM.

## Procrastination and Abdication of Personal Responsibility

*Procrastination* is voluntarily putting off doing what should be done in a timely fashion, despite good intentions and the recognition of the ill effects of the behavior (Balkis & Duru, 2007; Steel, 2007). Recent research has linked this behavior to low conscientiousness, self-regulatory failure, distractibility, poor organizational and time management skills, diminished achievement motivation, an intention–action gap, and task aversiveness (Balkis & Duru, 2007; Steel, 2007). It can be considered the psychological counterpart to organically based initiation problems.

*Abdication of personal responsibility* is the individual's inability or refusal to take ownership of, and experience a sense of duty about maintaining, his or her commitments. Clinical experience indicates that lack of responsibility is often related to Axis II personality disorders (e.g., antisocial), which can be preexisting (Hibbard et al., 2000). In addition, recent research has supported a relationship between blaming others for one's injury on the one hand, and poor psychological outcome and community productivity on the other (Hart, Hanks, Bogner, Millis,

& Esselman, 2007). In analyzing abdication of responsibility, the psychotherapist must thoughtfully weigh the relative contributions of an intentional inclination to shirk responsibilities with an inability to initiate and organize tasks, based on executive function deficits. Exploring the patient's preinjury personality and coping style is essential to this analysis. A very useful mantra for difficulties with procrastination and personal responsibility is "Just do it."

## BASELINE DETERMINATION OF ACCEPTANCE

As a patient develops awareness, the psychotherapist should begin to determine the patient's baseline level of acceptance. As stated previously, acceptance is predicated on a foundation of improved awareness. Therefore, it may be several weeks or even a few months before the psychotherapist is able to ascertain the patient's acceptance baseline. Establishing this baseline furnishes an entry point for addressing acceptance issues; it also assists the psychotherapist in identifying how "coachable" the patient is, and which tools and techniques will be most efficacious.

Table 5.1 identifies general guidelines for determining low, medium, and high acceptance. These should be viewed as points on a continuum, rather than as demarcated categories. Note that in the initial dialogue with the patient, the psychotherapist relies on what the patient says about acceptance, rather than on his or her actions. However, this functions as a reference point for interventions, especially compensation training. As shown in Table 5.1, the highly accepting patient is generally very aware of his or her specific deficits, as well as their impact on day-to-day functioning. He or she is open to information about coping tools and willingly integrates real-life experiences. These patients often have more intact executive functions, and can see the "big-picture" benefits of compensatory strategies. There is also usually a preinjury predisposition toward using organizational devices, in combination with a trusting approach to the therapeutic process. Such patients also have active "buy-in" from their families.

Patients with a medium baseline level of acceptance have a preliminary awareness of their deficits, buttressed by their experience of mild disappointments in real life because of their brain injuries. They communicate a tentative openness to new ideas and suggestions; they may be somewhat wary of the psychotherapy process, needing convincing and "proof" that the process can help. Often they have had some preinjury exposure to organizational tools, and their family members have at least a rudimentary appreciation of the value of compensation training. These patients have sufficient executive function skills to cope flexibly with their challenges.

Patients who initially demonstrate poor acceptance are sometimes in the acute phase of recovery and suffer from organic unawareness. Alternatively, they may have chronic injuries that have produced highly entrenched maladaptive habits. Therefore, both these groups of patients may display closed and even hostile reactions to the suggestion of injury-related sequelae and the need for compensations. They usually display a tenacious and rigid adherence to wishful or magical thinking, and reject factual information and/or the purveyors of that information (the psychotherapist or other helping professionals). Emotions often

**TABLE 5.1. Baseline Determinants of Acceptance**

| Low acceptance | Medium acceptance | High acceptance |
| --- | --- | --- |
| 1. Very poor awareness | Beginnings of awareness | Good awareness |
| 2. Defensive and uncomfortable demeanor with inquiry and the idea of compensations | Tentative openness and receptivity to inquiry and the idea of compensations | Open and receptive demeanor to inquiry and the idea of compensations |
| 3. Adamant rejection of collateral real-life data | Tentative openness to collateral real-life data | Full openness to collateral real-life data |
| 4. Chronic injuries that have produced highly entrenched maladaptive habits | Mild disappointments in real life; preliminary motivation to adapt | Ability to acknowledge and learn from real-life failures, with high motivation to change |
| 5. Poor preinjury utilization of organizational tools | Some preinjury willingness to use organizational tools | Good preinjury discipline and use of organizational tools |
| 6. Poor trust in the working alliance | Beginning trust and a developing working alliance | Strong trust and a fortified working alliance |
| 7. Severe executive function deficits, with poor initiation and follow-through | Milder executive function deficits; capacity for a flexible and systematic approach | More intact executive functions, including reasoning and flexible problem solving |
| 8. Poor family knowledge and "buy-in" | Some family knowledge and "buy-in" | Active family involvement and "buy-in" |

rapidly escalate, especially when the nature of the injury affects self-regulation, auditory perception, and/or comprehension. The psychotherapist's inquiries can be misinterpreted as signs of criticism and negativity, and these misinterpretations perpetuate a downward spiral of distrust and dissension. The psychotherapist should then begin to assess for possible psychological underpinnings to poor acceptance, including denial and/or disavowal. These patients also do not appreciate the necessity for adopting compensatory strategies. In fact, they may feel that compensations are "crutches" that will impede their healing process. Patients with frontal lobe injury, who show significant executive deficits in the realms of initiation, planning, reasoning, and follow-through, may give lip service to compensations but fail to follow through behaviorally. There is often an absence of preinjury discipline in using organizational tools. Finally, family members often undermine attempts to remediate acceptance problems—usually relying on poor coping skills, which are mirrored in their loved one.

## INCREASING ACCEPTANCE IN INDIVIDUAL PSYCHOTHERAPY

The heart of psychotherapeutic intervention for acceptance lies in candid yet empathic dialogue about a patient's psychological stance. As stated above, a hallmark of the acceptance process is the patient's coachability in adopting compensatory tools (Klonoff, Lamb, Henderson, Reichert, et al., 2000). Ideally, exploration of healthy coping techniques is intertwined with behavioral changes in the form of active use of compensations. Simple signs can tell the psychotherapist how the acceptance process is unfolding. Do patients bring their datebooks to sessions? Do they either initiate note taking or respond positively to mild cueing to take notes?

Patients often doubt or reject the value of memory compensatory systems (e.g., datebooks, watch alarms, or procedural checklists). Employing collaborative evidentiary techniques, the psychotherapist can then gently and respectfully construct situations in which to gather measurable and cogent "test data." Patients often appreciate such evidence of the realities and implications of brain-injury-related changes, and can gradually modify their outlook to accept these tools as beneficial and effective. Providing weekly percentages of their successfully completed memory assignments is one such technique, discussed further in Chapter 6. Dialogue about the relative merits of compensation training during cognitive retraining sessions also emphasizes their intrinsic value. Concrete and regular feedback from real-world situations also helps to reinforce the benefit of particular compensations. For example, school projects and test grades can confirm the value of detailed note taking and/or other adapted study techniques. When recommended tools result in successes, the collaborative efforts and working alliance are fortified.

In what follows, I describe manifestations of patients' struggles with acceptance, together with an eclectic array of possible psychotherapeutic interventions. Deciding which approach is most efficacious at any given juncture requires a psychotherapist to have a good "handle" on the nature and expression of the neurological correlates, clinical intuition, and keen perceptions of a patient's state of mind and psychodynamics. The patient's responsiveness will assist the psychotherapist in self-appraisal of the timing and likely success of any given approach.

### Acceptance Crisis: "Why Me?"

Psychotherapists will often need to tackle patients' lamentations of "Why me?" (Delmonico et al., 1998). This question is often precipitated by catastrophic reactions, or the stark contrast between life before the injury and life after. External feedback or self-recognition of a plateau in recovery, which signals imperfect healing, can also launch this crisis in acceptance. Other antecedents include depression and the profound sense of loss that emerges as organic unawareness abates. A psychotherapist's empathic listening, in combination with normalizing these feelings as predictable and understandable, will bolster and sustain a patient through this difficult transition. Written materials such as the book *When Bad Things Happen to Good People* (Kushner, 1981) can also serve to remind patients of the unpredictability of the universe, as well as the prevalence of human suffering.

In some situations, the patient feels responsible for his or her health predicament—perhaps because of ignoring personal health concerns, driving drunk, or other irresponsible behavior. Besides sorrow, there may be profound guilt and regret (Chamberlain, 2006), intensified by the burdens placed on others in the patient's environment (e.g., family, coworkers, supervisors). The psychotherapist must gently assist such a patient with self-forgiveness; otherwise, he or she may be lost in the mire of misery and self-hatred. Specific techniques include reifying values (see Chapter 4) and helping the patient rebuild a foundation of self-worth through meaningful activities, such as service to others.

### "Hindsight Is 40/40"

An integral part of the reconstitution process is working through feelings of regret. Often this is catalyzed by retrospective "what-ifs" or the "would-have, could-have, should-have" syndrome. Patients can sink into self-recrimination, which promotes second-guessing or overanalysis of past actions. At these times, the psychotherapist can introduce the metaphor "Hindsight is 40/40." The "40/40" reference is meant to emphasize the deleterious consequences of a preoccupation with self-blame, along with the sense of "double trouble." It also adds some subtle wit and momentary levity to a dialogue that is often steeped in hurt and remorse.

### "History Isn't Destiny"

Sometimes patients become locked in the past. This may be due either to organically based perseverative and rigid thinking, or to a tendency to ruminate about losses. Patients can also feel powerless and defeated by their circumstances; this "no way out" form of thinking hampers the patient from envisioning and navigating toward a constructive future. A reference to Henry Kissinger's proclamation "History isn't destiny" can be an effective tool in reversing or derailing this self-perpetuating mode of thinking. It often serves as a self-sustaining mantra in times of turmoil.

### "Snarky" Behavior

In my psychotherapy practice, the word "snarky" is often used to describe patients' expressions of discontent or irritation with feedback. As mentioned in Chapter 2, the term is a more palatable way of conveying to a patient his or her defensiveness and/or resistance. Using this "rehab lingo" in the moment conveys the psychotherapist's genuine and immediate observations, and assists the patient in self-monitoring behaviors that may alienate others and/or interfere with receptivity to feedback. The movie *Up* (Con et al., 2009) is a delightful yet poignant portrayal of "snarky" behavior. Exploration of Carl's (the main character's) crabby behavior reveals his underlying struggles with accepting and adjusting to losses—a predicament patients can well relate to.

### "Yeah, Buts"

A signature phrase associated with the unfolding acceptance process is "Yeah, but" (Klonoff, 1997). This represents a patient's attempt to normalize an organic deficit, minimize feedback, or justify a problematic course of action. When patients are delinquent in accomplishing a task or maintaining a commitment, they may blame others or external circumstances, and/or attempt to negate the significance of the event. Very often this phrase is used in regard to a specific neurocognitive problem (e.g., with memory, initiation, prioritization, organization, or follow-through). An articulate patient, in fact, can present a barrage of "Yeah, buts," leaving the therapist with a feeling that the patient has an answer for everything. To an observer, it can appear like verbal ping-pong. It can be very therapeutic to process the process of "Yeah, but" retorts, including tracking their frequency. This represents the here-and-now approach to treatment (Yalom, 2002), in which the therapist uses the context, immediate setting, and interpersonal communications to unearth and enhance the insight process. In the context of a strong working alliance and the psychotherapist's empathic understanding of the patient's frustrations, the patient may begin to express amusement at recognizing and self-monitoring the frequent use of this phrase. This can help the patient perceive the underlying behaviors (e.g., defensiveness, cognitive rigidity, and argumentativeness).

### The "Glass-Half-Empty" Syndrome

A pessimistic, negativistic outlook can be a major obstacle in the struggle to accept and adjust to the devastating effects of brain injury. This can take the form of the "glass-half-empty" syndrome or a "doom-and-gloom" attitude. No matter how elaborate and innovative the therapeutic suggestions may be, the patient will systematically criticize them or discount any potential merit they may have. The psychotherapist should first empathically join the patient, validating his or her feelings and not trying too quickly to talk the patient out of despair. Following that, the psychotherapist should gingerly provide evidence to the patient of a better outlook; diagrams and charts with positive data and achievements can be instrumental tools. Readings such as the essay "Welcome to Holland" (Kingsley, 1987) can also be effective in counterbalancing a negative perspective. Sometimes the patient can be enticed into a healthier perspective if the psychotherapist introduces contrary evidence as "Yeah, buts" in response to the patient's "Yeah, buts." When depression is feeding the patient's pessimistic perceptions, psychiatric intervention and psychotropic medication are warranted.

### "Try It, You'll Like It" and "I Think I Can, I Think I Can"

Because of cognitive rigidity and the inability to see the "big picture," patients may be convinced of their ineptness and incapacities. The psychotherapist may then employ "psychological arm-twisting" techniques, including visual aids, mantras, and metaphors, to cajole such a patient into considering new frontiers. This includes the take-home message from *The Little Engine That Could* (i.e., "I think I can, I think I can"; Piper, 1986), or the saying "Try it, you'll like it." For the patient with a more chronic injury, the phrase "Teach this old dog a new trick" can be a humorous yet valuable technique to undermine cognitive rigidity. Often a time-limited proposal (e.g., trying a compensation for 4 weeks) offsets some of the understandable skepticism and anxieties, and allows a patient time to contemplate and ease into new behaviors. It also enhances dialogue and reemphasizes the patient's role in the decision-making process. In all these ways, the psychotherapist's optimism and empathic resolve can guide and eventually propel the patient toward a more hopeful and empowered outlook.

### *"Devil's Advocate" and "Psychological Judo"*

Sometimes psychotherapists may feel like helpless bystanders when patients are adamant in pursuing a course of action that is not considered in their best interest, or even seems dangerous. Resistance and denial, coupled with organic unawareness and characterological factors (e.g., rule-breaking and risk-taking behavior), can raise ominous warning signs to which patients are indifferent or oblivious.

In these instances, psychotherapists have a couple of choices. First, they can take the "devil's advocate" position. This counterargument technique can assist patients in cogitating about viable alternatives, especially in situations where a patient exhibits "tunnel vision" secondary to executive function deficits. Diagrams, pros-and-cons lists, and pie charts are effective in articulating the various possibilities to be considered and can guide the patient toward healthier options. Alternatively, a psychotherapist can back off and yield the decision-making responsibility to the patient (i.e., "psychological judo"; see Gleser & Brown, 1988, for a review). In this latter case, the psychotherapist intentionally takes a more passive or neutral position during the dialogue process; ideally, this encourages the patient directly or indirectly to assume the responsibility and initiative for reconsidering his or her motives.

### *Cost–Benefit Analysis and "Planned Failures"*

Part of the acceptance process is assessing one's perspective and then undertaking stepwise decisions. Patients often struggle with uncertainty and fear of failure in making decisions. To assist them in clarifying and judging alternatives, patients can be guided to construct a cost–benefit analysis. This consists of listing what stands to be gained versus sacrificed, given a particular option. This not only illuminates the possible advantages and pitfalls of a quandary, but also affords patients valuable practice with the executive functions associated with judgment, prioritization, problem solving, and decision making. It also helps to preserve the working alliance, as generally, with support, the answers become relatively self-evident to patients.

Sometimes a patient (and/or family) insists on making an ill-advised decision, despite a preponderance of evidence that it is an unwise one. To preserve the working alliance, an opportunity to "test the waters," or a "planned failure," can be constructed. Most often this takes the form of a community-based activity (e.g., coursework or a job). The psychotherapist takes a sideline position, and allows the patient the dignity, the freedom, and ultimately the responsibility of making his or her own decisions. Such a failure experience can be a "therapeutic reality check" and help the psychotherapist and patient refine their treatment goals, while still preserving mutual hopefulness and goal orientation.

### *The "Full-Court Press"*

When a strong foundation of trust and open communication exists, the psychotherapist may resort to a more confrontational attempt to reach the patient and penetrate denial, disavowal, and extreme resistance. One common "red flag" is prolonged lip service about the intent to use compensations ("talking the talk"), but no active implementation ("walking the walk"). This can be dealt with by taking a much more proactive and directive stance; metaphorically, it is the psychotherapist's use of a "full-court press" approach. Specific concerns and recommendations are delineated, which invariably are predicated on the patient's agreeing to a psychotherapeutic "game plan." Frequent examples include committing to abstinence from nonprescription substance use or adherence to driving regulations. Note taking by the patient, in combination with diagrams, clarifies the dilemmas. Stories of prior patients who made similar poor choices with negative consequences, and/or conjoint meetings with a prior patient who learned from similar errors of judgment, can also positively influence the patient.

There is a fine line between communicating genuine productive worry and making a patient feel coerced or demeaned. It is imperative for patients to understand that ultimately their preferences and decisions are respected and accepted by the psychotherapist. This is the case even when patients appear to flagrantly disregard feedback. When judiciously employed, the "full-court press" technique can be instrumental in exposing heretofore psychologically inaccessible realms. Often a patient is more stirred by a psychotherapist's expression of emotion and sincere concern than by the specifics of the dialogue. This technique also reassures the psychotherapist that he or she has done the utmost on behalf of the patient's well-being. In good conscience, the patient can now be afforded the liberty to incorporate or reject ideas in the context of all possible supports and endeavors.

### *"Probation"*

The technique of probation is a last-ditch effort when all other attempts to remedy a patient's noncompliance have failed. Probation makes continued individual psychotherapy (or neurorehabilitation) contingent on meeting a set of behaviors for a period of time, such as 2–4 weeks. This approach is used only with patients who have significant characterological (vs. organic) problems and who are not motivated for, engaged in, or disciplined about their therapeutic responsibilities and commitments. In group environments, these patients can disrupt or contaminate the therapeutic ambience for other patients. Exploration of preinjury adjustment usually reveals that these patients have a significant history of deceitfulness, acting out, and/or irresponsible and adversarial behavior toward authority figures.

Because characterological problems (e.g., antisocial and narcissistic personality disorders) can coexist with organic memory and executive systems problems, the terms of probation should clearly document the necessary behaviors and possible consequences. Generally, the probation letter is shared with relevant family members, referring physicians, and cotherapists, in order to hold the patient most effectively accountable. Figure 5.3 is a sample probation letter. The tone is straightforward to convey the seriousness of the expectations; however, care should be taken that it does not appear punitive in either content or language. As with all therapeutic interventions, the "if, when, how, and why" of probation are best considered in consultation with other treatment team members or professional colleagues.

[Date]
[Patient's name]
[Patient's address]

Re: Probation

Dear _____ :

    This letter is a follow-up to your meeting with me earlier today regarding your participation in therapy. As we discussed, over the past _____ weeks you have demonstrated difficulties with responsible behavior, and have been noncompliant in interactions with your therapist(s). Problems includes the following: _____ [Examples: You have missed a number of appointments for unexplained reasons, and have been delinquent in telephoning in advance. Your effort on your datebook and Home Independence Checklist continues to be below your potential.]

    Because of the behavior problems described above, you are being placed on a _____ [e.g., 2-, 4-]week probation, effective immediately. As I explained, probation is a last effort to help you succeed in the psychotherapy/rehabilitation process and reach your stated goals of _____ [e.g., living independently, returning to productive work].

    On _____ [date], I reviewed with you a behavior contract that specifies appropriate behaviors. They are also described below. You must consistently demonstrate these behaviors to continue your participation in treatment.

    Specifically, during this probationary period, it will be necessary for you to demonstrate consistent motivation, follow-through, and engagement in your therapies and with your responsibilities at home. In addition, you must do the following:

1. Demonstrate forthright communications with your therapist(s) and patient peers.
2. Maintain socially appropriate language and conversational content with others.
3. Maintain weekly datebook scores of 80% or better.
4. Demonstrate consistent effort in all individual and group-oriented therapies.
5. Follow through with all program recommendations in a consistent and effortful manner.
6. Approach therapies in a businesslike and focused manner (e.g., be on time for appointments).
7. Follow through with your Home Independence Checklist and homework exercises.
8. Have weekly "milieu meetings" with your family, to review your progress in the psychotherapy/rehabilitation process.

    Each week, your performance in meeting these goals will be reviewed with you and your family. If you do not meet these requirements, you will be discharged from therapy, and other treatment resources will be provided. In the interim, if at any point you wish to discontinue attending and participating in therapy, I will fully respect your wishes and provide you with alternative resources.

    Thank you for your willingness to improve your participation in the psychotherapy/rehabilitation process.

Sincerely,

_____
Psychotherapist's signature
cc: Family
    Physician

**FIGURE 5.3.** Probation letter.

## "Things Take Time," "One Day at a Time," and the Tortoise and the Hare

For patients in the throes of the acceptance and adjustment process, a comforting mantra is "Things take time" (Hein, 2004). This helps to reduce the overwhelming anxieties patients can feel associated with the "what-ifs," such as "What if I can't work at my old job?" or "What if I can't attain the career I dreamed of?" The abbreviation "TTT" reminds patients that time is healing, and helps to ameliorate their understandable bewilderment, impatience, and/or anguish associated with uncertainty about the future. A related adage is "One day at a time," which also inspires patients to take small, manageable steps toward goals. Similarly, the metaphor of running a marathon, rather than a sprint (S. Myles, personal communication, n.d.), reinforces the pacing and perseverance needed to succeed. Finally, it can help to review the storyline and theme of the fable *The Tortoise and the Hare* (Aesop, 1984) in psychotherapy sessions. It has useful lessons for the therapeutic and recovery process after brain injury, which is typically incremental and, by definition, arduous.

## "I'm Not 100% Recovered"

With time, patients may come to realize that they will not make a full recovery. One helpful approach for the psychotherapist is to differentiate between "physiological" and "functional" recovery. Physiological recovery relates to the healing process associated with the actual brain damage. Recovery of function and brain plasticity is complex, and scientific knowledge about this is evolving (see Stein & Hoffman, 2003, for a review; see also Watson, 2007). Clinically, a generous margin of up to 2 years is recommended for functional recovery. In addition, therapists can help patients realize that recovery is multidimensional; some abilities will improve more than others, depending on the nature and location of the injury. A psychotherapist must help a patient accept that the physiological recovery process is beyond the patient's control as long as he or she follows a healthy lifestyle and does not further compromise brain function by making self-destructive choices (e.g., drug and alcohol use). One helpful image is that the brain injury sets the outside limits or parameters of the overall recovery process. Another helpful concept is that the psychotherapy process can facilitate, but does not dictate, the nature of or time frame for recovery.

The psychotherapist can emphasize that the patient's capability for functional gains is more self-determined; with the foundations of psychotherapy and rehabilitation, the patient can always strive for improvement through compensatory strategies. The creative search for alternative coping mechanisms to accomplish realistic goals is not time-limited. As discussed in Chapter 3, the movie *The Karate Kid* (Weintraub et al., 1984) is an excellent illustration of this process; with coaching, trust in the process, and self-discipline, new skills and accomplishments are achievable. Nonetheless, honest dialogue and the associated grieving process are inherent in the tumultuous acceptance voyage, and the psychotherapist must bear witness to the inevitable emotional roller coaster while supporting the patient.

### The "80/20 Rule"

A common consequence of executive system dysfunction is "black-and-white" thinking. After brain injury, patients may develop perfectionistic expectations of their recovery, which set the stage for disillusionment. The "80/20 rule" reminds patients that in every positive situation (the 80%), there are certain negatives (the 20%). The rule promotes more balanced thinking in the "gray zones," and helps patients to anticipate and cope with periodic setbacks and disappointments.

### "Prepare for the Worst; Hope for the Best"

In determining a course of action, patients need to consider a range of eventualities. The proverb "Prepare for the worst; hope for the best" is a helpful coping tool in psychotherapy to remind patients to consider and prepare for all possibilities, including potential impediments and/or failures. The short film *Partly Cloudy* (Reher & Sohn, 2009) is a charming illustration of this principle and also teaches resiliency, adaptability, and perseverance.

### The "Good-Enough" Outcome: Accepting the Silver or Bronze versus the Gold

The acceptance process involves the recalibration of future goals and aspirations. Helping patients accept "good-enough" outcomes, using the Olympics metaphor of silver or bronze versus gold medals, helps to combat perfectionistic, grandiose, and all-or-nothing thinking. Patients often develop an idealized hindsight view of their preinjury lives, ignoring the reality that even without brain injury, people don't always get what they want. This normalizes the inevitable disappointments and detours of life.

## INCREASING ACCEPTANCE IN GROUP PSYCHOTHERAPY

The sharing of experiences in group psychotherapy is vital for the acceptance process after brain injury. It has a supportive effect on the group members (O'Callaghan et al., 2006), who gain valuable feedback, inspiration, and perspective from their peers. In a safe and protected environment, patients can express their often intense emotions, while at the same time developing and practicing healthy coping techniques. The commonality of challenges and the quest for emotional relief bond the group.

Figure 5.4 lists group psychotherapy topics pertinent to the acceptance process. The first set of topics is grouped under the theme "Sources of Angst and Turmoil" (e.g., "Why me?" and life's unexpected changes). The group can explore specific terminology and constructs, such as "snarky," "commitment," "self-sabotage," "procrastination," or "resistance." A dictionary definition of such a term can facilitate discussion. The group can also provide a forum for therapeutic venting about difficulties with acceptance. This allows members to commiserate about built-up frustrations with the psychotherapy and rehabilitation process, often manifested as burnout or "rehabitis." As part of the group exchange, practical implications of acceptance are posed, including what information to disclose about the injury in the community, to whom, and how. This may involve construction of a group-generated pros-and-cons list. With careful monitoring of group dialogue, the psychotherapist can gain insight into each patient's underlying qualms about the acceptance process.

The group process is also powerful for reinforcing "Healthy Coping Techniques," a second theme of group topics. Frequently addressed topics include the purpose of consistent (and often lifelong) use of compensatory strategies and how patients feel about them. Another favorite topic is the role of psychotropic medication, its potential value, and whether or not to take it. Group dialogue on such topics helps patients work through differences of opinion and find "middle ground." This underscores the value of the working alliance and collaboration process.

A third theme, "Guided Exercises and Activities," furthers group involvement (see Figure 5.4). These are specific round-robin techniques that enable patients to reflect on and work through their personal acceptance hurdles. Examples include patients' situating themselves in the coping zones of the PEM; self-ratings of percentage of recovery in various domains; and self-ratings of determination. Other exercises include developing self-motivating personal mottos, and identifying and setting individual responsibilities by sharing "what's on my plate." Selected readings can give hope and inspiration. These include patient-chosen music lyrics; *Napoleon Hill's Keys to Success: The 17 Principles of Personal Achievement* (Hill, 1994); "A Letter from Your Brain" (St. Claire, 1996); *It's Not about the Bike* (Armstrong with Jenkins, 2000); and *When Bad Things Happen to Good People* (Kushner, 1981). Visits from prior patients who have excelled in their acceptance and recovery, but moreover, who can resonate with the current patients' anguish, are also extremely helpful activities.

## THREE EXTENDED CASES

### Sally: Optimal Acceptance

Sally was age 28 when she sustained a traumatic brain injury as a result of a horseback riding accident. She was unconscious at the scene and rapidly intubated. Upon her arrival at a trauma center, her Glasgow Coma Scale score was 7. CT brain scans revealed falcine subdural hematomas and subarachnoid hemorrhage. MRI of the brain showed multiple shear injuries in the frontal and temporal lobes, more prominent on the right side, consistent with diffuse axonal injury. Neuropsychological testing at 8 weeks postinjury revealed moderate deficits in the areas of speed of information processing, word finding, verbal learning and recall, delayed visual recall, complex attention, mathematical skills, and executive systems (e.g., abstract reasoning, strategy generation, and flexible problem solving). Sally's personality testing with the MMPI-2 (Butcher & Williams, 2000; Butcher, 2005), did not indicate any mood difficulties. Her profile indicated that she was cheerful, friendly, outgoing, and well adjusted overall.

Sally was invited to share background history in her initial consultation. She had been an equestrienne for many years; as a youngster and teenager, she had

**Sources of Angst and Turmoil**
- Definition of acceptance.
- Why me?
- Sources of postinjury stress and worries.
- Feelings of guilt, shame, and anger about one's injury circumstances.
- What if I don't make a 100% recovery?
- Feelings about specific injury limitations.
- Feelings about postinjury life changes.
- The definition and roles of "resistance," "self-sabotage," "negativity," "denial," "burnout," and "procrastination" in recovery.
- Am I "snarky" and why?
- The whats and whys about "Yeah, buts."
- What are my psychological "blind spots"?
- Sources of postinjury frustration and struggles: The "sick and tired" syndrome.
- General concerns, complaints, gripes, and "rehabitis."
- Purposes of and feelings about psychotherapy probation.
- Pros and cons of disclosure about one's injury.

**Healthy Coping Techniques**
- The purposes and benefits of group psychotherapy in the acceptance process.
- Trust and faith in the psychotherapy process: The role of the working alliance.
- Conflict resolution, negotiation, and "middle ground."
- The role of resiliency, commitment, compliance, attitude, motivation, self-discipline, and accountability in recovery.
- The "three P's": "Positive, patient, and persistent."
- Prior life-altering and life-influencing experiences.
- Healthy versus unhealthy coping techniques before and after injury.
- The role of spirituality.
- The whats and whys of compensations.
- The role of psychotropic medication.
- What's the "80/20 rule"?
- Feelings about "Things take time."

**Guided Exercises and Activities**
- Self-ratings (0–10; 0 = no problem, 10 = large problem) versus peer ratings versus the psychotherapists' ratings of acceptance and stress levels.
- Personal goal setting, and self-ratings of percentage of recovery (0–100%) in various domains.
- Which coping zone am I in, according to the PEM?
- Self-ratings (0–10; see above for scale) versus peer ratings versus the psychotherapists' ratings of "Yeah, buts" and "snarkiness."
- How full is my plate, and what's on it (individualized lists)?
- Personal challenges and mechanisms for accepting brain injury.
- My Olympic medal definitions for future success (gold, silver, and bronze).
- Self-ratings of determination.
- Personal choices of music lyrics depicting one's dilemmas and challenges.
- Reading and discussion of "A Letter from Your Brain" (St. Claire, 1996).
- Reading and discussion of "Welcome to Holland" (Kingsley, 1987).
- Reading *Napoleon Hill's Keys to Success: The 17 Principles of Personal Achievement* (Hill, 1994).
- Reading *When Bad Things Happen to Good People* (Kushner, 1981).
- Reading passages from *It's Not about the Bike* (Armstrong with Jenkins, 2000).
- Visits from patient "graduates": How have they coped and compensated over the long term?

**FIGURE 5.4.** Group psychotherapy: Acceptance themes and topics.

participated in dressage competitions and won a number of awards. This required many years of disciplined practice; often she awoke at dawn and rode 1.5 hours before school, and then 2–3 hours after school. She had a close and loving relationship with her family, especially her father, who supported and mentored this avocation. She was also an excellent student; she had consistently been on the honor roll during elementary and high school, and had graduated from college summa cum laude with a bachelor's degree in business administration. Her family described her preinjury personality as "upbeat, conscientious, and grounded." Nonetheless, Sally had experienced prior life traumas, and had shown exemplary ability to "bounce back." When she was 15 years old, her biological mother died of bone cancer, after a prolonged and debilitating struggle. Throughout this process, Sally demonstrated laudable dedication to her mother, and also drew strong sustenance from her religious affiliation. Afterward, she returned to riding competitions as a source of consolation and a sign of her resiliency. When her father remarried 3 years later, Sally again showed sensitivity and versatility in her reactions and coping behaviors. At the time of the accident, Sally coowned a small eclectic bookstore with a close friend. Her friend willingly took over the store responsibilities during Sally's convalescence. Her psychotherapist realized that Sally's preinjury emotional stability and accomplishments would serve her well in her current toils.

Sally initiated psychotherapy and cognitive therapies 10 weeks after her injury. Within the first few weeks, it became clear that Sally's acceptance of her predicament was high; this formed the baseline for treatment interventions. For example, she showed unusually good insight into her injury-related deficits. She was extremely motivated to address these problems and very trusting of therapeutic recommendations. She was adamant about returning to work, as she was passionate and prideful about her small store, which she and her friend had founded and nurtured into a popular and innovative cozy retreat.

Sally explained in individual psychotherapy that among her preinjury responsibilities were researching and ordering rare books and magazines and doing the business's bookkeeping. She had paid meticulous attention to detail, and had constructed multiple organizational protocols to streamline her workday. These preinjury aptitudes, in combination with her self-disciplined life approach, enabled her to make excellent use of psychotherapy, cognitive exercises, and memory compensations. She attacked her problem areas with gusto—often completing assignments ahead of time, and putting extra hours into homework and self-initiated computer, workbook, and other games to tackle her deficits. She was also a voracious reader, and she progressed from reading short stories to epic novels over the course of several months. She had committed to a 10-kilometer walk with friends in 6 months to raise money for diabetes, and self-initiated a "one-day-at-a-time" retraining program through her exercise club to rebuild her endurance and fitness for the activity.

Early in the psychotherapy relationship, Sally stated, "I don't want to dilly-dally about returning to work; I'll do whatever it takes." Her psychotherapist perceived Sally as a "worker bee"; her approach to life was to set subgoals and systematically fulfill them until she reached her main objectives. Individual psychotherapy capitalized on her resiliency, coachability, inner fortitude, pragmatism, and self-discipline. Collaboratively, she and her psychotherapist developed a tentative timetable for achieving various goals (i.e., living in her own apartment without family assistance, driving, doing part-time supervised work, and finally returning to full-time work). In group psychotherapy, she chose the *Snow White* music lyrics "Heigh-ho, heigh-ho, it's off to work we go" (Churchill, Harline, & Smith, 1937) to depict her enthusiasm about her work reentry.

At junctures, Sally became understandably perturbed and forlorn when she did not make progress to the degree or at the rate she expected. Her psychotherapist made several suggestions to ameliorate these feelings, including for Sally to reach out to her support network, as her religious beliefs and "church family" provided an emotional compass for her. She was also introduced to the movie *The Horse Whisperer* (Markey & Redford, 1998), which dealt with recovery from a riding accident. Sally also drew solace and inspiration from the storyline and themes. Gradually, through the therapist's attunement, Sally more freely expressed her feelings of loss and sadness over her life's detour. Her psychotherapist regularly verbalized that Sally could resume her business, which became a sustaining thought. She also constructed therapeutic opportunities for Sally to accumulate successes (e.g., cognitive retraining exercises), which were empowering. At the same time, her psychotherapist cautioned her that she might not make a 100% recovery in all areas.

A sign of Sally's improved coping capacity was her exceptional willingness to take full ownership of any and every compensation recommended to her. Her psychotherapist capitalized on this eagerness, and instructed her in devising and implementing procedural checklists for learning and recall difficulties in multiple settings. Overall, despite her frontal lobe injury, Sally was very coachable in appreciating the "big picture" of her therapy and its applicability to independent living and work. Specifically, by improving her abstract thinking, word generation, divided attention, and math, she could multitask, do proper calculations for invoices and order confirmations, and "think outside the box" at work. During her participation in her psychoeducation group, she was introduced to the PEM. Her personal rating of herself as in Phase 5 ("green") accorded with those of her patient peers and therapists, and reflected her highly adaptive coping style. With support and therapeutic guidance, Sally adopted the "just do it" attitude, counterbalanced with the insight and patience to recognize that "things take time" (Hein, 2004).

Overall, Sally's psychotherapy focused on providing her with psychoeducation and empathically supporting her step-by-step endeavors to reclaim her productive lifestyle. Sally expressed considerable appreciation for her degree of recovery, and, through dialogue, came to recognize how her preinjury tribulations had furnished her with the inner resiliency to face and overcome psychological humps. Because of Sally's natural leadership skills and perky personality, her psychotherapist recommended that she become involved in community education and other avenues for peer support. Sally was elated with this idea, and began a campaign to raise social consciousness about the effects of acquired brain injury. Her therapist not only helped coordinate a presentation at a local conference for survivors, but referred her to a government-based consumer board designed to help allocate monies to state rehabilitation programs.

About her psychotherapy, Sally wrote:

"I have been working on maintaining my overall mood and my adjustment to life now that it involves some difficulties. It's nice to get a second, outside opinion of things so that I do not jump the gun at work. I also continue to take notes in my sessions to help imprint the necessity to take notes at work, in meetings, on the phone, or in face-to-face communications. I want to personify a well-put-together person. By discussing my feelings and 'unloading' my frustrations, I won't cause strife at my office. I want to sustain a positive attitude to work at my full capacity and maintain important relationships with my family, coworker, and clients. My self-assurance is back!"

## Zoë: Irremediable Denial and Resistance

Zoë was age 28 when she suffered a severe traumatic brain injury as a result of a car accident. She was driving when the highly inebriated driver of another car hit her head on. Zoë's fiancé was killed instantly in the crash. Zoë was comatose for 2 weeks and spent 3 months recuperating in the hospital. Her MRI/CT scans showed bilateral small frontal contusions, a left parietal contusion, a small brainstem contusion, and diffuse brain swelling. She suffered from diplopia. Zoë also had a preexisting history of bipolar disorder, and persisted in her refusal to comply with medication and psychiatric treatment. Her parents minimized the diagnosis and symptoms, stating that she had a "flamboyant zest for life."

Zoë desperately wanted to return to her former employment as a pharmacist. She was referred for neuropsychological testing and psychotherapy by her rehabilitation physician, who was concerned that this was not a realistic vocational plan. Her neuropsychological evaluation at 2.5 years postinjury revealed adequate attentional and language abilities. However, she demonstrated severe deficits in the areas of working memory, verbal learning and recall, attention to visual detail, visuospatial skills, mathematical skills, visual recall, and executive functions (especially abstract reasoning, problem solving, multitasking, and impulse control). Behaviorally, she showed very poor communication pragmatics, including hyperverbality, socially inappropriate behavior, disinhibited comments, and bluntness.

The psychotherapist's baseline assessment of Zoë's level of acceptance indicated that it was poor, in part due to the severity of her executive system deficits. Zoë's psychological approach to her injury-related sequelae was dominated by avoidance and recalcitrance. Her entrenched maladaptive habits included refusing to use a datebook system, and instead relying on Post-its, which she stuck all over her home. Her family was also highly skeptical about the benefits of psychotherapy. As therapy progressed, Zoë often called in "sick" for appointments, when actually she was "sick and tired" of having to confront her injury-related realities. She refused to wear her prism glasses, rationalizing that her eyesight would become "dependent" on the glasses. She was also steadfastly unwilling to discuss her feelings about her fiancé's death, stating that she was "fine with it." All of these behaviors signified the depth of her denial, rooted in her deeply traumatizing experiences. Zoë's chronic behavioral and cognitive deficits, in combination with her persistent denial and resistance, raised substantial concerns about her ability to return to work as a pharmacist. Despite her psychotherapist's concerns, Zoë was unfazed, reemphasizing her dogged intention to return to her prior position.

Once the working alliance was established, Zoë showed tentative amusement at the psychotherapist's references to her as the "Queen of Yeah, Buts." Zoë appeared to have an excuse for every conceivable failure, becoming "snarky" and blaming others for her shortcomings. She dismissed her psychotherapist's recommendation in cognitive retraining to log the number of "Yeah, but" responses per session as a way to self-monitor and improve her "buy-in." She also refused to compensate for her memory difficulties and was vexed at the recommendation for psychiatric care. Substantial time and effort were spent in individual psychotherapy—including the "Try it, you'll like it" approach, psychological judo, and the devil's advocate position—to convince her of the merit of compensatory strategies. Diagrams, such as the one shown in Figure 5.1, were used to help illustrate the process. In other attempts to penetrate her cognitive rigidity, the therapist discussed with her the lyrics to the song "My Way" (Anka, Revaux, Thibault, & Frankois, 1969) and the metaphor of "teaching old dogs new tricks." Zoë was also invited to watch the movie *Grace Is Gone* (Cusack et al., 2007). The movie shows how the pain and angst associated with the abrupt death of a loved one can result in running away from this knowledge. With time, Zoë could recognize her coping style and could even laugh at the regularity of her "Yeah, but" retorts. Nonetheless, the denial and resistance behaviors persisted. It was as if by retreating back to her old work life, she could salvage the remnants of her historical "happy and fulfilled" self.

A pros-and-cons list of Zoë's work capabilities was made. The pros included her retention of knowledge in the field and her motivation; the cons included her diplopia and other neuropsychological/neurobehavioral deficits that were incompatible with the job of a pharmacist. She and the psychotherapist discussed the play *Peter Pan* (Barrie, 1904/1985) to illustrate the importance of "growing up" and taking on personal responsibility for her injury-related deficits. However, Zoë persisted in the fantasy that life would be "normal" as soon as she went back to work.

In group psychotherapy, Zoë was the brashest spokeswoman for gripes and "rehabitis." Her peers rated her with a high degree of "Yeah, buts" and "snarkiness," and as being in the "yellow" warning zone on the PEM, but she persisted in discounting and arguing with the feedback. She vehemently denied any psychological "blind spots." Her self-rating of her overall recovery was 90%, and her self-proclaimed mantra was "I know best."

Incidentally, Zoë's coping mechanisms closely mirrored those of her parents. They too were adamant that "where there's a will, there's a way," and they rejected the validity of the neuropsychological test findings. Their preinjury parenting style had been to indulge Zoë, so as to avoid conflict; this contributed to her feelings of invincibility and entitlement. The family members did not "buy into" the necessity or value of compensatory strategies. They were determined to prove her psychotherapist wrong, and expected a 100% recovery. They dismissed the feedback about Zoë's behavioral problems, stating, "She's always been this way; it's just her personality." The working alliance had disintegrated into a power struggle between Zoë and her psychotherapist.

In a last-stand approach, her psychotherapist tried the "full-court press" and called a family meeting to explicitly review the reasons Zoë was unready to return to work, warning them of the strong likelihood that she would be fired and jeopardize her license to practice. As part of the dialogue, Zoë and her parents were encouraged to take a "wait-and-see" approach and to invest her energies in compensation training. So as not to aggravate the situation further and eradicate the working alliance, the psychotherapist also encouraged Zoë and her parents to seek a second opinion. Soon after this meeting, they elected to terminate psychotherapy; however, the door was left open for resumption of treatment, should the need or desire arise.

## Lewis: The Acceptance Journey

Lewis was age 21 when he was involved in a single-car, rollover motor vehicle accident. He sustained a severe traumatic brain injury, with an initial Glasgow Coma Scale score of 4. Neuroimaging studies revealed a frontoparietal depressed skull fracture and left frontal parenchymal contusion. Acutely, he demonstrated significant expressive aphasia. Lewis underwent a neuropsychological examination at 8 months postinjury; the findings revealed moderate deficits in the areas of executive functions (anticipatory planning, problem solving, mental flexibility, impulsivity, and multitasking) and verbal learning and recall (with confabulation), as well as severe deficits in the areas of verbal working memory. Speech–language testing demonstrated residual deficits in the areas of reading comprehension, auditory comprehension, naming, and verbal formulation. At the time of the accident, Lewis had been drinking; although he was not cited in the accident, his blood alcohol level was .05.

Before the accident, Lewis intended to complete premedical coursework in the next year and then enroll in medical school. His preinjury grades were marginal; however, Lewis was convinced that he would have improved his grades enough to have been easily accepted into a medical school.

Lewis began individual and group psychotherapy as part of a complement of neurorehabilitation therapies. His initial self-awareness and acceptance of neurological problems were fair. He was beginning to recognize his deficit areas, including forgetfulness. At first he tended to minimize his problems, stating that they were no worse than those most of his friends had. However, he was receptive to further inquiry and showed beginning trust in the working relationship.

Lewis's coping style meandered between the adaptive ("green") and the warning ("yellow") zones of the PEM. After his psychotherapist reviewed the initial therapy assessments with Lewis, his mood shifted from benign euthymia to feeling depressed and overwhelmed. In addition, his girlfriend of 18 months abruptly ended their relationship. This precipitated an emotional crisis characterized by thoughts of "If only . . . " and "Why me?" His heartache and recriminations were fueled by guilt over his choice to consume alcohol the night of the accident. Constructive psychotherapeutic approaches included discussion of "Hindsight is 40/40" and "A Letter from Your Brain" (St. Claire, 1996). With the psychotherapist's urging, Lewis also agreed to see a psychiatrist, and soon afterward he began antidepressant medication. This enabled him to cope better with his multiple stressors. Lewis remarked that "Individual psychotherapy is making me aware of what I need to accept; it's like falling and hitting a pillow."

His psychotherapist incorporated data from cognitive retraining sessions to help Lewis appreciate his strengths and difficulties and compensate effectively for the difficulties, using note taking and double-checking to ameliorate problems with impulsivity and memory. He was ambivalent about these tools. One goal of the rehabilitation process for Lewis was preparing to resume university coursework. To this end, he worked with his speech–language pathologist and his psychotherapist. Lewis insisted on taking an upper-level biology class, despite the recommendation to begin with an easier online class. His therapists decided then to step back and treat the class as a "planned failure." It soon became apparent to observers that Lewis's study skills were substandard. Before the accident, he had studied minimally; he was therefore (overly) confident that he could revert to this approach without negative consequences. Further exploration in psychotherapy indicated that he had always been a procrastinator about school responsibilities. When he obtained a failing grade on his first biology quiz, he defaulted to a "Yeah, but" and blamed the lack of in-class teacher interactions, rather than his neuropsychological deficits and poor study skills. As a technique to help him reflect further on the pros and cons of this tendency, his psychotherapist asked him to look up the definition of the word "procrastinate" and write about the ramifications of this life approach. He wrote:

> "Procrastination means to postpone doing something as a regular practice. When I think about it, I put the 'P' in procrastinate. In the dictionary, my picture is next to the definition. All of my life I have waited to the last minute to do everything. Sometimes it does not affect my work, but other times it does completely. No matter how large the assignment is, I will still wait to the last minute and sometimes never finish. Even after the lesson, I still do not learn that procrastination is not the way to go . . . "

Another helpful therapeutic tool to dislodge his passivity was the story "God Will Save Me" (n.d.), which illustrates the dire consequences of the "do-nothing" approach versus becoming proactive about compensations. Lewis stated his resolve to better apply his study skills. Helpful mantras he was provided included "History isn't destiny," "Fly right," and "Show me the marks." Soon after this, Lewis was involved in two fender-benders within 3 days. He was miffed that his driving privileges were temporarily removed by his rehabilitation physician while he underwent another adaptive driving evaluation. To improve his "ownership" of these accidents, his psychotherapist assigned an essay as a vehicle for self-reflection. He wrote:

> "Last Sunday I was involved in a car accident. I do not have a 'Yeah, but' for this situation, but we all know how stupid tourists drive. Three days later, I got a ticket for rear-ending another driver. My therapist is saying that this

other accident was also caused by my brain injury because I was not paying attention. But I know for a fact it was not my brain injury that caused it; in a nutshell, there is no way that the brain injury can connect these events. Taking away my driving privileges is an inconvenience in every single way possible. Did I mention that the adaptive driving class will cost me $250, and it will be a waste of time?"

His psychotherapist and rehabilitation physician then constructed a "driving probation agreement" and had Lewis sign it. The contract spanned 6 weeks and stipulated that Lewis would not drive with others in the car; that he would be home by 8 P.M.; and that he would not use his cell phone while driving. Although he was initially irate and "snarky" about the recommendations, after several months Lewis came to appreciate that the psychotherapist's approach of "not turning a blind eye" (G. A. Lage, personal communication, n.d.) stemmed from a sense of legitimate concern. After deliberation, Lewis was assigned another essay to further the process of internalizing conscience, reliability, maturation, and self-regulation:

> "While I was under the driving probation period, I have become a much safer driver and formed many new habits by being very cautious everywhere that I drive. Whether it's not driving too late, or not rushing to my destination, I am working to be more internally self-policed and not wait for others around me to instruct me and supervise over my shoulder. Once I accomplish this goal, I will be able to move out on my own and live by myself."

Although Lewis's overall therapy engagement and self-awareness improved, it became apparent from both his pre- and postinjury academic performance that it was premature (if not actually unlikely) to expect that he would be accepted into medical school. Initially, Lewis engaged in avoidance and resistance behaviors, including minimizing the issues and glossing over his poor grades. In addition, he gave insufficient credence to his working memory problems and their potential impact on the practice of medicine. Lewis was asked to watch the movie *Little Miss Sunshine* (Friendly, Saraf, Turtletaub, Dayton, & Faris, 2006). He and his psychotherapist discussed the scene where the character Dwayne discovers that he is color-blind and can never gain admission to the Air Force Academy. This catalyzed Lewis's own epiphany, and sparked a poignant dialogue about his own personal deficiencies.

During group psychotherapy, Lewis was a lively member and vociferously expressed his opinions, particularly when working through his frustrations and disillusionment with the psychotherapy process and "imposed restrictions" (including his driving probation). During the period when he was displaying avoidance and resistance, his psychotherapist brought a broom and dustpan to group psychotherapy to stimulate a discussion about "sweeping problems under the rug." As Lewis's level of engagement in his rehabilitation and psychotherapy process further waned, the group listened to the song "Superman (It's not Easy)," as sung by Five for Fighting (Ondrasik, 2000), to spark dialogue. What emerged was how much Lewis's "playfulness and joking demeanor" were covering his inner sadness and grief. He stated: "I'm continually laughing; otherwise, I'll never stop crying."

Because Lewis had responded well to essay writing, he was asked by his psychotherapist to do a small research study on working memory. This encompassed the definition, cognitive indices, his own personal examples of problem areas, the neuroanatomical correlates, and appropriate strategies and compensations. This was an excellent exercise in awareness and acceptance; he was becoming his own best expert. He was asked to present this research in the psychoeducation group (see Chapter 3), as well as to his parents during a family meeting. This process empowered Lewis; he was developing the necessary insight and acceptance to evaluate and construct his future plans. It should also be noted that Lewis's parents had an outstanding working alliance with his psychotherapist, cultivated through individual family psychotherapy sessions, conjoint meetings with Lewis, and habitual attendance at the weekly relatives' group. Chapter 7 describes family involvement in greater detail.

Over the course of the next 3 months, Lewis voiced a willingness to explore other career directions as part of his acceptance process. His psychotherapist used the Olympic medal metaphor and identified a step-by-step progression into the field of health care. Although the gold medal was attached to being a physician, Lewis identified a feasible silver medal as being a physician assistant, and a bronze as working in the field of nursing. Applying the mantra "Try it, you'll like it," Lewis decided to enroll in prenursing coursework as a first step toward his objectives. A timely visitor to group psychotherapy had successfully returned to work as a nurse after overcoming similar psychological hurdles. He helped Lewis view his own glass as "half full." Now Lewis was pleased with his plans, and felt empowered by his improved psychological demeanor and tool kit of compensatory strategies.

Patients and their support network will benefit from a broad array of compensatory tools; these are described in the next chapter.

# CHAPTER 6

# Life Skills Training

$A$ primary goal of neurorehabilitation is the reacquisition of functional life skills needed for successful reintegration into the community (see Karlovits & McColl, 1999, for a review). Patients who achieve this goal will need less supervision, will have better safety awareness, and will be able to resume preinjury chores and duties in/for the home (e.g., shopping, meal preparation, laundry, gardening, and banking) (Klonoff et al., 2003). Physical, behavioral, cognitive, and perceptual deficits can all interfere with reattaining life skills after acquired brain injury (Dikmen, Machamer, Powell, & Temkin, 2003; Linden, Boschian, Eker, Schalen, & Nordstrom, 2005; Mazaux et al., 1997; Tate & Broe, 1999). Effective life skills training emphasizes remediation of multiple deficits, including attention, memory, initiation, planning, organizing, problem solving, deductive reasoning, flexibility, self-monitoring, multitasking, safety awareness, and judgment (Condeluci, Cooperman, & Seif, 1987; Goverover, 2004; Hart et al., 2003; Mazaux et al., 1997; Worthington & Waller, 2009). This is accomplished through task analysis, sequencing, overlearning, and generalization, as well as through teaching self-responsibility (Condelucci et al., 1987; Martelli, Nicholson, & Zasler, 2008).

This chapter describes the datebook and the Home Independence Checklist as key compensatory and psychoeducational techniques. Now the psychotherapist is functioning as a pragmatist—entering a patient's phenomenological world, and using collaborative evidentiary techniques to enhance independent functioning in the home and community environments. This knowledge is especially essential for the solo practitioner, who may need to proactively manufacture and oversee user-friendly tools for his or her patients and their support networks. Group psychotherapy and family therapies are also discussed in this context, to enable patients to experience a renewed sense of community and family life with the aid of outsiders' feedback and perspectives (Klonoff et al., 2003, 2008). This chapter also describes interventions to facilitate the reattainment of driving privileges. Additional aspects of community reintegration (those related to communication, social skills, and leisure activities) are addressed in Chapter 8.

## THE DATEBOOK

The datebook is the foundational compensatory tool after acquired brain injury (Klonoff et al., 2003; Sohlberg & Mateer, 1989). With it, patients can compensate for vexing cognitive deficits, including new learning and recall, as well as problems with organization, initiation, follow-through, planning, and prioritization (Klonoff et al., 2003; Mateer & Sira, 2008; Skeel & Edwards, 2009). As an externalized record of the past, present, and future, it enables patients to efficiently track and accomplish major responsibilities, including appointments, self-care, and other home-based chores and tasks (Klonoff et al., 2003). The datebook's unique composition enables a flexible and personalized approach (Sohlberg & Mateer, 1989; Tate, 1997), which enhances the ultimate utility and appeal of the system.

I recommend the FranklinCovey system (*www.FranklinCovey.com*). Items included in the datebook should be "month-at-a-glance" pages; two full datebook pages for each day; an address and phone number section; a medication card; personal information; a "today ruler" (i.e., a 1- to 2-inch-wide plastic bookmark); business card holders; and a small pencil pouch that also contains highlighters. Figure 6.1 displays a typical two-page-per-day datebook setup. Generally, it is helpful to have the daily pages for the preceding month, the current month, and the subsequent month in the datebook. Daily activities and appointments with designated times are entered under "Appointment Schedule" on the left page. More details about appointments and other things to do can be logged under "Prioritized Daily Task List," also on the left page. For clarity and organization, appointments and tasks should be numbered, and specific times for task completion should be written alongside. Highlighting the numbers serves as a good visual cue. Once a task is accomplished, it should be checked off; uncompleted tasks need to be carried forward to an appropriate day and time. The "Daily Notes" heading on the right page is for noting details about events of the day, assignments, telephone conversations, or journal entries. The "today ruler" is helpful to mark the current datebook page. To log future appointments or obligations, the patient should keep month-at-a-glance pages in the datebook for one preceding month (for reference), the current month, and subsequent months. On the first day of each month, the patient should transfer information on the month-at-a-glance pages to the daily pages.

Repeating or standing appointments and tasks should be put into the datebook for a few weeks at a time. Examples of standing daily tasks include taking medication, exercise, homework, and pet care. Repeating weekly tasks include loading the pillbox, doing laundry, completing a weekly meal plan, grocery shopping, preparing dinner, making social plans, and paying bills. Datebooks also need to contain relevant personal information, including emergency contact information and doctors' phone numbers.

**19** Thursday March 2009

S M T W T F S
1 2 3 4 5 6 7
8 9 10 11 12 13 14
15 16 17 18 19 20 21
22 23 24 25 26 27 28
29 30 31

February 2009 April 2009

✓ Completed
→ Forwarded
X Deleted
G⊘ Delegated
• In Process

**↓ ABC Prioritized Daily Task List**

✓ (1.) ✓ Tell Mara things I bought on Saturday.
✓ (2.) Give Mara Homework.
✓ (3.) ✓ Tell Mara my plans for my birthday.

**Daily Tracker**

Track expenses, e-mail, voice mail, or other information.

(1.) Mystery Book from the Book Store. New Purse – Perfume
(3.) Get together with family. Have lunch with friends.

© FranklinCovey. All Rights Reserved. • franklincovey.com • Original–Classic

**Appointment Schedule**

8
/9 Take prescription pills. Eat Breakfast. Get dressed. ✓ Take vitamins.
/10 Leave for therapy.
/10:30 Rec. Therapy
11 (2)(3)(3)
/11:15 Speech Therapy / Mara
/11:50 Millieu
/12 Lunch
1
1:30 Go to Drug Store.
/2 Take Dogs for a walk
/3 Pick up in Bedroom
/4 Go to Pet Smart
/5 Go to Airport
6
/7 Vitamins
/8 Veggie Burger & Rice
/9:00 Take Prescription Pills
11:45 Actual Bedtime

A loving person lives in a loving world.
A hostile person lives in a hostile world.
Everyone you meet is your mirror.
—Ken Keyes Jr.

**19** Thursday March 2009

**Daily Notes** 78th Day 287 Left Week 12

11:45 Speech Therapy – I had a clipboard with 10 directions to follow and complete, of which I completed seven of them on my own. It was an enjoyable experience, and another strengthing and learning experience. I really enjoyed working with Mara very much! She has a very nice & pleasant personality and I have come to really enjoy her company very much.

News Assignment –

As the Obama administration prepares to send more then a hundred federal agents to the U.S. Mexican Border Congressional Committees are holding hearings to learn more about the violent Mexican Drug Cartels. The death toll from drug related violence in Mexico last year surpassed 6,000, more then double the previous year. The bloodshed which historically has been confined to Mexico is escalating and migrating. In 2008 Phoenix reported 366 abductions, mostly tied to Mexican human smugglers and narcotics gangs.

Pepsi intake 40 oz.

© FranklinCovey. All Rights Reserved. • franklincovey.com • Original–Classic

**FIGURE 6.1.** A typical two-page-per-day datebook setup.

Sohlberg and Mateer (1989) have eloquently described the essential components of a functional memory book system and behavioral training techniques. They describe three phases of instruction: "acquisition," in which the patient attains basic competence with the notebook through familiarization training; "application," in which the patient learns when and where to utilize the new skills and applies them to suitable situations; and "adaptation," wherein the patient demonstrates the ability to adjust and modify skills to accommodate novel situations via training in naturalistic settings. All phases require instruction.

During the instruction phase, the patient is informed that there is no "wiggle room"; he or she must adhere to a regimented protocol for datebook usage to master the concepts. Key strategies include encouraging the patient to take detailed notes, following the "Who, What, When, Where," format. Often tasks will require a "planning" entry to remind the individual about an event or appointment later in the week (e.g., packing running shoes the night before for a physical therapy session). During the training process, the therapist should monitor specific datebook entries. This includes making sure that the patient has taken legible notes in sufficient detail; in addition, the therapist should track the time frames and descriptions in planning entries, and check that each due date also has a reminder. Patients should not get in the habit of repeatedly moving responsibilities forward, as these are likely to get lost or to be completed late. Successful use of the datebook requires daily habitual practice, including on weekends and holidays. For some patients with severe memory or initiation problems, it is necessary to supplement the datebook with other cueing devices (e.g., a watch alarm or a DataLink watch to remind them to access their datebooks). Patients with better memory and executive functions and a predilection for new technology may progress to using pagers, text messagers, personal digital assistants (PDAs) or other portable electronic devices, smartphones, web-based resources, cameras, location detection devices, or virtual reality procedures (Boman, Tham, Granqvist, Bartfai, & Hemmingsson, 2007; Green, 2007; Hart, Buchhofer & Vaccaro, 2004; Mateer, 2005; Wilson & Kapur, 2008; Worthington & Waller, 2009).

If such a professional is accessible, it is ideal to enlist an occupational therapist and/or speech–language pathologist in the training and implementation of specific datebook techniques, in order to reinforce datebook use. Group settings can also emphasize the various applications of the datebook. Figure 6.2 is a useful handout that explains the conceptual and practical applications of the datebook system. Family members and other meaningful support persons should be educated about the rationale, components, and procedures of datebook use. Most often these persons will need to attend educational sessions and maintain close dialogue with the psychotherapist regarding practical and psychological challenges as they arise. This allows for external support and reinforcement and successful generalization of the datebook system to nonclinic settings. Interestingly, some family members embrace the datebook system to such an extent that they themselves incorporate datebooks into their own daily routines. Then during family "milieu meetings" (described later), all parties can "synchronize their datebooks."

When the patient is at home, the datebook should be kept in a consistent location; each evening, time should be allocated to plan for the following day, including last-minute plans or new phone calls. Outside the home, the datebook should accompany the individual at all times. Expected datebook use skills include the following:

1. Initiating notes in the appropriate locations without external cueing (e.g., therapy schedule, doctors' appointments, work meetings, school schedule, and personal events and commitments).
2. Keeping information organized and the datebook tidy (e.g., no loose papers or papers stuffed into the front and back pockets of the datebook).
3. Spontaneously asking for clarification of instructions, as well as spontaneously opening the datebook at regular times throughout the day to take and review notes.
4. Demonstrating advanced planning skills and accepting 100% accountability for consistent and competent usage.
5. Obtaining at least four consecutive weekly datebook scores of >90% (described later).

1. Your therapy will help you become aware and acceptant of the benefits of a datebook to compensate for your memory difficulties. If you do not feel you need a datebook, you will not have the motivation necessary to use your datebook effectively and consistently. Consider it your "new best buddy."

2. Using the datebook successfully takes a lot of practice and commitment. It does not happen overnight. Remember, "Things take time."

3. Carry your datebook with you *at all times*. You never know when you will be asked to do something or need to write something down.

4. Put *important* information in your datebook (emergency contact information, doctors' phone numbers, etc.).

5. Log all memory assignments under the "Prioritized Daily Task List"; use the "Daily Notes" page for extra details. Make sure all notes are legible, complete, and organized. Follow the format of: "Who, What, When, Where." Place a highlighted number beside each memory assignment, and also at the designated time of day on the "Appointment Schedule."

6. Get into the habit of writing things in your datebook you want to remember. Write things down *as soon as you think of them*—in therapy, at home, and in the community.

7. Include personal events in your datebook, such as birthdays, anniversaries, graduations, summer trips, sporting events, and medical appointments. The more you personalize your book, the more you will use it!

8. Write all *standing memory assignments* in your datebook for a few weeks at a time. These can include reminders to call in prescriptions, take medication, go to exercise classes, or do other things you do routinely.

9. Even if you think you will remember, look at your datebook *regularly*! This includes first thing in the morning, before every therapy session, at lunch, before you leave a setting, when you get home, and at night in preparation for the next day. Make it a *habit*. Do not ignore your datebook at night or on the weekends.

10. If you have trouble checking the datebook, consider obtaining a watch alarm (e.g., a DataLink watch). Ask your therapists for suggestions about the best system for you.

11. Plan ahead, so that you will be more prepared and less stressed. Do you have an assignment/ project/paper due next week? Next month? Is tax time coming? Is your holiday shopping completed? Make sure to put a planning entry into your datebook to remind you to complete a task *before* it is due. The planning entry should specify *what* the task is, *when* it is due, *where* the task is due, and to *whom*.

12. Check off each memory assignment as soon as it is done. This helps you keep track of your accomplishments. If an item is not completed on a particular day, move it forward to a day and time when you can finish it.

*Examples of good datebook entries*

| September 12 | 9:50 A.M. | Turn in my journal to my therapist. |
| November 8 | 6:00 P.M. | Share my datebook score for the week with my family. |
| October 3 | 8:15 A.M. | Pick up my new HIC. |
| December 1 | 3:30 P.M. | After therapy, shop for, purchase, and wrap Mom's Christmas gift. |

*"The palest ink is better than the strongest memory."*—Ancient Chinese proverb

**FIGURE 6.2.** Datebook strategies.

The datebook represents a rich source of psychotherapeutic material, especially in the domains of awareness, acceptance, and realism (Phases 4–6 of the PEM). For example, to assess the patient's level of awareness of memory and executive function deficits, the psychotherapist can appraise the patient's perception of the purpose and need for the datebook system in the context of his or her injury-related deficits. In general, the size of the datebook corresponds to the severity of the memory/executive function deficits; therefore, even the size of the datebook the patient initially chooses is symbolic of his or her level of awareness. Patients often state that they will remember pertinent information and so do not need to use a datebook and/or take detailed notes. Alternatively, they may be convinced that the only way to remedy memory problems is to exercise their memories by trying to memorize information; compensation may be seen as a "crutch." Creating daily and weekly assignments, and then monitoring each patient's level of follow-through, will emphasize the relevance of the datebook system and enhance the awareness process. One useful technique is for the psychotherapist to furnish a number of memory assignments, and in subsequent sessions calculate the percentage of their completion with the support of the datebook (i.e., a datebook score between 0% and 100%). Such assignments can include instructing the patient to telephone the office at designated times to leave a message, bring in mementos from home, keep a daily journal, or complete other homework assignments. This data-driven approach facilitates the education process and allows patients to observe measurable progress.

The psychotherapist should also monitor the overall organization and tidiness of the datebook. One effective (and fun) technique is the "datebook shakedown," in which the patient turns the datebook upside down and shakes it, in order to demonstrate that no loose papers are hidden between pages. The psychotherapist can also help a disorganized patient "thin" the datebook when extraneous paperwork is housed unnecessarily.

Patients' willingness to incorporate the datebook into their daily routine is a hallmark of the acceptance process after acquired brain injury. Patients' attitudes about the datebook reflect either adaptive coping (the PEM "green" zone) or resistance behaviors (the PEM "yellow" warning zone). Some patients understand and can verbalize the value of the system on the intellectual level, but may reject it on a deeper emotional level. For these patients, the datebook may be a painful external stigma of their brain injury. Several approaches can increase such patients' acceptance of this tool. Describing the frequency of datebook use by "everyday people" with busy and productive lives will help normalize it. The psychotherapist's encouragement and reminders of the importance of the "two P's"—patience and practice—will also help patients appreciate that the datebook is the best way to ameliorate the feelings of frustration, embarrassment, and discouragement often associated with memory failures. Ideally, datebook use creates a positive feedback loop: The patient experiences feelings of mastery and emotional well-being, which further promote embracement of this compensation. Peer support and mentoring relationships with other patients who adeptly use a datebook system, and who excel in various community settings, will also reinforce a positive impression of the datebook.

In sum, the datebook provides the necessary structure to ensure the proper planning of daily activities, and thus to assist with prospective memory (Fluharty & Priddy, 1993). The datebook process provides patients with a sense of purpose, sharpens their focus, and serves as a "game plan" for improving and sustaining their overall level of productivity. The psychotherapist's role in emphasizing the consistent use of the datebook system is key to helping patients reach higher levels of efficiency and reliability, which result in greater confidence and self-efficacy in the home and community (including social life, work, and school). When date-books are employed effectively, patients become participatory and complementary members of their families, their social networks, and the community at large.

## CASE STUDY

Jessica was age 24 when she began individual psychotherapy. She had sustained a very severe traumatic brain injury 10 years previously, at age 14, as a back-seat passenger in a car. Her brother, who was driving, was killed instantly. Jessica was thrown from the vehicle and suffered severe bilateral brain contusions in the frontal and temporal lobes, with subsequent bilateral subdural hygromas. She was comatose for 20 days and was discharged home to the care of her parents 2 months later. At that time there were minimal outpatient therapies available, and Jessica received a few months of physical therapy. She remained at home, and her parents provided as much tutoring and retraining as possible, helping her eventually to graduate from high school through special education classes. They even "job-shadowed" her so that she could maintain minimum-wage positions. Eventually, Jessica was referred by her neurologist for psychotherapy, as her aging parents were in failing health and beginning to find the totality of her care overtaxing.

Jessica came to her initial appointment with a small notebook filled with heaps of loose papers. Notes were taken sporadically and erratically in the book, without corresponding dates. Jessica stated that she had used the notebook for several years and clutched it as if it were a transitional object. The psychotherapist made a mental note of the chaotic condition of the book, and was resolute about addressing this issue in upcoming sessions, once a preliminary working alliance was established.

A neuropsychological examination was performed at the same time that the individual psychotherapy sessions began. Results revealed relative strengths in the areas of basic attention, speed of thinking, academic skills (reading, writing, and spelling), and motor dexterity. Jessica demonstrated severe short-term memory impairments in the verbal and visual domains, including verbal encoding deficits and confabulation. She also demonstrated mild to moderate executive system dysfunction, including higher-level planning and decision making, mental flexibility, and multitasking. Personality testing and clinical observation suggested that Jessica was very depressed about her limitations, especially her memory and the consequent need to rely on her parents for constant cueing and reminders. She appreciated their level of dedication to her; on the other hand, she was acutely aware that as a young adult, she was deprived of the freedoms and age-appropriate responsibilities she felt entitled to. Her confidence was very poor, and she was continually second-guessing herself about what she had or had not said or done. Her tendency to confabulate added to the confusion; she and her parents were often baffled and detoured by her erroneous recollections.

Jessica had a rudimentary understanding of her memory difficulties, but she significantly underestimated their severity and impact on daily functioning. Several approaches were taken to improve her awareness and acceptance of her current neurological status, as well as the potential advantages of compensatory strategies. First, the core results of the neuropsychological evaluation were reviewed with her and her parents; the psychotherapist emphasized the nature and extent of the memory problems, in the context of good academic skills. The concept of "confabulation" was introduced to Jessica and her parents, to explain her intrusion errors on verbal memory tests.

It was recommended that Jessica engage in individual psychotherapy twice per week, as well as group psychotherapy and weekly family psychotherapy visits. The dual emphasis was on (1) training her to use the Home Independence Checklist (described later) and a sophisticated datebook system, and (2) addressing her depression and low self-esteem. Initially, Jessica stridently opposed replacing her current notebook with a "new and improved" model (i.e., she was in the "yellow" warning zone of Phase 5 of the PEM). She tried to convince the psychotherapist that she would be unable to transfer to an alternative system because of its unfamiliarity and novelty. She frequently employed "Yeah, but" responses when therapeutically confronted with her avoidance and resistance behaviors. She stated that she had always used her own system, and that others in her environment were content to cue and support her memory. She felt that the bigger, more detailed system was cumbersome and a "hassle." Her psychotherapist explained that not attempting the datebook system was like signing up for swimming lessons, but refusing to get into the pool. This helped Jessica realize that she needed to be flexible and brave about trying this new technique. She agreed to experiment with completing memory assignments with and without the datebook system; this helped to improve her awareness and acceptance of its necessity. At the psychotherapist's urging, Jessica also participated in a conjoint session with another psychotherapy patient who had a similar neuropsychological profile. This patient demonstrated her datebook protocol and explained the virtues of her superior system for enhancing her autonomy and strivings. This made Jessica more enthusiastic about using a similar system.

Group psychotherapy was a potent outlet for Jessica to discuss her underlying feelings of resistance to her datebook. The group sessions included the associated topics of self-perceived emotional and cognitive reasons for not using a datebook (e.g., organic unawareness, denial, divided attention, lack of initiative); the pros and cons of using a datebook; self-evaluation of postinjury listening and note-taking skills; "good" and "bad" datebook habits; the role of planning in datebook utilization; and the emotional challenges posed by the consistent and protracted use of the datebook, including feeling stigmatized. In the context of her therapeutic venting, peer input and reinforcement helped Jessica work through her inner conflicts and struggles.

Over the next several weeks, a gradual transfer to the new datebook system was accomplished. To help reassure Jessica that she would not sacrifice the material in her old notebook, selected meaningful material was rewritten in a specific section of her new book. Colored paper was also used in the new datebook as a visual cue for separate sections (notes for doctor appointments, journal entries, etc.). Jessica was happy with the colorful additions and began to enjoy using the system; her neatness and organizational skills were substantially improved. She was given several datebook assignments per week (e.g., taking notes at doctors' appointments, completing homework, and purchasing a birthday card for her mother). Her realization that she was attaining the necessary skills reinforced the value of the process. As one of these assignments, she and her parents were instructed to watch the movie *50 First Dates* (Ewing & Segal, 2004), as a depiction of the contrast between Jessica's life now that she was using the datebook and the perplexity and mishaps experienced by the main character, who has no organized system to consult. As Jessica made progress, her parents were encouraged to write her a letter as a visual reminder that they were proud of her improvement and her newfound independence.

As depicted in Phase 5 of the PEM, Jessica's datebook mastery was her "dress rehearsal" for her new life. She was now ready for her "second chance," so her psychotherapist helped her pursue part-time work in the community. She was a very sociable young lady who enjoyed interacting with the elderly. Together, the therapist and Jessica found a position for her in a senior care center, reading and engaging in other activities with the inhabitants. She was trained to use her datebook systematically to record the names of her clients, as well as the rules to the games and activities. She also was given a laminated copy of a map with directions to and from work, until she had memorized the route. Eventually, she became the coleader of a calisthenics class. She compiled a list of exercises in her datebook to facilitate this process. Her self-esteem continued to improve, and she expressed a sense of pride and triumph in her enhanced self-reliance and productivity.

One year after starting psychotherapy, Jessica wrote her psychotherapist:

> "I just want to pay recognition to a very special anniversary day—and that's today. It's the 1-year anniversary since I've started coming to see you. I know this because I have it written in my datebook—which is detailed and organized, thanks to you. You've taught me that I'm not the weak child–teenager I used to be, but the strong, independent, confident woman I am today."

Two years after her discharge, Jessica was invited to group psychotherapy, and also began to meet conjointly with "fresh" psychotherapy patients and the psychotherapist. As a mentor, she continues to proclaim the importance and advantages of her refined datebook system. For example, she "loves" the datebook and perpetually carries it with her. She happily depends on it to anchor her time lines both prospectively and retrospectively. In comparison to her early feelings of angst and exasperation, she now feels effective, organized, and independent. She recognizes and appreciates how much this tool has boosted her confidence. She also incorporates new pertinent subsections on an as-needed basis, with the input and assistance of her parents (e.g., updated responsibilities at her work site, relevant checklists and maps, and her current gym exercise program).

## THE HOME INDEPENDENCE CHECKLIST

The Home Independence Checklist (abbreviated in the rest of this chapter as the HIC) is one of the most effective tools for assisting patients in becoming as self-sufficient as possible in the home (Klonoff et al., 2003). The HIC helps a patient organize his or her day, recall specific details for completing home tasks, and remain focused on each activity (Klonoff et al., 2003). As such, it is a vital compensation for deficits in the areas of attention, concentration, memory, executive functions, and sequencing. The HIC also allows measurement of the patient's progression from reliance on others to unsupervised and empowered self-reliance; it thus serves as a concrete representation of the patient's contribution to family life as a "team player."

The psychotherapist should take an instrumental role in establishing the use of the HIC system, especially if he or she cannot collaborate with professionals from other treatment disciplines. However, if collaboration is feasible, it is advisable to enlist an occupational therapist to set up and monitor the use of the HIC. Such a therapist has expertise in translating physical, visuoperceptual, and cognitive deficits into functional implications in the home and community environments (Landa-Gonzalez, 2001). Home visits can then include the psychotherapist on an as-needed basis. These visits can provide real-world observational data that cannot be easily replicated during in-clinic sessions. Participation by family members or other housemates is mandatory, to help all parties develop meaningful parameters.

The rationale and benefits of the HIC must first be discussed in individual psychotherapy sessions to maximize compliance. Benefits include enhancing the patient's feelings of self-efficacy and self-worth, contingent upon improved mastery of personal responsibilities. Given patients' difficulties with executive functions (e.g., abstract reasoning, flexible thinking, seeing the "big picture") and memory, putting the rationale and expectations in writing is advisable. Figure 6.3 is an example of a document explaining the HIC's purpose and procedures.

Next, the psychotherapist (or occupational therapist if one is participating) must identify the household responsibilities to be addressed, based on input from the patient and relevant third parties (family members or roommates). Salient areas include general household chores (e.g., dusting, vacuuming, laundry); medication management; meal planning and preparation; and bill paying. Whenever possible, the patient should select those tasks that produce maximum emotional satisfaction; this will increase the patient's enthusiasm about using the HIC. The checklist is often divided into daily, weekly, and monthly responsibilities, to provide the necessary structure and visual reminders. At first the responsibilities are placed in a grid format, in which the patient must mark off that he or she has completed the tasks. The psychotherapist's mantra "Do it; mark it" reminds the patient to mark off each item on the grid before moving on to the next task. He or she is also cautioned not to "back-check" (i.e., go back later and try to recollect what was accomplished), as this can introduce errors secondary to faulty recollections, and may encourage a nonsystematic or deceptive element.

The HIC should be kept in the front of the patient's datebook, or posted on the refrigerator for easy access and as a visual reminder. As the patient makes

## Purpose

The purpose of this handout is to help you and your support network understand the Home Independence Checklist (HIC). Your HIC is designed to help you compensate for problems in the areas of attention, memory, sequencing, and executive functions (such as initiation, planning, and problem solving). The goal is for you to be able to perform your daily tasks consistently and successfully. Your HIC will also help you adhere to your daily schedule, which will provide you with the necessary structure to achieve a successful daily routine. This promotes improved self-reliance, self-esteem, and productivity at home.

Use your HIC as a compensatory memory strategy to help you stay focused on the task at hand, to organize your day, and to become self-sufficient with daily home management skills such as these:

- General household management (making your bed, sweeping, mopping the floors, doing laundry, etc.)
- Medication management
- Meal planning and preparation
- Completing homework
- Bill paying
- Leisure activities
- Home exercise program/gym exercises

## Procedures

Together, your therapist, you, and relevant family member(s)/other person(s) will develop a list of activities that reflect your current skill level and responsibilities in the home. As you begin to use your HIC, verbal cues or reminders from a family member or significant other are generally required and are encouraged. This allows you to learn to use your HIC, following the proper protocol for "errorless learning." However, there is a fine line between the other person's cueing you to refer to your HIC and telling you what task to perform. The other person's role is to "cue, not do." Verbal cues and reminders will slowly diminish as your use of the HIC becomes routine and consistent. Your therapist will work directly with you and your family regarding how and when to provide verbal cues. Keep in mind that the tasks should be completed efficiently and accurately. You need to adopt the "Do it; mark it" approach, in which you check off each step immediately after its completion before going on to the next step. You should not "back-check" the list; that is, you should not go back to mark a task as done when it was not completed. Similarly, you should not check off a task before the task is completed. Remember, the ultimate goal is for you to regain as much independence as possible.

Your HIC is to be completed *daily*, 7 days per week. After each task is completed, your family member or significant other may be asked to "sign off" on the task, noting whether it was done accurately and on time. All parties will decide in the therapy sessions whether and, if so, when your family member/significant other should sign your HIC. You will hand in your completed HIC at each appointment, and it will be scored by your therapist. You will receive a weekly percentage score, indicating the proportion of tasks you have performed successfully. Credit will not be given if a task is checked off that has not been done, or if the task was not done on the designated day or time. The goal is for you to achieve 90–100% on your HIC each week. With time and practice, your progress on your HIC will lead to enhanced responsibilities and a sense of mastery.

**FIGURE 6.3.** Home Independence Checklist (HIC) description and protocol.

---

progress and the completion of tasks becomes automatic, the patient can make the transition to a list of chores on his or her "today ruler" in the datebook, or can even perform the tasks solely from memory.

The HIC is also an effective tool for structuring, and reminding the patient to complete other daily and weekly responsibilities to enhance his or her neurological recovery and quality of life. Examples include an exercise schedule (both home exercise programs and gym visits) and a food log (for a patient working on nutrition and weight management). Food documentation is particularly helpful for the patient's physician and/or a treating dietician. The patient can also log his or her bedtime, which is beneficial to review as part of psychotherapy sessions, to be sure the patient is sufficiently rested and is not experiencing sleep problems; such problems may be symptomatic of other concerns (e.g., poor time management, depression, or anxiety). Figure 6.4 is a sample HIC.

The psychotherapist needs to monitor how successfully the patient is able to use the HIC in the home. The percentage of properly completed tasks should be calculated and discussed with the patient (and significant others) as part of each psychotherapy session, to facilitate follow-through and accountability. Target scores based on the concept of "errorless learning" (Martelli et al., 2008; Mateer, 2005; Sohlberg & Mateer, 2001; Wilson, Baddeley, Evans, & Shiel, 1994; Wilson & Kapur, 2008), should be agreed upon, and the patient should be properly instructed about the expectations for task completion and recording protocols in a step-by-step manner that ensures success. For example, initially the patient may be expected to complete 70% of tasks successfully, with the expectation that over a 4- to 6-week period the target score will become 90+%. This provides explicit clarification of the expectations. Consistent and successful completion of the HIC is one form of tangible and affirmative evidence to the patient (and family) that he or she is competent to be left unsupervised in the home.

## IMPLEMENTATION CHALLENGES WITH THE HIC

### Cognitive and Physical Factors

Frequently there are challenges and periodic failures during the implementation process of the HIC. The psychotherapist must then investigate where and why there was a breakdown. First and foremost, the HIC format and protocol must be commensurate with the patient's skills and goals. A common cause of malfunctions is an HIC that is too lengthy or complex; a patient may become overly exhausted, confused, or forgetful when attempting to complete such a checklist. Other frequent causes of problems include decreased initiative or poor visual scanning (in reading the specific items). Once the psychotherapist ascertains the underlying cause for the problems with the HIC, he or she can rectify the situation by adapting the format, length, or demands of the process. Adaptations can include using picture icons instead of written instructions for an aphasic patient, or incorporating items that are within a patient's cognitive and physical capabilities (e.g., short and precise wording; no chores that would endanger a patient with hemiparesis and/or balance difficulties).

Patient _____

Week _____

Date _____

| MORNING TASKS | MON | TUE | WED | THU | FRI | SAT | SUN |
|---|---|---|---|---|---|---|---|
| 1. Breakfast/cleanup | ___ | ___ | ___ | ___ | ___ | ___ | ___ |
| 2. Review datebook | ___ | ___ | ___ | ___ | ___ | ___ | ___ |
| 3. Take meds | ___ | ___ | ___ | ___ | ___ | ___ | ___ |
| **AFTERNOON TASKS** | | | | | | | |
| 4. Review datebook | ___ | ___ | ___ | ___ | ___ | ___ | ___ |
| **EVENING TASKS** | | | | | | | |
| 5. Help prepare dinner 3×/week | ___ | ___ | ___ | ___ | ___ | ___ | ___ |
| 6. Assist with dinner cleanup daily | ___ | ___ | ___ | ___ | ___ | ___ | ___ |
| 7. Review datebook | ___ | ___ | ___ | ___ | ___ | ___ | ___ |
| 8. Complete homework assignments | ___ | ___ | ___ | ___ | ___ | ___ | ___ |
| 9. Physical therapy stretches/ exercise of the day | ___ | ___ | ___ | ___ | ___ | ___ | ___ |
| 10. Take evening medication | ___ | ___ | ___ | ___ | ___ | ___ | ___ |
| 11. Record bedtime | ___ | ___ | ___ | ___ | ___ | ___ | ___ |
| **WEEKLY TASKS** | ___ | ___ | ___ | ___ | ___ | ___ | ___ |
| 12. Clean room 1×/week | ___ | ___ | ___ | ___ | ___ | ___ | ___ |
| 13. Clean bathroom 1×/week | ___ | ___ | ___ | ___ | ___ | ___ | ___ |
| 14. Do laundry 1×/week | ___ | ___ | ___ | ___ | ___ | ___ | ___ |
| 15. Fill your pillbox 1×/week | ___ | ___ | ___ | ___ | ___ | ___ | ___ |
| 16. Load/unload dishwasher 3×/week | ___ | ___ | ___ | ___ | ___ | ___ | ___ |
| 17. Go to the gym 3×/week | ___ | ___ | ___ | ___ | ___ | ___ | ___ |
| 18. Plan and prepare two meals independently over the weekend | ___ | ___ | ___ | ___ | ___ | ___ | ___ |

_____     _____
Patient's signature                          Family member's/significant other's signature

**FIGURE 6.4.** Sample Home Independence Checklist (HIC).

### CASE STUDY

Laila initiated individual psychotherapy at age 25; she had sustained a severe traumatic brain injury as a result of a motor vehicle accident at age 17. Her initial CT scan indicated bilateral temporal lobe contusions and shearing injury in the frontal lobes. The neuropsychological and language deficits resulting from her injury included severe memory problems, slowed speed of information processing, problems in executive functions (including decision making, self-monitoring, and multitasking), and moderate to severe aphasia (including difficulties with both verbal expression and reading skills).

Initially, Laila was provided an HIC with assigned tasks in prose form. However, secondary to her aphasia, she became confused and overwhelmed when attempting to read the HIC. Her mother, with whom she lived, had to read each item to her in order for Laila to understand the instructions. This was very time-consuming and only served to increase Laila's dependency on her mother, defeating the purpose of the HIC. Therefore, in therapy, the HIC was simplified by replacing the prose with picture icons (e.g., a broom to signify sweeping). Laila's level of emotional distress rapidly lessened, and she enjoyed success in independently consulting her checklist.

## Attitudinal Factors

Other barriers to successful HIC use include attitudinal factors, such as lack of motivation to complete chores and home activities. Reasons for this include gender bias, such as when male patients with traditional values do not want to assume a "homemaker" role. Patients who have never been accountable for household chores may also resist using the HIC. Effective psychotherapeutic techniques include educating patients about the impact of their deficits on family members, as well as the importance of give and take in significant relationships. This is especially important for patients with executive function deficits, who may react with a more self-centered attitude, and who often have difficulties with cognitive rigidity and seeing the "big picture." Discussing the concept that "The volume is turned up" (see Chapter 3) on preexisting characterological tendencies (e.g., dependency) can also help a patient with his or her maturational process. Incorporation of symbolic and personalized mottos and mantras may likewise help the patient refocus his or her energies on collaboration with his or her loved ones.

### CASE STUDY

Zachary was a 54-year-old married man who suffered a subarachnoid hemorrhage and right internal carotid artery aneurysm clipping. Postsurgery complications included a stroke with vasospasms and hydrocephalus, for which he underwent insertion of a ventriculoperitoneal shunt. Zachary began individual psychotherapy and marital counseling 6 months after his stroke. Among the initially identified concerns were decreased initiation and follow-through with household tasks. This was most obvious and troubling to his wife, Hazel, who was weary and beleaguered with the expansion of her household responsibilities. Because of her husband's dependent status and her precipitously augmented household responsibilities, she had had to quit her job in order to provide round-the-clock supervision for her husband.

Before his neurological insult, Zachary had shared in limited household chores, primarily confined to outdoor responsibilities (e.g., yardwork and pool maintenance) and bill paying. However, Zachary's postsurgery motor apraxia, left-sided weakness, and problems with balance, endurance, and heat sensitivity prevented him from doing demanding outdoor physical chores. He was also unable to manage bill paying or other more complex financial tasks, secondary to problems with memory, visual scanning, and mathematical calculations.

Initially, Zachary was totally opposed to increasing his contributions to indoor chores, stating that these were Hazel's responsibilities. He maintained traditional beliefs about role definitions within the marriage, and he felt demeaned by and irritated about doing what he referred to as "menial" household tasks (e.g., folding laundry, dusting).

Individual psychotherapy and conjoint sessions were devoted to helping Zachary make the necessary cognitive shift to acknowledge that in the "big picture" it was critical for him to establish a more equitable relationship with his wife and reduce her daily burdens. As a roadmap of the process, the psychotherapist discussed adaptive versus problematic coping and behaviors, using the PEM to guide the discussion. Several other techniques were employed to help Zachary accept redefining his role in the household. Before his injury, he had been a personnel director for a large corporation. As part of his work vernacular, Zachary was very fond of catch phrases, many of which he had used to motivate employees. These included "Every adversity has a seed of greater benefit;" "Repetition makes perfection," "Use it or lose it," and "Lend a hand; lift a heart." Zachary was also very enthusiastic about *Napoleon Hill's Keys to Success* (Hill, 1994) and had used them in training seminars. His psychotherapist adapted several of these principles to his situation at home, including "definiteness of purpose," "going the extra mile," "personal initiative," "self-discipline," and "teamwork." These mantras helped remind Zachary of his behavioral impact on his wife.

Because Zachary had retained a strong sense of humor, he and Hazel were asked to watch the movie *Failure to Launch* (Rudin & Dey, 2006) as a light-hearted illustration of the detrimental impact of overdependency on others. Zachary found this film highly entertaining. After answering the probing questions in Figure 6.5, he could more clearly perceive the importance of self-sufficiency in nurturing meaningful relationships. This represented a turning point in his psychotherapy, and Zachary agreed to follow an HIC and perform several indoor household chores. With psychoeducation, time, and practice, he came to appreciate that these tasks were improving his motor apraxia, left-sided motor weakness, and physical endurance, as well as enhancing the quality of his marital relationship.

Zachary's testimonials in group psychotherapy reinforced the importance of the HIC. Other patients also described how they regained control over their daily routines; they noticed that family members ascribed more authority and credibility to them as a result.

(Short answers: 2–3 sentences for each question.)

1. Did you like the movie? Yes _____ No _____ Why or why not?

2. What do these statements mean?

   a. (Question:) You live with your parents?
      (Answer:) Is that a problem?

   b. Walking your path vs. sitting on a rock near the path.

   c. Goal: Happy and perfectly functional.

3. What is the theme or message of the movie?

4. How was the family affected by the son's choices?

5. How does this message relate to your psychotherapy and recovery?

**FIGURE 6.5.** Psychotherapy questions for *Failure to Launch.*

## *Other Psychological Factors*

Psychological factors other than attitude can interfere with patients' use of the HIC. These include depression (manifested as low energy and/or inertia), as well as catastrophic reactions when the patient observes that a household task is much more taxing than it was before brain injury. In the latter case, patients may withdraw from the process or make self-deprecating comments about the quality of their efforts. In these circumstances, the psychotherapist should emphasize that use of the HIC leads to self-empowerment and self-reliance. Starting with a few meaningful components on the HIC, and then adding items as a patient experiences success, helps to ameliorate feelings of helplessness and discouragement. Helpful supplements to enhance open-mindedness include the mantras "Try it, you'll like it," or "I think I can, I think I can" from *The Little Engine That Could* (Piper, 1986). The psychotherapist's anecdotes about past patients' achievements, or conjoint sessions with, more seasoned patients who have profited from the HIC can inspire novice patients to take action.

### CASE STUDY

Anita was age 42 when she suffered a massive right intraparenchymal hemorrhage in the right parietotemporal area. She underwent an emergency right frontoparietal temporal craniotomy for evacuation of the hemorrhage. After her stroke, Anita suffered from left-sided hemiparalysis and a left homonymous hemianopsia. Anita began individual psychotherapy at 4 months poststroke. Her goal was to improve her level of independent functioning, so as to be able to move from a group home to living with her sister in an apartment.

Before the stroke, Anita was very athletic and prided herself on her physical agility and prowess. She had engaged in "extreme" sports and traveled widely around the world. Anita was understandably very depressed and disheartened at first about her poststroke physical limitations. Every activity she attempted took extensive time and seemingly infinite patience. Her rate of progress felt impossibly slow, and the goal of self-sufficiency in an apartment seemed untenable; she would often cry during psychotherapy sessions and felt hopeless about her potential to advance. The HIC became a powerful therapeutic tool, as it gave tangible evidence of weekly changes and growth. To counteract her catastrophic reactions, the psychotherapist at first devised an HIC with only a few items pertaining to basic self-care. As Anita mastered these, other items were gradually added. However, the psychotherapist was mindful about the pace and the rate of expansion, as well as the complexity of tasks.

Her psychotherapist also encouraged Anita's regular weekend visits to her sister's apartment. Conjoint sessions were conducted to educate and support Anita and her sister in their venture. Anita's preinjury tenacity and adventurous spirit enabled her to embrace and use helpful coping techniques; the success of these enhanced her emotional resiliency and made her much more hopeful about conquering her infirmities. Group psychotherapy was a helpful adjunct to the individual and conjoint psychotherapy sessions: Anita and other patients participated in a layered goal-setting exercise, identifying their current barriers to independence and their perceived time frames for goal attainment. All of these interventions bolstered Anita's confidence, and within 6 months she was living amicably with her sister.

### Role of the Family/Support Network

A third party will usually need to judiciously oversee the patient's completion of the HIC. This involves taking time to observe, monitor, and (when necessary) intervene on behalf of the patient. As patients progress toward more independent functioning in the home, some significant others will require assistance in being less overprotective and "letting go." Reminding significant others to "cue, not do" is an important mantra; the concept that they are on "standby" to remind the patient to use the HIC in a systematic manner is also helpful.

Alternatively, some significant others may overestimate patients' ability to initiate tasks, problem solve, or remember to complete the HIC, and so may adopt a detached, distracted, or peripheral role. They can then become irritated or disappointed when the process fails in the home. In these cases, the psychotherapist needs to ascertain the practical and psychological barriers to successful completion and prescribe beneficial compensations. This may involve helping the patients' loved ones muster the necessary physical and psychological energies to assume the appropriate monitoring and cueing role for the patients' implementation of the HIC. Figure 6.6 is a Significant Others' Checklist, which articulates how and when family and friends should be assisting their loved one.

### CASE STUDY

Zachary's wife, Hazel, had considerable initial difficulty in assisting and cueing her husband when he was using the HIC. She had a tendency to be very distracted and would try to multitask (e.g., to work on the computer in a different room and casually remind him of activities from a distance). Hazel also tended to query Zachary about the HIC, rather than take the time to provide standby assistance, which he needed during early phases of the implementation process. She would then become very dejected and exasperated with him when he omitted or overlooked his responsibilities.

Several separate individual psychotherapy sessions were conducted with Hazel. In them, she was able to articulate and share her feelings of loss over her husband's decreased capabilities. With guidance, she began to realize that her behaviors were steeped in avoidance, and thus were hindering Zachary's progress. Through exploration of her grieving process in psychotherapy, Hazel eventually realized that her own emotional adjustment to his circumstances was a critical precursor for optimally assisting him in his recovery and rehabilitation. She was then able to adjust and contribute to her husband's use of the HIC.

The case of Zachary and Hazel demonstrates how individual psychotherapy sessions, as well as conjoint meetings with the patient and significant other(s), provide vital psychoeducation and emotional support regarding the value and application of the personalized HIC. This maximizes the overall harmony in the home.

| | Spouse | Teenage Children | Mother/ Father | Adult Sister/ Brother | Extended Family | Friend | House-mate |
|---|---|---|---|---|---|---|---|
| Remind _____ to use his/her datebook in the A.M. and P.M. | | | | | | | |
| If you ask _____ to do or remember something, please make sure he/she has written it down immediately in his/her datebook. Ask _____ to read it back to you to make sure he/she has all of the correct information. | | | | | | | |
| Cue _____ to record in the datebook *what* he/she does each day and his/her thoughts and feelings. | | | | | | | |
| Cue _____ to always take notes in the datebook during doctors' appointments, volunteer work, and meetings. | | | | | | | |
| Cue _____ to review any notes he/she wrote (e.g., a note about a change in his/her work schedule). | | | | | | | |
| Cue _____ to schedule his/her weekly chores in the datebook. | | | | | | | |
| Cue _____ to fill his/her pillbox on Sunday; assist with refills. | | | | | | | |
| Cue _____ as he/she does housecleaning if he/she appears to be getting "stuck" in the middle of a task. | | | | | | | |
| Cue and assist _____ with his/her scrapbooking activities. | | | | | | | |
| Assist _____ as he/she completes three exercises/day at least 3 times a week. | | | | | | | |
| Encourage _____ to walk 3+ times a week with someone. | | | | | | | |
| Cue _____ to regularly schedule rides for volunteer and leisure activities. | | | | | | | |
| Assist in making sure _____ obtains a monthly transit pass. | | | | | | | |

The goal is to *cue* _____ to do the tasks. Please don't *do* them for him/her. Thanks.

**FIGURE 6.6.** Significant Others' Checklist.

## "MILIEU MEETINGS" FOR THE HOUSEHOLD

Regular "milieu meetings" with family members or housemates constitute an ideal method for delineating and coordinating personal and shared responsibilities within the household. These meetings should be scheduled once or twice weekly, and a procedural checklist can be used to make sure the salient topics and concerns are addressed. The therapist should educate the patient and family about the protocol and merits of these meetings, and should also include some "mock" meetings as part of psychotherapy sessions. It is imperative that the patient take notes in his or her datebook during the meetings, to provide a permanent record and visual prompts for follow-up. Among the common pitfalls are that family members may not monitor closely enough what and where their loved one is writing in the datebook, or may not allow enough time for him or her to complete the entries before progressing to the next agenda item.

Figure 6.7 is a sample procedural checklist for the "milieu meeting" agenda. The agenda can be logged into the patient's datebook as a recurring entry; alternatively, a separate form with listed topics can be photocopied and inserted at specified time intervals directly into the datebook. It is often helpful to include a space on the agenda where topics for upcoming psychotherapy sessions can be suggested and recorded. This is helpful when an impasse occurs or when tensions escalate. This enlightens the psychotherapist about real-life failures in communication and/or practical problem solving. Family members are encouraged to use their own datebooks or PDA systems to help coordinate schedules and address mutual priorities. The success of the "milieu meetings" is contingent on full commitment and regular attendance by all relevant parties; preparation on the part of family members and the patient regarding pertinent issues; and uninterrupted focus and constructive contributions during the process. Setting realistic and consistent meeting days and times is also crucial for maximum follow-through.

## DRIVING

The ability to drive after brain injury is pivotal to reclaiming independence and self-reliance. Multiple brain regions have been identified as underlying various aspects of driving behavior, including the premotor, orbitofrontal, parietal, lateral occipital, insular, subcortical, and cerebellar regions (Spiers & Maguire, 2007; see Tamietto et al., 2006, for a review). Research studies indicate that postinjury deficits in visuoperceptual/visuospatial abilities, visual memory, working memory, motor skills, sustained and divided attention, speed of information processing, and executive functions (e.g., multitasking, impulse control, planning, problem solving, and route finding) can hinder driving or preclude it altogether (Brouwer, Withaar, Tant, & van Zomeren, 2002; Lundqvist, Alinder, & Rönnberg, 2008; Mazaux et al., 1997; Novack, Alderson, Bush, Meythaler, & Canupp, 2000; Sundet, Goffeng, & Hofft, 1995; Tamietto et al., 2006; see Brenner, Homaifar, & Schultheis, 2008, for a review). Awareness of impairments and self-regulation have also been identified as indicators of success in a postinjury return to driving (Lundqvist &

1. **What phone calls need to be made this week?**
   (Examples: calls to schedule appointments, obtain medication refills, conduct household or school-related business, etc.)
   If none, check here: _____

   a. _____
      Document in datebook when call is to be made.

   b. _____
      Document in datebook when call is to be made.

2. **What specific household tasks need to be done?**
   a. _____
      Document in datebook when task is to be done.

   b. _____
      Document in datebook when task is to be done.

3. **Meal planning**
   a. _____
      Document in datebook when meal is to be prepared.

   b. _____
      Document in datebook what meal is to be prepared.

   c. _____
      Add missing ingredients to the shopping list.

4. **Social events planned for the week:**
   a. _____
      Document in datebook when this event will take place.

   b. _____
      Document in datebook when this event will take place.

5. **Finances:** Give an update on checking and savings account balances. Discuss any outstanding bills.

6. **School:** Discuss school schedule, assignments, tests, and supplies to be purchased.

7. **Topics for next psychotherapy appointment:**
   a. _____
      Document in datebook.

   b. _____
      Document in datebook.

8. **Transfer appointments from "Month at a Glance" onto daily pages.**

**FIGURE 6.7.** Sample "milieu meeting" agenda.

Alinder, 2007; Schanke & Sundet, 2000). Patients' overall neurological status (e.g., seizure status) must be taken into account as well. In addition, patients' preinjury driving record relates to their postinjury driving performance (Klonoff et al., 2006). The personality trait of conscientiousness has been identified as a predictor of driving style and rate of car accidents (Tamietto et al., 2006); this trait is sometimes preserved after injury. Figure 6.8 lists fundamental physical, visual/visuoperceptual, cognitive, and emotional/behavioral components to be evaluated for postinjury driving capacity.

Despite the research cited above, there is no consensus about the predictors of successful postinjury driving (Galski, Ehle, McDonald, & Mackevich, 2000). Therefore, the psychotherapist faces multiple ethical and pragmatic challenges when formulating a clinical judgment about a patient's potential to drive. States vary in their requirements for a return to driving after acquired brain injury. It is the psychotherapist's professional responsibility to know the state's regulations and to share this information with the patient and family (and, if necessary, other medical professionals when they are unaware of the provisions).

In my experience, one of the biggest psychological "blind spots" for patients is underestimating the impact of their neurological sequelae on driving capacity, due to organic unawareness. This is especially the case when patients have sustained visual field impairment or other significant visuoperceptual deficits (e.g., visual neglect). Reviewing the germane skill domains in Figure 6.8 with the patient is an effective psychoeducational and awareness tool for stimulating dialogue. The patient's identification of his or her relative strengths and difficulties should be compared to data and observations derived from testing and therapeutic interventions. Cognitive therapy in the form of computerized driving programs (e.g., Driver-ZED) can also bolster the psychotherapist's impartial and informed recommendations, by providing a concrete demonstration to patients of their strengths and shortfalls for driving.

Whenever possible, an adaptive driving evaluation by professionals trained to assess driving potential after acquired brain injury should be pursued (Schultheis, Matheis, Nead, & DeLuca, 2002). It evaluates the patient's neurological status, practical knowledge, and operational abilities. This provides objective feedback to the patient and assists in the decision making about the patient's readiness to drive. The psychotherapist also often serves as the liaison among the rehabilitation doctor or the releasing physician, the patient and family, external evaluator, and the state department of motor vehicles, especially when obstacles or delays impede the process. Helping to translate and streamline the myriad steps required to return to driving can reinforce the working alliance between the patient and psychotherapist.

## CASE STUDY

Jeremy was a 40-year-old married man who, at age 32, had sustained a severe traumatic brain injury as a result of a motor vehicle accident. He suffered multiple open skull fractures and facial lacerations, and a CT scan demonstrated left parietal and bifrontal subarachnoid hemorrhages. His admitting Glasgow Coma Scale score was 8.

## Physical Components

- Motor abilities and reflexes in arms and legs
- Neck range of motion
- Vestibular skills
- Sitting balance and head control
- Sensation of movement and touch
- Eye–hand/eye–foot coordination
- Physical reaction time
- Endurance
- Hearing

## Visual/Visuoperceptual Components

- Acuity
- Double vision
- Depth perception
- Visual field impairment
- Visual neglect
- Night vision
- Visual processing and scanning
- Figure–ground perception
- Visual closure
- Visual memory
- Visual discrimination
- Visuospatial abilities

## Cognitive Components

- Sustained and divided attention and concentration
- Distractibility
- Mental fatigue
- Speed of thinking
- Auditory processing
- Short-term memory
- Problem solving/decision making
- Planning
- Route finding and topographical abilities
- Multitasking
- Judgment

## Emotional Components

- Frustration tolerance
- Irritability
- Impulse control
- Preinjury personality (e.g., conscientiousness)

**FIGURE 6.8.** Factors to assess for driving after brain injury.

After his accident, Jeremy participated in traditional rehabilitation therapies for approximately 2 years. He progressed to volunteering in an elementary school and drove for 4 years. He stopped driving after a neuropsychological examination determined that he was too cognitively impaired (although he had no history of accidents). Jeremy relocated to another state and was referred for individual psychotherapy by his rehabilitation doctor, secondary to severe depression, poor parenting skills, family tensions, and lack of a productive lifestyle.

Jeremy began psychotherapy 8 years after his injury. At the outset, the psychotherapist performed repeat neuropsychological testing; this revealed moderate deficits in speed of information processing, attention and concentration, verbal learning and recall (with confabulation), visual memory, and visuospatial skills. He showed moderate to severe deficits in his executive functions and nondominant simple motor speed. His mood was characterized by significant depression and anxiety. He was considerably dependent on family members. An associated occupational therapy assessment revealed moderate deficits in visuoperceptual skills and bilateral fine motor coordination. A physical therapy assessment revealed minimal deficits in lower-extremity strength, and mild to moderate deficits in his lower-extremity range of motion and stamina.

A major goal of individual psychotherapy was to reduce Jeremy's level of overreliance on family members, especially his wife. This had contributed to considerable burnout on their part, and had fostered a cycle of withdrawal and low self-esteem in Jeremy. He also felt bereft about having lost his driving privileges, and identified the resumption of driving as a top priority of his therapy. The psychotherapist undertook to advocate for Jeremy and coordinated with his occupational and physical therapists to further remediate his physical and visuoperceptual deficits. His occupational therapist conducted biweekly computer sessions with the simulated driving program (Driver-ZED), and helped Jeremy move successfully through the various levels of complexity. His psychotherapist also initiated applicable cognitive retraining activities as part of the treatment regimen, to instruct Jeremy in meaningful compensations that would generalize to driving skills. Examples included "keep the pace" and using his nondominant hand more readily in bimanual tasks. His psychotherapist also consulted his rehabilitation doctor about starting Jeremy on medications to increase his alertness and concentration, as well as an antidepressant to ameliorate his psychomotor retardation and diminished mental energy.

In group psychotherapy, various driving-related topics were addressed. These included exploration of the group's emotional reactions to the postinjury loss of driving privileges; existential and practical reasons for desiring a return to driving; the underlying skill sets (using Figure 6.8), including ratings of the patients' perceived deficit size (0 = none, 10 = severe); associated therapeutic interventions; the purpose, benefits, and components of the adaptive driving evaluation; and postinjury compensations to reduce accidents. Jeremy also utilized peer input and support to discuss his frustrations with his personal predicament of having lost his driving privileges after driving for several postaccident years. Part of the group discussion focused on "social consciousness," or the importance of personal and public safety behind the wheel. The encouragement from the other patients, who had successfully returned to driving after brain injury by taking incremental steps, inspired Jeremy to persevere with the process. The group also heard testimony from a patient visitor with cognitive deficits similar to Jeremy's. After failing the adaptive driving evaluation during the acute phase of recovery, this patient had been able to pass it 2.5 years later. This highlighted the importance of a persistent and hopeful attitude.

After 5 months and sufficient progress in Jeremy's psychotherapy and adjunct therapies, his psychotherapist helped coordinate an external adaptive driving test. Jeremy passed this examination and gleefully resumed driving on a gradual basis, first locally and then for longer distances. This process greatly enhanced Jeremy's self-esteem and sense of autonomy, and further fortified the working alliance.

Patients' compensatory tool use and driving status both have an impact on their social system—their families. The next chapter addresses how brain injuries affect a patient's support network; relevant therapeutic interventions are described.

# CHAPTER 7

# Family Life

*with* Edward Koberstein

## THE IMPACT OF BRAIN INJURY ON THE WHOLE FAMILY

Research and clinical observations have documented acute and enduring emotional sequelae for the family after a loved one's brain injury. Understandably, these include depression and anxiety (Boyle & Haines, 2002; Kreutzer, Marwitz, & Kepler, 1992; Lezak, 1978; Mintz, Van Horn, & Levine, 1995; Ponsford, Olver, Ponsford, & Nelms, 2003). Some researchers have identified a sense of "never-ending crisis" and "episodic loss reactions" as typical postinjury consequences for family members (Davis et al., 2003; Williams, 1991). Other signs of upheaval and adversity for family members include psychosomatic disorders, interpersonal discord, financial burden, maladaptive role changes, feeling trapped, and social isolation (Boyle & Haines, 2002; Lezak, 1978; Mintz et al., 1995; Williams, 1991).

Sources of more significant family stress include greater severity of brain injury; poorer neuropsychological functioning, awareness, impulse control, and planning and other executive function skills; inability of the patient to empathize with caregivers; and decreased family income (Anderson, Parmenter, & Mok, 2002; Machamer, Temkin, & Dikmen, 2002; Sander et al., 2003; Wells, Dywan, & Dumas,

**Edward Koberstein, BSc,** is affiliated with the Center for Transitional NeuroRehabilitation, Barrow Neurological Institute, St. Joseph's Hospital and Medical Center, Phoenix, Arizona.

2005). Research has identified patients' improved control of their emotions and behaviors as the most salient predictor of caregiver well-being and life satisfaction (Ergh, Hanks, Rapport, & Coleman, 2003; Harris, Godfrey, Partridge, & Knight, 2001; Testa, Malec, Moessner, & Brown, 2006; Wells et al., 2005).

Family dynamics can contribute to caregiver stress. Sander et al. (2003) have reported that preinjury emotional distress and/or unhealthy family functioning increased families' vulnerability to injury-related stresses and decreased their postinjury coping. Testa et al. (2006) reported that family dysfunction at a 1-year follow-up was best predicted by family dysfunction at the time of hospital discharge. Pearlin, Mullan, Semple, and Skaff (1990) devised a multidimensional scheme for caregiver stress; this scheme included preinjury factors (e.g., socioeconomic status and resources), as well as the level of vigilance by the caregiver (secondary to the loved one's dependency needs), level of conflict, and loss of sense of self in the caregiver.

The nature and causes of emotional distress in family members are also related to the specific relationships between family members and the injured loved ones. Some have postulated that a spouse faces greater challenges and obstacles than a parent, including the intangibles of living with a person who is likely to be different from the individual he or she married. There are also societal pressures on spouses not to grieve for their losses or divorce their injured mates (Lezak, 1978; Webster, Daisley, & King, 1999). Other challenges include stresses associated with the reallocation of roles and loss of a reciprocal relationship (including financial decision making), as well as changes in sources of income, running the household, and caring for the children (Curtiss, Klemz, & Vanderploeg, 2000; Florian & Katz, 1991; Gosling & Oddy, 1999; Mauss-Clum & Ryan, 1981; Webster et al., 1999; Wedcliffe & Ross, 2001; Wood, Liossi, & Wood, 2005). Changes in the sexual relationship and loneliness are also commonly reported (Florian & Katz, 1991; Gosling & Oddy, 1999; Wedcliffe & Ross, 2001).

The emotional and practical reverberations of a brain injury within an entire family system (including children and siblings) are often underrecognized, given the constant needs of the injured party (Gan & Schuller, 2002; Perlesz, Kinsella, & Crowe, 2000). Common problems include emotional distress, bewilderment, insecurity, loneliness, helplessness, conflict, anger, neglect, abandonment, and diminished quality of life (Aniskiewicz, 2007; Degeneffe, 2001; Florian & Katz, 1991; Gan et al., 2006; Lezak, 1978). Parents face their own unique problems, including extended parenthood (Degeneffe, 2001).

In contrast, other researchers have reported positive experiences and limited stress for caregivers (Machamer et al., 2002), including lower divorce rates and relatively stable postinjury marital relationships (Klonoff et al., 2006; Kreutzer et al., 2007). Factors contributing to better postinjury coping by caregivers include reduction in self-appraised burden; belief in self-efficacy and empowerment; self-reliance; reciprocal communication and affective relations between the injured loved ones and family members; and social support, especially when the support system is caring, trustworthy, and uplifting (Douglas & Spellacy, 2000; Ergh et al., 2003; Hanks, Rapport, & Vangel, 2007; Harris et al., 2001; Man, 2002; Pearlin et al., 1990; Verhaeghe, Defloor, & Grypdonck, 2005).

## THE FAMILY'S ROLE IN THE PATIENT'S RECOVERY

Both research and the clinical literature have stressed the importance of collaboration and cooperation between the treating therapist(s) and family members—not
only to maximize the family's own emotional well-being (Sohlberg et al., 2001),
but to ensure the best possible outcome for their loved one (Bowen, 2007; Klonoff
et al., 1998; Klonoff, Lamb, & Henderson, 2001; Mauss-Clum & Ryan, 1981; Sander
et al., 2002). Establishing a positive working alliance with the family is generally
the most consequential precursor (and in some cases the only hope) for developing and maintaining the working alliance with the patient (Klonoff & Prigatano,
1987; Sherer et al., 2007). Often the patient is ambivalent about, suspicious of, or
resistant to psychotherapeutic recommendations, especially early in the treatment
process. This is especially the case with painful, disappointing, or ego-dystonic
recommendations, including psychotropic medication or alternative career directions. It is often only when the family members can intervene and ally with the
therapist(s) that the patient begins to develop any trust in the treatment process.
In this way, the family members constitute an essential curative factor for their
loved one (Gleckman & Brill, 1995). When family members' perceptions and goals
conflict with those of the therapist(s), the patient will be influenced away from the
treatment process.

In some situations, a patient does not have family members available to
participate in the psychotherapy process. One option is to involve family members via telephone consultation, either separately or conjointly with the patient,
depending on the patient's preference. Alternatively, the patient may be alienated
from his or her family for a variety of reasons. In these instances, we encourage
the patient to involve whoever represents his or her support system in the psychotherapeutic process, through both face-to-face meetings and attendance at the
family group.

The working alliance with the family is enhanced when there is mutual
trust and when the family feels listened to, valued, and supported by the treating
professionals (Lefebvre, Pelchat, Swaine, Gelinas, & Levert, 2005; McLaughlin &
Carey, 1993; Testani-Dufour, Chappel-Aiken, & Gueldner, 1992). A positive working alliance heartens families to share their personal and sometimes divergent
observations about the patient's mood, adjustment, and productivity outside the
treatment environment (Klonoff & Prigatano, 1987). Then family members are better equipped to encourage their loved one to generalize newly acquired behaviors
and skills to the home and community environments, including work or school
(Klonoff et al., 1998, 2001).

Central components of the psychotherapy process include psychoeducation
for the family about the consequences of the injury, as well as provision of information about available resources (Gan et al., 2006; Gleckman & Brill, 1995; Man,
2002; Padrone, 1999; Williams, 1991). Other authors have advocated for educational
workshops, family therapy, marital counseling, support groups, and respite care
(Degeneffe, 2001; Gan et al., 2006; Perlesz et al., 2000; Tyerman & Booth, 2001).
Rotondi, Sinkule, Balzer, Harris, and Moldovan (2007) have differentiated priorities for the educational process, depending on the point on the spectrum of

recovery that the patient and family have reached. This necessitates a multimodal treatment approach, focusing on information, support, and anticipatory guidance; provision of problem-solving, communication, coping skills, stress management, and behavioral management techniques; access to community resources; practical adaptations in the home; and facilitation of life planning (Gan et al., 2006; Holland & Shigaki, 1998; Rotondi et al., 2007; Solomon & Scherzer, 1991; Testani-Dufour et al., 1992).

In the holistic clinic where the first author (Klonoff) practices, family members are given a binder of approximately 40 handouts when they begin psychotherapy. These include pertinent research articles and inspirational readings. The materials provide valuable information that diminishes their confusion and angst. Other clinicians have also emphasized the importance of educational materials for family members (Morris, 2001; Sinnakaruppan & Williams, 2001; Verhaeghe et al., 2005; Wilson & Kapur, 2008).

## FAMILY INTERVENTIONS

This section provides a brief overview of the types and goals of family interventions.

### Psychotherapy for Family Members

Psychotherapy for family members (without the patient) is designed to help them cope emotionally with the consequences of their loved one's injury. Very often at the outset of therapy, the family members feel frustrated, overwhelmed, exasperated, depressed, guilt-ridden, and helpless and/or hopeless about the future. The assumptive world that grounded them and provided their sense of reality has been shattered (Kauffman, 2002). Psychotherapy sessions provide a private and safe outlet for them to express their feelings, unhindered momentarily by outside responsibilities and stresses. Multiple techniques are utilized to help them explore their inner feelings. For example, family members are invited to bring in mementos and pictures from their past to facilitate the grieving and mourning process. This can catalyze important exploration of paralyzing feelings (e.g., undue second-guessing). Keeping journals can give them a vital outlet for working through their psychic pain, as well as a way to chronicle sometimes forgotten or minimized tangible evidence of progress. Recommended inspirational readings (e.g., Crimmins, 2000; Woodruff & Woodruff, 2007) can replenish the family's sense of hope and optimism about the future. Lastly, adopting the "one day at a time" philosophy allows the family members to set "bite-size," manageable subgoals, which will help them to avoid becoming overwhelmed or trapped in misgivings.

As noted earlier, a primary goal of individual psychotherapy for family members is to provide psychoeducation about the nature and extent of their loved one's brain injury. A detailed understanding about the underlying "whys" of their loved one's behavior equips them to provide constructive suggestions or interventions. Psychoeducational topics usually include memory, executive functions, and common behavioral sequelae, including catastrophic reactions. In particular, family members benefit from instruction about the nature and extent of their loved one's memory problems, and from practical descriptions of how these deficits manifest themselves in the home and community environments. Related to this, the family members are taught all of the strategies or compensations their loved one is using (see Chapter 6). Helping family members appreciate the practical complications arising from executive function deficits is also fundamental. This includes translating medical terminology into user-friendly phrases, such as "tunnel vision" for difficulties with abstract reasoning; "black-and-white thinking" for metacognitive deficits; "get up and go" for initiative; "my way or the highway" for cognitive rigidity; and "being fixated" for perseveration. Family members' grasp of the unique precursors and manifestations of catastrophic reactions in their loved ones is also essential for harmonious interactions. Finally, resource reading and attendance at educational conferences can be helpful for family members.

### Conjoint Therapy

Conjoint therapy with the family members and the patient helps each party appreciate the others' perceptions and feelings. Any mix of patients and family members is appropriate (e.g., patient and spouse, patient and parents, or patient and siblings). It is advisable to ascertain in advance whether the patient and family members have the emotional control and coping strategies for discussing difficult issues; otherwise, more preliminary dialogue should occur between the psychotherapist and each party prior to conjoint meetings.

Conjoint therapy is most efficacious once a working alliance with all parties has been established. This allows the participants to reach the necessary comfort level with the psychotherapist before discussing delicate issues with each other. Generally, to facilitate the dialogue and prevent unproductive escalation of feelings, it is best to identify agenda items in advance and, if possible, to conduct some preliminary discussion with each party.

Conjoint therapy increases patients' awareness of the impact of their cognitive, emotional, and psychosocial deficits on their families. The psychotherapist also has the opportunity to directly observe the interaction between a patient and family members, and to educate the family members about the pace, timing, and complexity of information they impart to their loved one.

Conjoint therapy sessions focus on practical techniques. Clinical experience indicates that family members manage their multiple responsibilities best when they have their own sets of compensatory tools. These include datebooks of their own. These not only help them organize their own days, but also normalize datebook use for their loved one. When family members and the patient all have datebooks, they all should take notes in psychotherapy appointments and during family "milieu meetings" (as discussed in Chapter 6). This helps remove any stigma the patient may attach to note taking. Written behavioral contracts and chore checklists for multiple family members and the patient are other excellent organizational tools. These serve to remind everyone of the importance of give and take, and of being a "good citizen" within the family structure.

## Marital Therapy

Marital therapy is often warranted when one spouse has sustained a brain injury and when both spouses remain committed to the marriage. There should be an agreement to this effect between the spouses before starting therapy. If there is no commitment, the noninjured spouse should be referred to outside resources for his or her own psychotherapeutic needs.

Themes that generally emerge in marital counseling include various effects of the patient's personality and role change on the spouse (e.g., the impoverishment of emotional and sexual intimacy, due to the patient's inability to relate on as deep a level emotionally and/or cognitively as before). Given the need to cue, direct, and guide the patient, the spouse often feels that he or she has adopted the role of a parent. This skews the balance and interrelatedness of the partnership.

As in conjoint therapy, most fundamental issues should first be addressed separately with the patient and spouse prior to their meeting together. Both should have the behavioral control to manage intense emotions. The therapy should incorporate a psychoeducational component that is problem- and solution-focused. Specific ground rules generally need to be established, in case either party tends to blame the other for the problems. Therefore, the emphasis of sessions should be on how each party can take personal responsibility for self-directed change. For the patient, the emphasis is on reclaiming as many responsibilities as possible and improving his or her level of sensitivity and empathy toward the partner. Helping the couple adjust to the role changes, many of which are permanent, is another principal focus of the therapy. A helpful diagram is one depicting a seesaw, which represents the imbalance of the patient's self-focus relative to the needs of the spouse. On each end of the seesaw, each party can document his or her specific personal commitment to creating a new, healthy equilibrium in the relationship. Ultimately, if the marriage is to survive and flourish, the partners will need to design a new relationship and find meaning and happiness in their current circumstances.

In some couples and families, of course, there are prominent preexisting problems that are only compounded by the effects of the brain injury. The psychotherapist may elect to involve a family or marital counselor in such cases, especially if the depth and breadth of the problems exceed the psychotherapist's training or comfort zone.

## Family Group

A family group is a forum to provide education, emotional support, and peer mentoring to adult family members (at least 18 years old) whose loved ones are actively engaged in the postacute stage of treatment and recovery. The group can comfortably accommodate up to 20 members and should be facilitated by at least one clinical neuropsychologist or psychotherapist. Sessions last 90 minutes each and meet regularly (e.g., weekly). Professional input and peer exchange build families' skill sets, and also validate and support their challenges and their emotional ups and downs. The family group represents a critical resource for families to build camaraderie and feel less alone. Light snacks and drinks are provided to the family members, to create a nurturing and supportive atmosphere. The format for family group is most effective when sessions are organized into three 30-minute segments: didactic lectures, support, and round-robin updates.

## Didactic Lectures

The first 30 minutes of each group session are devoted to didactic lectures. One possible format is to have therapists from multiple disciplines (e.g., neuropsychology, occupational therapy, physical therapy, speech–language therapy, recreational therapy, dietetics, social work, and vocational counseling) rotate into the group weekly and present educational material from their areas of expertise. This diversified set of topics will broaden the families' knowledge base and facilitate their adaptation. Topics fall into three categories: general education about the ramifications of brain injury; typical psychological adjustment challenges for the family; and useful coping techniques for the family.

The "nuts-and-bolts" educational category teaches families the specifics of injury sequelae in the cognitive, emotional, physical, and interpersonal domains. The PEM (see Chapter 1, Figure 1.2) is a key device for informing families about challenges commonly associated with the therapeutic process. The group educators also emphasize the benefits and components of various compensatory strategies. Members of each family are fully introduced to their loved one's "tool kit," which will ultimately reduce the stresses and burdens on the family. Figure 7.1 lists selected educational lecture topics. Figure 7.2 addresses concerns related to community reintegration, to equip the families for this transition process.

---

- Overview of basic neuroanatomy
- Postinjury personality and emotional changes
- The PEM
- Catastrophic reactions
- Seizures and treatment
- Memory problems
- Executive system problems
- Datebook system
- Home visits and the Home Independence Checklist
- Nutrition after brain injury
- Physical difficulties and home exercise programs
- Cognitive retraining
- Changes in identity and sense of self
- Communication pragmatics and socialization
- Sexuality and intimacy
- Factors to assess for a return to driving
- Efficacy research and long-term work outcome after brain injury
- Considerations before terminating psychotherapy

---

**FIGURE 7.1.** Family group lectures: Selected educational topics about brain injury.

- Reintegration into work and school settings
- Driving and transportation
- Hobbies and leisure interests
- Alcohol and drug use
- Social isolation and quality of life
- Community resources

**FIGURE 7.2.** Family group lectures: Selected topics about community reintegration after brain injury.

A second category of topics consists of common psychological adjustment challenges that family members themselves face. It also incorporates informational material, with an emphasis on frequent sources of upheaval (e.g., role changes, financial burdens, and interpersonal conflicts with their loved ones). Common manifestations of families' distress are defined and discussed, including feelings of loss and "Why us?"; the concept of "catastrophic reactions by proxy" (see the case of Nathan, Aaron, and Irwin, below); hypervigilance and overprotectiveness; managing "walking on eggshells" and "Yeah, buts"; and breaches in the working alliance. Family members' existential concerns are also addressed, including redefining their values and life priorities. A similar model focusing on the family's experience, the family experiential model (FEM) of recovery, helps to structure the discussion. The FEM is described in more detail later in this chapter. Figure 7.3 provides a sample of topics related to families' psychological adjustment.

Psychological adjustment also includes coping techniques. Figure 7.4 summarizes therapeutic recommendations to enhance families' coping, which are often reviewed as part of the family group. A very important self-care concept is "dignity of risk" (M. Pepping, personal communication, n.d.). That is, persons with brain injury have an inherent right to preserve their sense of dignity and

- The FEM
- "Catastrophic reactions (CRs) by proxy"
- Hypervigilance and overprotectiveness
- Feelings of loss and "Why us?"
- Self-recrimination
- Role changes
- Financial stresses
- Impact on immediate and extended family members
- Managing "walking on eggshells" and "Yeah, buts"
- Managing behavioral conflicts
- Causes of burnout
- Enhancing the working alliance between families and therapists
- Redefining values and life priorities

**FIGURE 7.3.** Family group lectures: Selected topics about psychological adjustment for families.

**Self-Care Techniques**

- "Dignity of risk"
- "Division of labor"
- Setting personal priorities and saying "no"
- "One day at a time"
- Respite time and pleasurable activities
- Meaningful hobbies and work
- Regular medical follow-up (for the family and loved one)
- Proper self-care
- Psychotropic medications
- Spirituality
- Inspirational readings, movies, etc.

**Practical and Time Management Suggestions**

- Crock-Pot or other slow cooker to streamline meal preparation
- Budget and financial assistance from trained professionals
- Prepaid credit cards
- Transportation resources
- "Milieu meetings"

**FIGURE 7.4.** Family group lectures: Selected psychological coping techniques for families—What helps?

self-determination, even if this translates into choices that their families disagree with or have trepidations about. The idea that there is dignity in risk helps families cope with the anxieties involved in "letting go" of their loved ones—which includes permitting them to make their own mistakes.

The psychotherapist should be mindful of family burnout. Examples include members' feeling overwhelmed and irritated by their loved one. It is at this juncture that "division of labor" becomes paramount; this means that more support is needed from friends and other family members, if possible. Sometimes the family needs to consider hiring a professional caregiver to reduce the burden on the main family caregiver. In some situations, family members can "trade off" the responsibilities for their loved one; this allows a knowledgeable outsider to reinforce healthy habits. Strategies that help avert burnout include life simplification techniques, such as setting personal priorities and learning to say "no" to low-priority or stress-inducing requests. An "occupational hazard" of the caregiving role is the tendency to resist sharing or delegating responsibilities, including rejecting others' offers of assistance. The family caregiver may develop a belief system predicated on guilt or insecurity about focusing on self-care. It is notable that family members are generally more willing to accept these types of recommendations from one another during therapeutic group interactions, as they are more adept at recognizing the warning signs and can impartially offer permission to each other to alter their routines.

Regular respite breaks are essential for family members to maintain their well-being and sustain their long-term emotional resources (Klonoff & Prigatano, 1987). This includes vacations (even short ones), involvement in enjoyable hobbies, social activities with friends, and mental health days (e.g., a spa or golf day). Some family members have found that pets are a source of enjoyment and healthy distraction. Family members and their loved ones also need community-based work activities that provide personal fulfillment. These not only will provide an opportunity for healthy separation from one another, but will enhance everyone's quality of life.

Family members can reduce their own health problems and those of their loved ones by scheduling regular medical appointments. Often family members sacrifice their own physical health needs (e.g., for adequate sleep and a healthy diet), thereby jeopardizing their physical and emotional resources (McPherson, Pentland, & McNaughton, 2000). Regular exercise and relaxation techniques (e.g., yoga classes, diaphragmatic breathing, and imagery) help the family members "unwind" and recalibrate emotionally. In some circumstances where family members become overwhelmed, anxious, or depressed for prolonged periods of time, with deleterious effects on their ability to cope with day-to-day responsibilities, psychotropic medication (prescribed by their treating physicians) can be a beneficial adjunct to other treatment interventions. Family members often report that major sources of solace are their spiritual beliefs and religious affiliations.

Group dialogue with the guidance of the psychotherapist can enhance families' strategizing. Creative and practical techniques to reduce their daily stressors include streamlining meal preparation by using a Crock-Pot or other slow cooker; hiring an outside expert to assist with financial management; and using prepaid credit cards to limit patients' unwanted spending (see Figure 7.4). Family members often report that having to transport their loved ones all around the community is a chief source of stress and energy depletion. Use of community-based transportation services (e.g., state-funded transport, taxis, hired drivers) can greatly reduce this highly time-consuming responsibility. Finally, as described in Chapter 6, regular family "milieu meetings" can streamline the communication and organizational structure of the household.

## Support Group

The second 30-minute segment of the family group is devoted to peer support, facilitated by clinical neuropsychologists or psychotherapists. This affords families the opportunity to share their personal woes, fears, and consternations, while receiving empathic understanding from others who "walk in their shoes." These discussions often become emotionally charged, with family members frequently tearful about their circumstances. Frequently this is the only opportunity families have to discuss their own predicaments. Some feel hesitant to share their personal trials and tribulations, and will lapse back into talking about their loved ones. They are then gently encouraged by the facilitators to focus on their own personal and emotional needs. A primary aim of the support component of the family group is to help family members accept realistically attainable goals for their loved ones. This process is furthered when various family members compare and contrast their perceptions from differing points on the rehabilitation continuum. Specifically, family members whose loved ones are in (the PEM) Phases 5 or 6 of the continuum can both identify and commiserate with family members of patients just beginning the rehabilitation or psychotherapy process, and can also help to uplift them in times of upheaval. The sharing of humorous personal anecdotes is a positive emotional release and adds levity to the dialogue. Another powerful healing tool is the group's resounding enthusiasm when family members share their personal psychological insights and accomplishments.

Another possible forum for emotional support for family members is a mixed meeting with them and their loved ones, carefully facilitated by the psychotherapist. Open dialogue about the families' angst and turmoil can be an "eye-opener" for patients, who then better appreciate how their injuries reverberate through the family unit. To avoid nonproductive escalation in emotions, it is advisable to review topics of discussion and possible "hot buttons" with each group prior to such a meeting.

### Round-Robin Updates

In the final 30-minute portion of each family group session, if feasible, additional multidisciplinary therapists join the group and provide updates regarding each patient in a round-robin format. These weekly updates on patients' progress and challenges keep their families "in the loop." The process also provides all families with a broader view of the recovery and rehabilitation process. Through these updates, families in an early phase of the recovery process are given previews of later challenges and triumphs.

## THE FAMILY EXPERIENTIAL MODEL OF RECOVERY

As mentioned earlier, the FEM is a potent clinical treatment tool for family group meetings, as well as for psychotherapy with family members. The FEM conceptualizes the phenomenological experience of family members whose loved ones have sustained a brain injury (Klonoff et al., 2008). It incorporates feedback we obtained from 87 family members—49 from a holistic milieu-oriented treatment orientation, and 38 from the community, where few or no neurorehabilitation therapies were provided (Klonoff et al., 2008). The model was developed to give family members their own voice about their experiential reactions; the language was chosen to resonate with families' often intense and tumultuous emotions. Figure 7.5 presents a modified version, which illustrates the stages and coping patterns family members experience after brain injury.

The FEM is an instrumental visual aid that can be used as a foundation for discussion about a family's experiences and coping styles. Because it depicts the totality of the rehabilitation and recovery process, the family gains a holistic overview that puts their own journey in perspective. The model format also normalizes family members' experiences. The FEM serves as a roadmap to positive outcomes, as well as a warning about wrong turns and dead ends (Klonoff et al., 2008).

As seen in Figure 7.5, the family members' experience mirrors the chronology of their loved one's recovery, proceeding through the same seven phases—from life as it was before the injury (Phase 0) through to treatment termination and the postrehabilitation future (Phase 7). Phases 4–6 describe the families' experiences in a holistic treatment environment, or in any setting where the emphasis is on improving their capacity for awareness of, acceptance of, and realism about their loved one's injury. The Loved One's Condition column at left depicts the clear interrelationship between the family's emotional status and the patient's medical, physical, psychological, and functional status. The dotted lines between columns from Phase 3 to Phase 7 depict the porous nature of these phases. Families revisit earlier phases on an episodic basis, based on new revelations and experiences.

The bottom three rows of the figure represent the family's emotional reactions. Using the same traffic light color-coding system as the PEM, the rows represent coping styles: adaptive adjustment ("green" = light gray); a warning zone ("yellow" = darker gray) of ominous coping difficulties, with the potential for adverse effects on the family's short- and long-term adjustment; and a period of disintegration ("red" = darkest gray), in which the family is unable to cope with the realities of the injury and deteriorates into a state of crisis and dysfunction. The arrows between the coping zones symbolize the predictable and normal fluctuations in the family's adaptability, resiliency, and overall adjustment, secondary to the patient's and family's complex predicament.

The following two cases illustrate the FEM and the psychotherapeutic techniques used to intervene with families. The first case describes a family mired in coping difficulties ("yellow" warning zone), which ultimately degenerated into a period of disintegration ("red" zone). The second case illustrates a family with a more adaptive ("green") coping style.

## TWO EXTENDED CASES

### A Struggling Family

Melanie, age 35, was married with two young children—a daughter age 4, and a son age 6—when she sustained a severe left-hemisphere stroke. A CT scan showed a left deep-brain hippocampal lesion. An MRI showed a left posterior communicating artery infarct with thalamic involvement. Before her injury (Phase 0), she was a stay-at-home mom and was fully responsible for running the household. Her husband, Jack, was an executive for a large bank, who worked long hours and traveled extensively. Jack later shared in a psychotherapy session that there were serious preexisting marital problems, and that he had been contemplating divorcing his wife immediately prior to her stroke. During Phases 1, 2, and 3, Melanie's care and recovery were very complex; she had severe problems with aphasia. She was right-handed before the stroke; the stroke left her with right-sided hemiparesis, which affected both her arm and leg. She was also wheelchair-bound for ambulation. After the acute hospitalization, Melanie was transferred first to an extended care facility because of her severe cognitive and physical deficits, and then to a hospital inpatient neurorehabilitation unit. In total, she was hospitalized for 3 months and then discharged home.

In Phases 2 and 3, Jack was very overwhelmed by the abrupt and drastic disruption to his personal, family, and professional life. Starting in the intensive care unit (ICU) and throughout Melanie's hospital stay, he was overtly dissatisfied with her care, often resorting to verbal altercations with the nurses ("yellow" warning

Discharge

| | PHASE 0 | PHASE 1 | PHASE 2 | PHASE 3 | PHASE 4 | PHASE 5 | PHASE 6 | PHASE 7 |
|---|---|---|---|---|---|---|---|---|
| | Preinjury | Time of Brain Injury | Early Adjustment | Seeks Help | Starts Outpatient Therapy | Retraining | Therapy Transition | Future ∞ |
| | | | | | AWARENESS | ACCEPTANCE | REALISM | |

**Reference Point**
Life as it was.

**PHASE 1 — Sudden Impact of Brain Injury**
- Constant vigil at bedside.
- Family misses loved one; core loneliness.
- Members become "instant experts" on loved one.
- Family is in "crisis mode."

**PHASE 2 — Initial Problems**
- Meandering in a foggy reality.
- Family orchestrates and facilitates loved one's care needs; undertakes "insurance trauma."
- Family wants loved one to "beat the odds" and expects instant results.

**PHASE 3 — How to Cope**
- Reality of 24/7 care sinks in.
- Family receives brunt of loved one's dependency and negativity.
- Physical, mental, and emotional exhaustion.

**PHASE 4 — Confronting Reality**
- Family learns appropriate vocabulary and terminology (e.g., "CRs by proxy").
- Unpredictability about the future.
- Members recognize they need help and are not alone.

**PHASE 5 — Compensations**
- Family mourns the losses.
- "Things take time."
- Members learn compensations for themselves and the patient.
- Family gains perspective and accepts "new" loved one.

**PHASE 6 — Approaching Discharge**
- Family observes patient's new freedoms and independence.
- Family prepares to assume more post-program responsibility.
- Juggles work schedule, finances, and caregiving.

**PHASE 7 — The Real World**
- Family and loved one maintain collaborative dialogue.
- Things aren't the same, but everyone can live a meaningful and productive life.
- Life is evolving.

**Lower band (LOVED ONES / E'S):**

PHASE 1
- Fleeting composure vacillating with emotional chaos.
- "Why us? Why them? What if?"
- So many questions, so few answers.
- On "automatic pilot."
- Life is surreal.

PHASE 2
- Family sacrifices personal needs in favor of patient's care.
- Family succumbs to intense emotions, with islands of resiliency.
- Worries something else "bad" could happen, but trusts the professionals.
- Family lovingly encourages the patient.

PHASE 3
- Parent/spousal role switches to role of caregiver/advocate.
- Family transforms feelings of helplessness into proactive behavior.
- Members realize they need further outpatient treatment for "injury aftermath."

PHASE 4
- Tentative yet hopeful.
- Family increases awareness and constructively manages profound yet universal feelings.
- Sense of relief or respite while loved one attends therapy.

PHASE 5
- Family copes by learning and supportive compensation training and goal setting.
- Emotional bonding and camaraderie in family group.
- Members resolve to "count their blessings."

PHASE 6
- Mutual realism about loved one's community reintegration.
- Family develops confidence and constructively manages trepidation about discharge.
- Family finds inner strength and courage through facing adversity.

PHASE 7
- Family intuitively evolves new strategies for quality of life.
- Door is always open for further help.
- Family assumes balanced roles with respite and social support network.

**LEGEND**
- L O V E D
- O N E' S
- ☐ Phases
- ☐ Coping Zone
- ☐ Warning Zone
- ■ Crisis Zone
- ---- Rotation
- ↔ Fluctuation

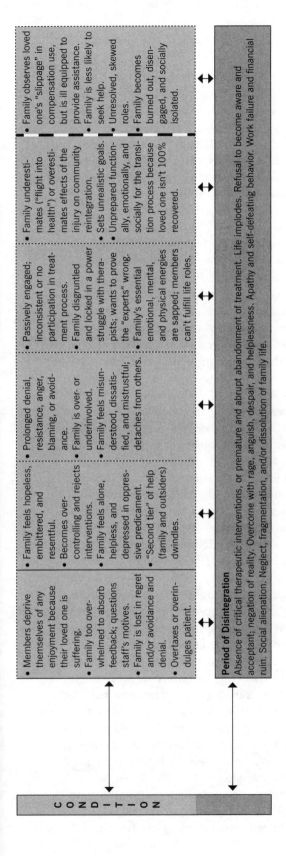

**FIGURE 7.5.** Family experiential model (FEM) of recovery after brain injury.

zone). He refused to listen to concerns raised by medical personnel regarding the seriousness of her condition and its prognosis; he was convinced she would be back to "normal" in no time. While Melanie was on the inpatient neurorehabilitation unit, he was also observed by the therapy staff to be overly taxing of his wife; his demeanor was demanding and demeaning. His follow-through with recommended adaptations and equipment for the home was poor; he was convinced that in a short time she would be walking, fully functional, and competent with her prestroke parenting duties. Jack became overcontrolling; he fired multiple in-home nurses and therapists. Because of his surliness and resentment, he also quickly alienated other family members and friends who offered their assistance. Over the next 4 months, the situation deteriorated. He became more depressed, overwhelmed, and alone, oppressed by his sole responsibility for his wife. He became desperate to find additional outpatient rehabilitation (Phase 3).

Even after Jack enrolled Melanie in an outpatient rehabilitation clinic (Phase 4), his mood was still dominated by petulance and exasperation ("yellow" warning zone). Twice-weekly individual psychotherapy sessions were immediately instituted to try to ameliorate the situation. Jack spent the early sessions bitterly complaining about the perceived "failings" of the preceding rehabilitation attempts. The psychotherapist attempted to establish a working alliance predicated on empathic listening (trying to "walk in his shoes") and assistance with practical problem solving to reduce his daily stressors. The latter included suggestions for delegating the responsibilities by hiring a constant caregiver, as well as arranging his wife's transportation to her rehabilitation. Although these early interventions provided him with some psychological relief, he soon began to blame the new therapy team for his wife's slow progress. He was resistant to suggestions for installing adaptive equipment in the home to assist with bathing and functional activities in the kitchen (Phase 5 "yellow" warning zone). During home visits, he refused to sit with the occupational therapist for longer than a few minutes; he was continually distracted by phone calls and work-related projects. He refused to see the relevance of the compensations and began to complain that the therapists did not have his or his wife's best interests at heart, because she was not showing a rapid enough recovery. Even when he did agree to follow recommendations, he never implemented them. For example, he quickly grew intolerant of and disgruntled with the detail-oriented and time-consuming aspects of the datebook and Home Independence Checklist, both of which he described as "nitpicky." Jack became increasingly hostile and distrustful of the treatment process, and actively fought further therapeutic suggestions for his wife (e.g., psychotropic medication). The psychotherapist instituted regular family meetings involving key treating therapists, to provide Jack with as much practical education as possible and to "brainstorm" regarding feasible solutions to problems, given Melanie's prognosis. For example, the occupational therapist invested considerable extra time in streamlining and articulating written protocols with "helpful hints," which she tried to review and help institute at the weekly home visits.

Jack reverted to some unhealthy coping styles, also characteristic of the warning zone of coping. At times he would criticize Melanie, to which she retaliated with "snarky" retorts. He would escalate the tensions by becoming furious with her. Then, when exasperated with Melanie, he would share his concerns with the psychotherapist, but would refuse to involve his wife in the dialogue process. This keeping of secrets disempowered his wife in their marital dialogue and made the psychotherapist uncomfortable about colluding with Jack in this manner. The focus was then shifted to helping Jack develop the confidence and tools to address his concerns directly with Melanie. This included encouraging him to take a more supportive and diplomatic approach to feedback. Gradually, some modest progress was made—first in conjoint sessions, and eventually with some carryover to the home environment.

The psychotherapist urged Jack to attend the weekly family group, hoping that peer mentoring and support would ease his woes. However, he refused after the first 2 weeks, stating that he felt it was a waste of his time to discuss personal feelings in a group environment. Nevertheless, his emotional, mental, and physical energies were totally depleted. His children were also suffering in the process; he did not have the emotional reserves necessary to nurture them.

The psychotherapist then suggested that Jack solicit additional family support to help with parenting responsibilities in the home and ease his workload. He invited his mother, Loretta, to come and stay with him. When the psychotherapist met with Loretta, it soon became apparent that Jack and his mother mirrored their coping styles. Their approaches to Melanie's illness were identical: They were both in deep denial about the severity of her problems, and minimized the serious implications for her long-term functioning in the home and community. They both resorted to blaming, and ultimately became locked in an intense power struggle with, the psychotherapist and treatment team. They put their energies into proving the "experts" wrong and maintaining an unrealistic and idealized view of Melanie's prognosis.

The movie *Ordinary People* (Schwary & Redford, 1980) was recommended to Jack and Loretta. The psychotherapist hoped that the themes and raw emotion of this movie would provide a somewhat neutral but clinically insightful vantage point, and would help Jack and Loretta in their self-exploration process. The film portrays the destructiveness of the fictional mother's denial, avoidance, repressed anger, and blame (indicative of the Phases 4, 5, and 6 "yellow" warning zones). The mother is ashamed to discuss problems with others, stating, "If we have problems, we solve them in the privacy of our own home." Her preoccupation with wanting to "get back to normal" hampers the healing process and exemplifies her problems with acceptance and realism. Mirrored familial coping styles are depicted beautifully in this film, as the maternal grandmother takes an identical approach to her daughter's, commenting, "I thought we were all done with that." Because of the fictional mother's refusal to seek help, she is consumed with underlying despair, and is unable to grieve adequately for her son's death or to adapt effectively to her tragic circumstances. Jack and Loretta rejected and scoffed at the symbolic representation.

Sadly, the therapeutic situation deteriorated further, and the family plunged into a period of disintegration ("red" zone). Melanie was not making the necessary gains, and the insurance funding became precarious. At the same time, Jack was experiencing severe work stresses and was reprimanded about his work absenteeism and distractibility. He therefore abandoned all additional attempts at therapeutic intervention and precipitously withdrew his wife from the treatment milieu. After the withdrawal, Jack soon became utterly burned out by the enormity of Melanie's needs; he did not have the emotional or pragmatic supports or resources in place to cope. Because of the abrupt cessation of her therapies, Melanie also plateaued in her recovery and became severely depressed and agitated, illustrating the interface between the loved one's and family's condition. Within 1 month, Jack sent his wife out of state to live with her sister, fragmenting the family unit.

Unfortunately, the psychotherapeutic/neurorehabilitation process was outwardly unsuccessful in this case. Some consolation was gained from the belief that "therapists can only help the patient as much as the family will let them" (G. A. Lage, personal communication, n.d.). After team conferences and much therapeutic soul searching, it was concluded that the best efforts had been made to establish a meaningful working alliance, and it was hoped that the "seeds were planted" regarding the benefits of psychotherapy, marital counseling, and compensation training. Information about additional community resources (including names of psychotherapists, alternative therapy sites, and support groups) was sent to Jack, together with an invitation to recontact the clinic in the future if he desired additional assistance.

### An Adaptively Coping Family

Irwin, a 21-year-old male, sustained a severe traumatic brain injury from a motor vehicle accident, which was caused in part by his speeding and driving recklessly. The initial brain scans indicated bilateral frontal subdural hematomas. He underwent bilateral frontal craniotomies for evacuation of the subdural hematomas, and then required a right frontal craniotomy with removal of the bone flap. Irwin developed multiple complications while in the hospital, including a methicillin resistant *Staphylococcus aureus* infection, respiratory failure, and a subclavian deep-vein thrombosis.

Irwin was admitted to an outpatient program at 10 months postinjury (Phase 4). He then underwent a comprehensive assessment. In psychotherapy sessions, the written report outlining the sobering findings of the evaluation was reviewed in detail with Irwin; his father, Nathan; and his brother, Aaron, 4 years his senior. The psychotherapist then shared the treatment team's recommendation that to maximize recovery and functional improvement, the length of stay could extend up to 6 months.

Nathan and Aaron began family psychotherapy as part of Irwin's rehabilitation. They met weekly with the psychotherapist and also attended the weekly family group. The FEM was used as a psychoeducational tool and a mechanism to facilitate self-exploration and healing. In early sessions, the psychotherapist empathically listened to their story. Importantly, much of this had to be placed in the context of Phase 0 ("Life as it was"). Irwin's parents had divorced when he was young, and he and Aaron had been raised by his father. Nathan worked in law enforcement, and as part of his job was called to many accident sites where other young men had been critically injured or killed. His experience of this part of his job was now changed from that of objective "notifier" to the horrifying experience of the "notified." Aaron, who was studying psychology in order to become a therapist, was in a similar position; he too had to come to terms with his role reversal from the "treater" to the "treated." Their heartrending account informed the psychotherapist about their phenomenological stance in life; clearly, both Nathan's and Aaron's assumptive worlds had been shattered. Because of their stations in life, the therapist also realized the importance of functioning as their "copilot," so as not to be overbearing with advice about their quest for emotional relief.

The psychotherapist intuited that Nathan's and Aaron's grim description of the night of the accident was pivotal in their grieving process, and encouraged them to delve into these agonizing memories. They lamented how they were notified in the middle of the night and catapulted into "crisis mode" (Phase 1). They recounted how both of them "practically lived" at the hospital in social seclusion, especially because Irwin almost died several times from medical complications. Nathan adopted a constant bedside vigil, praying and bargaining with his God if only his son would survive. Aaron was miserable and bereft, seeing the shell of his younger brother lying in bed connected to life only by tubes, unable to speak or move. The family's daily lives were turned upside down; both Nathan and Aaron took immediate leaves of absence from work and school. Empathic listening in the protective haven of the psychotherapy office provided them their very first opportunity for emotional catharsis.

The father and brother bemoaned how the early realities of brain injury began to sink in, once Irwin was transferred to the inpatient neurorehabilitation unit (Phase 2). They felt perpetually sleep-deprived, and meandered in a foggy reality. Nonetheless because of their loving "hands-on" support, they alternated sleeping over every night, and ardently tutored Irwin in his cognitive and physical exercises ("green" adaptive coping zone). Although medical professionals had prepared Nathan and Aaron for the worst outcome, they believed in their hearts that Irwin was special and would "beat the odds." The psychotherapist reflected back to Nathan and Aaron that clearly their devotion to Irwin was laudable, and emphasized that their emotional resiliency would continue to be a source of sustenance. She framed this in the context of their new journey as "a marathon, rather than a sprint."

Nathan then described how after 3 weeks, Irwin was discharged home with minimal follow-up therapies because of insurance limitations (Phase 3). The realities of 24/7 care cascaded upon Nathan and Aaron. Irwin could not be left unattended because of his severe cognitive, emotional, and physical challenges. Behaviorally, he was profoundly unaware, impulsive, irritable, and depressed. The family's schedule upheaval continued. Aaron was forced to quit university and tend to Irwin's constant needs, while Nathan returned to work in a limited and modified capacity. Bills were mounting up. The father and brother also became targets for Irwin's extreme catastrophic reactions. Nathan and Aaron were reluctant to give Irwin feedback, often "walking on eggshells." The three of them were completely isolated within the home ("yellow" warning zone). Nathan and Aaron became physically, emotionally, and mentally exhausted. They did not have the ability or the resources to help Irwin, and they were devastated and overwhelmed by the magnitude of the situation. Nathan had then contacted Irwin's rehabilitation physician to search for help ("green" adaptive coping zone). Their stark depictions highlighted their feelings of helplessness and desperation; the psychotherapist then reassured them both that they were not alone in their distress and that they did not have to have all of the answers themselves. Their relief, and their appreciation for having new and strong "shoulders to lean on," were palpable.

Nonetheless, profound psychological distress abounded at the outset of psychotherapy (Phase 4). It was evident to the psychotherapist that Nathan's and Aaron's total attention and energies revolved around Irwin, at the expense of their own needs. Their psychological condition fluctuated in tandem with Irwin's psychological and rehabilitation status. When Irwin was having a good day, so were they; when he was not, they became panicky and overwhelmed. They had also developed an anxious habit of calling Irwin multiple times per day. Months after the accident, they were still keeping a constant nighttime vigil, consumed with fears that he would be hurt in some other way and they would not be there for him. This roller coaster of emotions (i.e., fluctuation between the adaptive and warning coping zones) reminded the psychotherapist to be cognizant of Nathan's and Aaron's feelings about the unpredictability, vulnerability, and fragility of life. Psychotherapy was therefore aimed at creating an atmosphere where they felt that their loved one was safe and where they themselves felt comfortable and comforted. This atmosphere included Irwin's new therapy environment, as well as the suggestion (which they eventually accepted) of respite care with trustworthy friends. The psychotherapist also provided additional education to reduce unlikely worries. Then they could gently be helped to "let go" and set healthier boundaries, so as not to smother Irwin.

The psychotherapist focused her energies on teaching Nathan and Aaron adaptive coping strategies. One apparent strength that she capitalized on was Nathan's and Aaron's hunger for knowledge. Multiple educational materials, research articles, and books by survivors of traumatic brain injury were shared and discussed with them. They eagerly absorbed all of this reading material, and they appreciated being treated as active, informed, and vital members of the treatment team.

Nathan and Aaron were also introduced to new and relevant terminology to help frame their personal challenges. For example, the concept of "catastrophic reactions (CRs) by proxy" was described, to capture Nathan's and Aaron's acute awareness and painful reminders of the decline in Irwin's capabilities. For example, the injury had put an end to brotherly one-on-one basketball games and to computer and video game competitions. As a threesome, they were also unable to enjoy camping and hunting trips, as they did before the accident. The concept of CRs by proxy served as an anchor for these experiences, which ultimately helped them make sense of their feelings.

In addition, Nathan's and Aaron's profound feelings of disappointment, sadness, and loss were explored as part of the psychotherapeutic process (Phase 4 "green" adaptive coping zone). The circumstances of Irwin's accident—speeding and driving recklessly—were especially egregious in the context of his father's and brother's commitment to "righting wrongs." Understandably, they were perturbed by and sometimes resentful of Irwin's thoughtlessness. The psychotherapist's energies now turned to helping them forgive Irwin for his actions, reminding them that "hindsight is 40/40" (see Chapter 5). Of several recommended outlets, Nathan chose a journal; his writing spurred the therapeutic dialogue, introspection, and coping process. Aaron preferred music lyrics and filled several psychotherapy sessions with somber selections that poignantly depicted his anguish. To infuse a different perspective, at one point the psychotherapist suggested that Aaron listen to "Everybody Hurts" as recorded by R.E.M. (Berry, Buck, Mills, & Stipe, 1992) as a reminder of the universality of suffering. Nathan and Aaron also needed to invest their psychological energies in forgiving themselves; they were consumed with feelings of "would have, could have, should have" and "if only." The psychotherapist also encouraged the "one-day-at-a-time" approach, with a focus on the here and now (Yalom, 2002), rather than retrospective rumination. With time and forethought, Nathan and Aaron each wrote a heartfelt letter to Irwin—describing their newfound feelings about his injury and recovery, and also emphasizing their pride in his accomplishments, his "second chance" at life, and their enduring cohesiveness as a family. They were invited to read these in a family session, where many collective tears were shed. Ultimately these letters were magnificent healing tools for all parties. Nathan and Aaron gradually became hopeful about the future for Irwin, as well as for themselves.

In Phases 5 and 6, Nathan and Aaron navigated through the mourning process and embraced the realization that "things take time" as a way to instill patience. Psychotherapy focused on how the family members (as well as their loved one) could rebuild their lives. Reading portions of *The Art of Happiness* (Dalai Lama & Cutler, 1998) as part of the psychotherapy sessions helped Nathan gain a perspective on his core personal values. He began to consider returning to full-time work, and reinvesting in "saving and protecting" the public as well as Irwin ("green" adaptive coping zone).

Irwin's brother struggled more. At times, Aaron wandered psychologically into the "yellow" warning zone of coping with intense survival guilt, which kept him from any gratifying pursuits. He had difficulty keeping loyalty and self-sacrifice from becoming self-punishment and self-deprivation. One helpful tool was reading, with the psychotherapist, Wally Lamb's (1998) novel *I Know This Much Is True*. The novel helped sensitize Aaron to the possibility of extreme caregiver burnout. The book's main character is saddled with lifetime caregiving responsibilities for his brother, who has schizophrenia. He ultimately becomes filled with rage, despair, and disillusionment because of the never-ending responsibilities. Through psychotherapy, the main character is able to explore and resolve his feelings of guilt, avoidance, and rage. Aaron was able to see how his own personal life circumstances were mirrored in the novel. Eventually, with the psychotherapist's urging, he returned to his university; he was assisted in identifying a manageable course of studies, and in balancing his caregiving responsibilities with his own personal needs and aspirations.

Once the acceptance "storm" subsided, the family's healthy coping strategies enabled them to actively learn about and support Irwin's use of compensatory strategies ("green" adaptive coping zone). This included monitoring Irwin's use of his datebook and chore checklists, as well as providing transportation for him, since he remained unable to drive. The psychotherapist also furnished pragmatic suggestions to streamline Nathan's and Aaron's daily responsibilities, including use of their own datebook systems and weekly "milieu meetings" to discuss issues as they arose and coordinate schedules. Nathan's and Aaron's spirits were further bolstered by the bonding and sense of camaraderie they experienced in the weekly family group. As an exercise, the whole group watched the movie *Life. Support. Music.* (Metzgar, 2008), which reinforced the families' empowerment through devotion and collaboration with their loved ones. Sharing challenges and victories with others also provided the outlook integral to accepting Irwin for who he was now. Nathan and Aaron could now look to the future and "count their blessings."

As the therapeutic process turned down the home stretch, Nathan's and Aaron's confidence were strengthened by witnessing the gains in Irwin's freedoms and independence. Through conjoint sessions with Irwin, Nathan, and Aaron, mutual realism developed about each party's involvement and strivings within the family unit and the community. As discharge approached, all family members drew on their inner strength and courage, emboldened through their successes in facing and overcoming adversity (Phase 6 "green" adaptive coping zone).

Since Irwin's discharge, Nathan and Aaron have maintained good friendships with other participants from the family group. They regularly get together for meals and visits. Nathan and Aaron continue intermittent psychotherapy and attend an aftercare group for families (see Chapter 9). All parties are actively involved in work and/or school. The family has reconstituted itself, and its members are enjoying meaningful and fulfilling relationships with each other, their extended family, and friends (Phase 7 "green" adaptive coping zone). Nathan volunteers at a hospital ICU, supporting and mentoring parents of freshly injured young adults. He has written to Irwin:

> "I am a better person than I was. Life is so much more precious. I made a deal with God that if I could continue to be your dad I would give back to the world. . . . I love being your father and would not trade anything that has happened for an 'easier life.'"

The next chapter returns to a focus on patients and their need to relearn communication and social skills after brain injury. Adequate interpersonal skills are vital for successful reintegration into the community.

# CHAPTER 8

# Communication and Social Skills

Deficient social skills after brain injury have a negative impact on quality of life, life satisfaction, and psychosocial outcome, especially social reintegration (Corrigan, Bogner, Mysiw, Clinchot, & Fugate, 2001; Klonoff, Snow, & Costa, 1986; Mammi, Zaccaria, & Franceschini, 2006; Morton & Wehman, 1995; Pierce & Hanks, 2006). Social isolation and a scarcity of hobbies and recreation are often persistent problems, causing even greater disruption in the chronic stages of recovery than in the acute stages (Andrews, Gerhart, & Hosack, 2004; Dikmen et al., 2003; Inzaghi, De Tanti, & Sozzi, 2005; Klonoff et al., 1986; Middelkamp et al., 2007; Morton & Wehman, 1995; see Oddy, 2003, for a review). Patients themselves have described both pictorially and in poetry their feelings of loneliness and isolation after brain injury (Douglas, 2007; Klonoff, 2005). Reduced community reintegration has been associated with a variety of factors, including emotional/behavioral changes (e.g., depression, anxiety, aggressiveness, paranoia, disinhibition, impulsivity, moodiness, and irritability) (Inzaghi et al., 2005; Winkler, Unsworth, Sloan, & Caplan, 2006).

Higher-level language and executive function deficits affect conversational competency and impede social interaction. These include deficits in initiation; abstract reasoning; word retrieval; interpretation and use of social communication; discourse organization, continuity, and coherence; response relevance; selected and divided attention; and comprehension of language nuances (e.g., jokes) (Corkery & Fairweather, 2009; Godfrey & Shum, 2000; Snow, Douglas, & Ponsford, 1998). Several researchers have described how frontal lobe damage can cause behavioral alterations (e.g., lack of empathy, rigidity, concrete thinking, shallow affect, and childlike behavior) that result in impaired social competency and relations (Becker & Vakil, 1993; Miller, 1991; Warriner & Velikonja, 2006).

Patients recovering from brain injury encounter a number of social challenges, including difficulties with communication pragmatics, friendships, dating/romantic relationships, and leisure activities, as well as substance abuse issues. This chapter discusses these challenges and how to assist patients in overcoming them. Neurorehabilitation should focus on reestablishing meaningful leisure—the "play" and social aspects of recovery—to enhance community adjustment and quality of life (Morton & Wehman, 1995; Prigatano, 1989; Steadman-Pare, Colantonio, Ratcliff, Chase, & Vernich, 2001; Tomberg et al., 2005; Worthington, Matthews, Melia, & Oddy, 2006). This process often starts with evaluating and treating problems with the pragmatics of communication.

## THE PRAGMATICS OF COMMUNICATION

Social communication impairment is prevalent after acquired brain injury (Coelho, Youse, & Le, 2002). This often consists of difficulties with the "pragmatics" of communication, defined as the subtle social rules governing the use of communication, or the skills and abilities related to conversational exchanges (Cummings, 2007; Friedland & Miller, 1998; Wiseman-Hakes, Stewart, Wasserman, & Schuller, 1998). Communication pragmatics include three main components: (1) using language for different purposes, such as greeting, informing, demanding, promising, and requesting; (2) adapting or changing language according to the listener/situation, or giving sufficient background information to a listener who needs it; and (3) following the rules of conversation, such as turn taking, topic maintenance, rephrasing when misunderstood, appropriate facial expressions, and appropriate physical distance between speakers (American Speech–Language–Hearing Association, 1997–2005; Wiseman-Hakes et al., 1998). Communication pragmatics integrate linguistic components (e.g., syntax, phonology, and semantics) and broader cognitive skills (including memory and information processing) with the linguistic and conversational contexts of interactions (Friedland & Miller, 1998). They thus entail a complex interplay among cognitive abilities, self-monitoring of language skills, awareness of social rules, and emotional control (Dahlberg et al., 2007). Prior research has implicated the frontal lobes and right hemisphere in the pragmatics of communication (see Channon & Watts, 2003, for a review). Because patients generally lack insight into the social impact of their behaviors, they often lack the capability and/or motivation to monitor their interaction styles.

Pragmatic communication problems can cluster at two extremes: either a paucity or a surplus of speech and communication. Figure 8.1 lists common pragmatic communication difficulties after acquired brain injury. A dearth of postinjury communication is caused by several factors, often related to frontal lobe dysfunction. Patients with poor initiation skills have difficulty commencing conversations, including introducing themselves and greeting others, or sustaining turn taking during conversations (Coelho et al., 2002). Frontal lobe damage also often produces flattened affect, which hinders the engagement of the listener (Stuss, Gow, & Hetherington, 1992). Or patients may report a scarcity of topics or ideas; this is associated with deficits in higher-order conceptualization and/or thought formulation, word-finding deficits, and reduced speed of information processing

- **Vocal Difficulties**—Difficulty monitoring volume, tone, and/or rate of speech.

- **Impaired Thought Organization**—Difficulty organizing one's thoughts in preparation for clear communication.

- **Reduced Active Listening**—Difficulty maintaining a concerted effort to pay attention to the speaker.

- **Impaired Nonverbal Communication**—Inability to "read"/interpret social cues.

- **Impaired Topic Maintenance**—Difficulty adhering to the topic of conversation and/or preparing the listener for a topic shift.

- **Hyperverbality**—Using excessive words and information when speaking or answering a question.

- **Tangentiality**—Difficulty staying on topic.

- **Poor Turn Taking**—Difficulty maintaining a balance in discourse and not interrupting conversations.

- **Impaired Situational Use of Language**—Difficulty with monitoring and appropriately responding to the environment.

- **Impaired Age-Appropriate Communication**—Reduced awareness of actions and words, based on age and level of maturation.

- **Poor Etiquette**—Lack of use of polite language; inappropriate behaviors or responses.

- **Impulsivity**—Speaking or acting without thinking.

- **Disinhibition**—Inability to inhibit or control inappropriate social behavior.

- **"Snarkiness"**—Irritability, grouchiness, low frustration tolerance.

- **Egotistical Behavior**—Self-centeredness and difficulty seeing others' points of view.

- **Flat Affect**—Decreased facial expression and range of feelings/animation.

- **Lack of Initiation**—Difficulty starting a conversation.

**FIGURE 8.1.** Common pragmatic communication difficulties after brain injury.

(Friedland & Miller, 1998). Working memory deficits can interfere with patients' ability to track conversations and engage in active listening (Channon & Watts, 2003). Patients may also struggle with multitasking, due to challenges associated with the pace and flow of the discussion. Often individuals will need direct questions or prompts from their counterparts to extend the dialogue, and to keep interactions focused and meaningful (Coelho et al., 2002; see Dahlberg et al., 2007, for a review). Patients may also display reduced comfort with vocalizing in groups for other underlying reasons. For example, patients with speech production difficulties (e.g., dysarthria) often become much more self-conscious about conversing with others.

Frontal lobe damage can also produce an array of pragmatic communication difficulties that manifest as an excess of speech. These include hyperverbality and tangentiality (i.e., poor topic maintenance). Patients can be perceived as displaying "empty speech" (Galski, Tompkins, & Johnston, 1998), or speech that to others sounds vague, unfocused, and rambling. Disinhibition, impulsivity, and inappropriate comments (including swearing, insults, or bluntness) can result in exchanges that are considered offensive. Decreased perceptiveness, disorganized output, and poor self-monitoring (see Dahlberg et al., 2007, for a review) can also alienate or weary the listener.

Other worrisome social behaviors often emerge after frontal lobe injury. Patients tend to become more self-centered, in part related to their difficulties with flexible thinking (Stuss & Benson, 1984). This translates into an inability to show empathy, or "put themselves into the shoes of others." This tendency can become habitual, given the extensive attention justifiably lavished on these patients because of their disabilities. When self-centeredness is manifested as demanding and inconsiderate behavior, it can trouble and even overwhelm families, friends, and other social contacts. Patients may also display more childlike behavior, appearing immature in social interactions. This is often manifested in poor social etiquette and the inability to recognize and adapt to the social and communication requirements of varying settings (e.g., casual vs. formal). Verbal exchanges infused with unwarranted emotionality (e.g., "snarkiness") are another pragmatic complication after acquired brain injury; these can cause conversation partners to "walk on eggshells" so as to avoid further unpleasant escalations.

## TREATING PRAGMATIC COMMUNICATION PROBLEMS IN INDIVIDUAL PSYCHOTHERAPY

An essential task of individual psychotherapy after acquired brain injury is to help patients recognize and self-monitor pragmatic communication difficulties (Phases 4 and 5 "green" adaptive coping zone of the PEM). Identifying and discussing these communication issues can be quite perplexing and disturbing to patients, and may violate their self-concept. A strong working alliance with sufficient preparation must precede any intervention, so as not to offend a patient. The psychotherapist should strongly consider enlisting the participation of a speech–language pathologist, given his or her expertise in this field. It is helpful to provide neutral information first, in the form of generic handouts (e.g., Figure 8.1) or journal abstracts, to help ease the patient into the discussion.

One helpful tool to improve patients' awareness of communication deficits is a self-evaluation of germane pragmatic communication behaviors (see Figure 8.2). The completed self-appraisal can then be discussed as part of individual psychotherapy. Observations and ratings by significant others (family members, friends, etc.) can also be incorporated. Because of patients' organic unawareness of deficits, the psychotherapist should provide patients with specific examples of problems. This is an excellent exercise for developing awareness.

Conversational exchanges during individual psychotherapy sessions can be a rich source of pragmatic communication events and mishaps, both verbal and nonverbal. The psychotherapist who listens perceptively can discern subtle and sometimes flagrant difficulties. They often emerge on a smaller scale in a session than in other contexts, due to the structure and confines of the psychotherapeutic exchange. In an unstructured, unrestricted setting, these pragmatic communication problems can be exacerbated and alienating. Once a solid working alliance has been established, video recording is an ideal tool to demonstrate to patients their communication style and social impact on others. In session, I advise the following procedures: The psychotherapist should (1) prioritize identified behaviors, starting with the simplest and least threatening; (2) provide immediate feedback, with specific examples; (3) be kind, yet clear, direct, and consistent; (4) use role play to model appropriate substitutes for problematic behaviors; (5) compliment the patient when improvements are observed in the targeted behaviors; and (6) assist the patient in clearly documenting both the nature of the problems and useful compensations.

A patient can construct a personal list of strengths, difficulties, compensations, and goals (see Figure 8.3), with the input and assistance of the psychotherapist. This is an excellent exercise for developing both awareness and acceptance. This list should then be updated on a regular basis, based on clinic- and community-based observations and feedback. The patient should carry this list in the datebook, so that he or she can consult it and incorporate compensations while in community social settings. In this way, it serves as a tangible and accessible reminder.

With the patient's permission and readiness, involvement of family and friends in providing constructive input and helpful reminders can become invaluable for in-session dialogue and rehearsal. Usually this step is undertaken once significant others have reached a comfort level in providing feedback, and once the patient is comfortable receiving feedback from his or her "advisory board." As patients recognize and learn to remediate problematic behaviors, they are usually heartened by improvements in social relations.

Patients' difficulty with "snarkiness" is a common focus of individual psychotherapy sessions. There are several underlying reasons for the emergence of this behavior. For example, it may be a defensive reaction to feedback about injury-related deficits (see Chapter 5). In the context of communication pragmatics, "snarky" behavior often emerges as a form of catastrophic reaction when others reject or avoid patients in social situations. This is especially common when young

Please indicate to what extent you observe these behaviors in yourself since your injury. Circle 0 if you have no problem; 1 if it is mild; 5 if it is severe.

0  1  2  3  4  5     1. I have difficulty starting a conversation.

0  1  2  3  4  5     2. I have difficulty keeping a conversation going.

0  1  2  3  4  5     3. I tend to be more talkative.

0  1  2  3  4  5     4. I tend to be less talkative.

0  1  2  3  4  5     5. I talk about inappropriate subjects.

0  1  2  3  4  5     6. I act inappropriately in social situations.

0  1  2  3  4  5     7. I speak more bluntly.

0  1  2  3  4  5     8. I get off topic when I talk.

0  1  2  3  4  5     9. I tend to interrupt or dominate conversations.

0  1  2  3  4  5     10. I speak with too much detail or in a roundabout manner.

0  1  2  3  4  5     11. I show less range of feeling; I'm less animated.

0  1  2  3  4  5     12. I tend to focus on myself; I'm less involved in listening.

**FIGURE 8.2.** Communication Pragmatics Questionnaire.

Date created: _____

My personal strengths in communication pragmatics include:

1. _____
2. _____
3. _____
4. _____
5. _____

My personal difficulties in communication pragmatics include:

1. _____
2. _____
3. _____
4. _____
5. _____

My personal goals are:

1. _____
2. _____
3. _____
4. _____
5. _____

My compensatory strategies to reach my goal are:

| Difficulty | Compensation |
| --- | --- |
| 1. _____ | _____ |
| 2. _____ | _____ |
| 3. _____ | _____ |
| 4. _____ | _____ |
| 5. _____ | _____ |

Progress toward my goal:

| Date | Progress |
| --- | --- |
| _____ | _____ |
| _____ | _____ |
| _____ | _____ |
| _____ | _____ |

**FIGURE 8.3.** Communication pragmatics strengths and difficulties.

adults attempt to rejoin their preinjury social circle; patients often sense uneasiness or emotional distancing in their peers. Alternatively, patients can become overwhelmed in hectic social situations because of supersensitivity to noise and crowds, and/or discomfort with unpredictable events. Within close relationships (e.g., dating, family), patients may also erupt with "snarky" retorts, triggered by emotional vulnerability and low frustration tolerance. In addition, "snarky" interactions can result from auditory misperceptions, cognitive distortions, and suspiciousness after temporal lobe injury.

Helping patients recognize the underlying causes of "snarkiness" is the first step in ameliorating this behavior. Patients can be educated about "snarky" responses as manifestations of frustration, shame, or disillusionment due to catastrophic reactions. Patients can then be guided to identify antecedent events that cause these flareups, and given specific recommendations for recalibrating their thinking. This can include taking a "time out" when feeling irritable, and/ or writing journal entries about troubling thoughts. Another coping mechanism is to develop an external cueing system. For example, the therapist and family members should alert the patient when they feel they are "walking on eggshells." They can also arrange to give the patient a subtle time-out hand signal when they observe an escalation in emotionality. Sometimes humor can defuse the situation when there is a sound working alliance. Family members and other significant social connections should be educated about the underlying reasons for "snarky" behavior, and should be encouraged to "pick their battles" with the patient to avoid unnecessary agitation and conflict. They can also be educated in the "sandwich technique" of giving constructive feedback between positive statements. Selected psychotropic medications can be a helpful supplement to psychotherapy, especially when the patient lacks the internal regulatory mechanisms to exert the necessary self-control of this behavior.

A communication pragmatics log (see the case of Brady, below, for an example) is a technique that helps patients become more accountable for their behaviors. It also functions as an awareness and acceptance tool and training device. With the patient's permission, a rater completes the log by observing and recording the presence or absence of appropriate and inappropriate social communication behaviors. This can be done in therapeutic settings by a therapist and, when possible, at home or at social events by a family member or other support person. As with all therapeutic interventions, the patient must have the emotional insight, capacity, and motivation to cooperate with this process; otherwise, the process will disintegrate into a power struggle or avoidable emotionality.

## CASE STUDY

Brady was age 23 when he sustained a severe traumatic brain injury as a result of a motorcycle accident. His initial Glasgow Coma Scale score was 5, and radiographic studies indicated a right frontotemporal hematoma, left temporal subdural hemorrhage, and shear injury in the cerebellum and midbrain. His background history was significant for attention-deficit/hyperactivity disorder, for which he was treated with Ritalin and Adderall in elementary and high school. Prior to his injury, Brady was an English major in college and had achieved high academic honors. A neuropsychological assessment was conducted at 6 months postinjury; the results were consistent with moderate verbal learning and recall deficits and with moderate executive function deficits, particularly affecting impulse control, strategy generation, flexible thinking, and multitasking. Personality testing on the MMPI-2 indicated impulsivity and oppositional characteristics, and clinical exchanges suggested that Brady's postinjury symptom picture was an exacerbation of preinjury behaviors (i.e., "volume turned up") (see Chapter 3). Brady also presented with mild dysarthria and ataxic gait.

Following the evaluation, Brady initiated individual psychotherapy and was seen on a weekly basis. Clinical observation of Brady during the early individual sessions suggested problems with sensitivity to social mores and poor overall communication pragmatics (Phases 4 and 5 "yellow" warning zone of the PEM). He was easily angered and would make "snarky" comments to the psychotherapist, as well as to his parents, with whom he lived. He showed acting-out and rule-breaking behavior—for instance, refusing to follow through with household chores and insisting that it was easier for his mother than for him to do these activities, because of his memory difficulties. Tensions would then often escalate between Brady and his parents, and they viewed him as hostile, self-centered, and demanding. His difficulties with emotional dysregulation also affected social relationships. His girlfriend of 3 years had ended their relationship just prior to Brady's initiating therapy, stating that his volatility, bluntness, and overall insensitivity to her had become intolerable.

Brady clearly had feelings of self-loathing and low self-esteem, secondary to his dysarthria. He was encouraged to pursue speech–language therapy, which he began in conjunction with his individual psychotherapy. Sessions focused on improving his speech intelligibility, articulation precision, prosody, and voice through speech and breathing exercises, overarticulation, and a slower rate of talking.

The psychotherapist's observation of Brady's pragmatic communication skills revealed problems with disinhibited comments in the form of sarcasm and off-color jokes or comments. He was also very inflexible and impolite in his social interactions. His emotions would easily escalate during individual psychotherapy sessions: He would shake with anger, raise his voice, and refuse to engage in mutual dialogue with turn taking and consideration of the psychotherapist's perspective. Sometimes he would "pick fights." Brady was often suspicious of the motives of others, especially his parents, whom he viewed as unfair and unsympathetic to his needs and feelings. Overall, his clinical presentation revealed significant pragmatic communication deficits, consistent with frontal and temporal lobe dysfunction.

Because of his organic unawareness, Brady was perplexed about the social alienation and isolation he was experiencing. However, he gradually developed a trusting and constructive working alliance with the psychotherapist and was highly motivated to improve his social skills, especially after the dissolution of his romantic relationship. Brady's education about pragmatic communication difficulties included didactic material, self-ratings, and compilation of a strengths-and-difficulties checklist (see Figures 8.1, 8.2, and 8.3). Particular emphasis was placed on his challenges with active listening skills, poor etiquette, impulsivity, disinhibition, "snarkiness," and egotistical behavior. Collateral information was obtained from his family, including specific examples of argumentative behavior in the home. He was introduced to the mantra "Stop, look, and listen" as a way to "put on the brakes" and self-evaluate his interaction style.

Brady also collaborated with his psychotherapist and speech–language pathologist in developing a communication pragmatics log, which identified specific appropriate and inappropriate behaviors (see Figure 8.4). As specific examples of poor communication pragmatics arose during the sessions, the psychotherapist

| Appropriate | Inappropriate |
|---|---|
| 1. Stay cool, calm, and collected; disengage and take a "time out"; practice active listening | 1. Avoid "snarky" behavior; raising my voice, arguing, resisting suggestions |
| 2. Stop, look, and listen; be "professional" | 2. Avoid childlike behavior, verbal tantrums |
| 3. Stick with the "big-picture" topic | 3. Don't "nit-pick" or argue semantics (e.g., wording vs. concept) |
| 4. Put myself in the recipient's shoes; remember the "Golden Rule" | 4. Avoid off-color jokes, making fun of people, insults or sarcasm, being unkind |
| 5. Focus on being polite and respectful; be a "mensch" | 5. Avoid rude comments, swearing |
| 6. Meet others halfway; practice give and take; "go with the flow" | 6. Don't be critical or judgmental; avoid rigid or "black-and-white" thinking |

| Did I demonstrate appropriate communication pragmatics? Date: _____ |||
|---|---|---|
| Time | Comments | Initials |
| 9:00–10:00 A.M. | Y / N | |
| 10:00–11:00 | (Y)/ N   Better listening skills in Communication Pragmatics Group | BH |
| 11:00–12:00 | Y /(N)  Black and white thinking about the Home Independence Checklist | DPG |
| 12:00–1:00 P.M. | Y /(N)  Off-color joke during lunchtime | PSK |
| 1:00–2:00 | Y /(N)  Snarky retorts to psychotherapist when given constructive input | PSK |
| 2:00–3:00 | (Y)/ N   Respectful to speech–language pathologist | BH |
| 3:00–4:00 | Y / N | |
| 4:00–5:00 | (Y)/ N   Flexible about running errands | Mom |

etc.

**FIGURE 8.4.** Brady's communication pragmatics log.

and Brady used the log to process these, with the psychotherapist role-playing more appropriate behaviors. For example, Brady threatened to "tell off" and then "write off" a new friend after the friend canceled a social event at short notice because of illness. Brady's level of self-centeredness and inflexibility interfered with his ability to see the "big picture" and show a sense of empathy toward others. The psychotherapist would often play the "devil's advocate" to challenge Brady to reconceptualize issues from the opposite vantage point. Homework assignments included a written composition contrasting varying perspectives on issues (e.g., Brady's vs. his parents' vs. the psychotherapist's view of the pitfalls of being the "center of the universe"). The therapist also suggested that Brady bring in drafts of e-mail exchanges with friends, to be reviewed before they were sent. This was a practical exercise to generalize healthy communication habits to outside communications.

To assist Brady in diffusing his volatility and emotionality, he was encouraged to think of the television program *Dragnet* and focus on "just the facts." This mantra was a self-monitoring technique that reminded him to adopt some emotional distance and respond in a more neutral, objective manner. All of these exercises were conducted to help remediate his executive function deficits in the social milieu. With time, a shorter communication pragmatics list was developed and placed in his datebook:

1. Think before I speak.
2. Other people's feelings are as important as mine.
3. What goes around comes around (e.g., kindness, compassion).

The psychotherapist also explored psychodynamic issues as part of Brady's communication setbacks. As stated above, Brady had been very bright before his traumatic brain injury, and prided himself on his quick wit and intellectual prowess. He described himself as "intellectually arrogant," and would react to others with disdain when he could outsmart them. After his brain injury, Brady was acutely aware of his cognitive shortfalls; his way of dealing with his narcissistic rage was to verbally attack, "pounce" on, and ultimately demean others, to eradicate his feelings of humiliation and despair (Klonoff & Lage, 1991). His preoccupation with others' imperfections (particularly his parents') distracted him from facing and adapting to his altered abilities.

A diagram of his self-defeating cycle was presented to Brady (see Figure 8.5). His provoking and inflammatory behavior precipitated defensive reactions or hurt in others. This gave him temporary feelings of power, control, and victory, but it also alienated others, which ultimately increased his feelings of rejection and loneliness. The cycle was continually regenerated and intensified over time, particularly because he was not consciously aware of it. Brady was helped to recognize that his underlying feelings of insecurity and inadequacy were being displaced as superficial arrogance, whereas sensitivity to others was the optimal solution. He also came to recognize that his excessive need for admiration, his lack of empathy, and his sense of entitlement were creating destructive consequences. Once Brady reached a better understanding of the underlying reasons

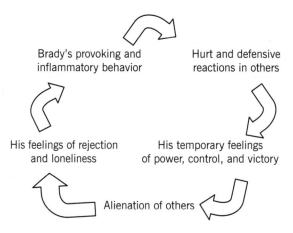

**FIGURE 8.5.** Brady's self-defeating communication cycle.

for his disruptive and self-destructive behavior, his commitment to altering these behaviors intensified significantly. His ability to show self-forgiveness for his depleted capabilities ultimately translated into forgiveness and tolerance of others' imperfections.

The insight-oriented psychotherapy also focused on his family of origin and the underlying reasons for his "snarkiness" and rebelliousness at home. Brady's father had been very lenient during Brady's formative years, and Brady had developed antiauthority and rule-breaking behavior at an early age. His postinjury memory deficits required him to be much more regimented and disciplined, in direct contrast to his preinjury nonconformist, "free-spirit" lifestyle. His parents recognized the need for structure (e.g., the datebook, pillbox, and Home Independence Checklist), but when they attempted to impose this structure, Brady became enraged. Therefore, individual psychotherapy sessions were used to help Brady accept these tools and refrain from "killing the messenger" when his parents provided necessary cues and supports.

Essays on pertinent topics were assigned, including the meaning and value of tolerance and self-discipline. Given Brady's knowledge of literature, suitable quotes and literary passages were incorporated in his therapy. For example, Brady brought in the following quotation from Oscar Wilde's *The Picture of Dorian Gray:* "As it was, we always misunderstood ourselves, and rarely understood others" (Wilde, 1891/1998, p. 97). This launched a pithy existential discussion about alienation and emotional detachment versus relatedness. Brady admittedly had real difficulty controlling his postinjury impulsivity and agitation. He was seen by a psychiatrist and was prescribed a low dose of risperidone, which helped him control his agitation and tendency to misperceive the actions and intentions of others.

Family sessions were instrumental in setting proper ground rules in the home. His parents were given specific guidelines to reduce tensions, including "picking their battles"; disengaging from bickering once Brady started to show signs of agitation; keeping communications clear and concise; finding the middle ground and avoiding ultimatums and polarization; adopting an attitude that "the punishment fits the crime" when transgressions and conflicts arose; and using the sandwich technique to give feedback politely when their son was demeaning or needlessly sarcastic.

Overall, Brady utilized his individual psychotherapy sessions effectively to raise topics of concern. He matured nicely in his social communication style through these acquired insights and adaptive coping techniques (reaching the Phases 4 and 5 "green" adaptive coping zone of the PEM). Once he returned to college, he became more sensitized to nonverbal communication signals; through continued psychotherapy, he gradually made good progress in refining his humor and self-monitoring his sarcasm. With therapeutic urging, Brady also became involved in volunteer activities with a local organization to assist the elderly by delivering meals to their homes. This greatly increased Brady's empathy for others. It also provided real-life practice in communication pragmatics, which further polished his skills. Once he was comfortable doing so, Brady shared more about his neurological history with his supervisor in this organization, and voluntarily solicited her perceptions of his social skills and interactions. Lastly, his psychotherapist also counseled Brady to enroll in a communications class at the college, which provided additional practice in and education about appropriate communication pragmatics.

## ADJUNCT GROUP THERAPIES FOR INCREASING SOCIAL SKILLS AND LEISURE ACTIVITIES

### Communication Pragmatics Group

Therapeutic group exchanges are ideal for ameliorating deficits in communication pragmatics (Braverman et al., 1999). A communication pragmatics group can be formed to provide psychoeducation, peer input, and skill reacquisition. Preferably, this group should be facilitated by the psychotherapist/neuropsychologist and a speech–language pathologist. If possible, this group should be held weekly for a designated time period (e.g., 8–12 weeks), to provide regular opportunities to learn and rehearse new techniques. Figure 8.6 is a purpose sheet to familiarize patients with the intent of the group. Purposes include (1) increasing patients' awareness of communication pragmatics; (2) improving their ability to self-monitor and modify communication behaviors; and (3) helping them to discriminate between effective/appropriate and ineffective/inappropriate communication behaviors within particular social environments. Specifically, patients practice expressing ideas appropriately, improve their comprehension skills, and role-play interactions in social situations. Patients are encouraged to share their self-appraisal rating scales and their lists of pragmatic communication strengths and difficulties with the group. This facilitates peer and staff input, as well as supplemental psychoeducation.

During this group, patients can practice improving the pragmatics of their communication with a number of exercises. Figure 8.7 is a list of pragmatic com-

**Purposes**

1. To increase our awareness of appropriate and inappropriate communication behaviors.

2. To learn to self-monitor our communication behaviors.

3. To learn to modify our communication behaviors appropriately within different social environments.

**Why Is This Group Important?**

The way we communicate and interact with people will affect the way they respond to us.

**Activities**

1. To practice expressing ideas appropriately.

2. To practice better comprehension skills.

3. To practice interacting appropriately.

**Target Behaviors**

1. Nonverbal communication

2. Initiation

3. Disinhibition

4. Hyperverbality

5. Getting to the point

6. Tangentiality

7. Social appropriateness

8. Flat affect

9. Egotistical behavior

10. Thought organization

11. Turn taking

12. Topic maintenance

13. Active listening

14. Rate of speech

15. Volume of speech

**FIGURE 8.6.** Communication pragmatics group purpose sheet.

---

1. *Topic:*     Conversing

   *Exercise:*  Role-play and video-record impressions of a movie you saw with a friend.

2. *Topic:*     Nonverbal communication

   *Exercise:*  Role-play various nonverbal communications (e.g., eye contact, hand gestures, and proximity); watch excerpts from the movie *Hitch* (Lassiter et al., 2005).

3. *Topic:*     Pragmatics when eating

   *Exercise:*  Video-record and discuss a community outing at a restaurant.

4. *Topic:*     What to say in difficult situations

   *Exercise:*  Role-play and video-record someone offending you about your deficits.

5. *Topic:*     Conflict resolution

   *Exercise:*  Role-play and video-record disagreements between friends about what restaurant to eat at.

6. *Topic:*     Appropriate forms of humor

   *Exercise:*  Review video-recorded examples of appropriate and inappropriate joking, and discuss.

7. *Topic:*     Meeting new people

   *Exercise:*  Role-play and video-record meeting someone new at a party.

8. *Topic:*     Appropriate topics and active listening skills, including nonverbal signs

   *Exercise:*  Role-play and video-record a first date.

9. *Topic:*     Pragmatics during game playing

   *Exercise:*  Video-record a game of Scrabble between patients.

10. *Topic:*     Appropriate e-mail correspondence

   *Exercise:*  Write an e-mail to a friend you haven't heard from in a while.

11. *Topic:*     Teamwork/sportsmanship

   *Exercise:*  Play a Wii game together.

12. *Topic:*     Pragmatic behavior at doctors' appointments

   *Exercise:*  Role-play and video-record an interaction at your doctor's office.

**FIGURE 8.7.** Pragmatic communication topics and exercises.

munication topics and relevant exercises. For each topic, a didactic presentation should be given, including the definition of each concept, neuroanatomical correlates, a list of "dos and don'ts," and suggestions for personalized compensations. Patients can then use these guidelines in their social interactions. Observations of patients' interactions by the group facilitators provide excellent "grist" for the psychotherapy "mill." Patients can also benefit from round-robin discussions, where they provide examples of relevant topics based on their social activities (e.g., attending a party over the weekend and meeting new people). These topics also lend themselves well to homework (e.g., self-reflection exercises about a social situation that transpired over the weekend). Role playing and video recording are therapeutic tools for developing appropriate pragmatics of communication, especially in casual conversations or when the video recording takes place in candid situations. Patients can obtain actual experience and clear-cut feedback regarding their social interaction styles, so as to refine their skills. Therapists can also easily role-play or model appropriate and inappropriate interaction styles for patients to critique. Overall, this blend of psychoeducation and experiential exercises provides invaluable practical experiences and bolsters patients' confidence and competency in various social settings.

## Current Events Group

Meaningful social exchanges can be daunting for patients after brain injury. Often they can focus on little besides their injury, and others may view them as narrow or boring conversationalists. Some emphasis on current events can be included as part of a communication pragmatics group, as part of individual psychotherapy, or in a current events group (Klonoff, Lamb, Henderson, Reichert, et al., 2000). Speech–language pathologists make excellent coleaders for this type of group. Encouraging patients to keep abreast of news and events outside their personal lives not only improves their social comfort, but supplies topics to talk about in social settings. Patients with memory difficulties can be encouraged and/or assisted by family members to write short daily news summaries in their datebooks, to help prompt them about current events (see Figure 6.1 in Chapter 6 for an example).

In the group setting, patients can be invited to bring in news articles or noteworthy topics of their choosing. Alternatively, articles can be provided by the group facilitators. Patients can gain valuable practice in conceptualizing and expounding upon the main ideas of each article, as well as sharing opinions in a socially sensitive manner. Group exchanges also provide the psychotherapist with direct observation of patients' listening skills, tolerance for dissenting opinions, and other pragmatic communication skills (Klonoff, Lamb, Henderson, Reichert, et al., 2000). Patients can be given supplemental homework assignments to discuss the news items as part of family meals or social events. Family members' or friends' input regarding the patients' thought formulation and delivery style can then be incorporated in follow-up therapy sessions. Patients often report positive reactions to this therapeutic intervention, as they develop a useful structured repertoire of meaningful conversational topics to share with others.

## Community Outings

Often patients' former leisure activities are inaccessible after brain injury, due to cognitive, physical, and functional limitations. Patients may also be much more self-conscious in the community, especially if they present with overt physical and/or expressive language deficits, which can baffle the general public. Some therapeutic settings incorporate community outings to target community reintegration and social skills (Braverman et al., 1999; Klonoff, Lamb, Henderson, Reichert, et al., 2000). Ideally, a recreational therapist, speech–language pathologist, physical therapist, and occupational therapist collaborate on these outings. Inclusion of the psychotherapist gives him or her invaluable opportunities to witness patients' behavior, interpersonal interactions, and overall mood and adjustment outside the confines of the treatment room. Importantly, patients are also exposed to leisure and cultural venues with which they are often unfamiliar. They can then pursue these outlets in their own free time. Favorite pastimes include sports events, bowling, museums, unique restaurants, zoos, and picnics.

Community outings in the context of neurorehabilitation provide a protective and structured form of reacclimation to social activities. At the same time, they can improve patients' leadership and cognitive skills, including time management, directionality, receptive and expressive language skills, and other salient executive functions critical for meaningful social relationships (e.g., flexible problem solving, judgment, decision making, initiation, follow-through, and impulse control).

One beneficial format is to assign a different "job" to each patient going on the outing, and then to provide each patient with the requisite therapy to master this role, including functional compensations (e.g., checklists). These jobs can include leading the group, being the time keeper, making phone calls, handling the expenses, and creating the map to the destination. Before each outing, patients should meet in a therapeutic planning group to decide on a destination (Klonoff, Lamb, Henderson, Reichert, et al., 2000). The process of discussing options and arriving at a consensus is an important communication pragmatics exercise; it provides training applicable to many other social interactions and milieus, including friendships, dating, and event planning. Patients should be encouraged to identify specific and personalized goals for each outing. Group feedback sessions after the outing provide a setting to address areas of concern and upgrade compensations. The psychotherapist's involvement in the group also provides each patient with an opportunity to observe positive modeling behavior, practice pragmatic communication skills, address behavioral concerns, and incorporate pretaught compensations (e.g., the datebook). All of this yields worthwhile observations to be processed in follow-up sessions.

### CASE STUDY

Brady had the opportunity to participate in a current events group and community outings as part of his therapy schedule. The current events group provided him with practice to improve his articulation, decrease his tangentiality, and expand his narrow and rigid thinking. When potentially "hot" topics were raised (e.g., politics, religion), he would escalate into an argumentative and sometimes insulting stance. His psychotherapist attended these groups, and Brady was also video-recorded as part of the group interactions. Specific ground rules for discussion were developed for Brady, including monitoring his tendency to interrupt, criticize others, raise his voice, roll his eyes, shake his fist when upset, and tip back in his chair. Peer input, review of videos, and observational data from his psychotherapist enhanced Brady's level of awareness and appreciation of his social impact on others, and marked improvement was noted over 12 weekly sessions.

Initially during community outings, Brady was somewhat socially withdrawn and did not contribute ideas to the planning sessions. He was socially awkward and had difficulty generating topics of discussion while on the outings. His gait was quite ataxic, and he was noticeably unsteady navigating in small spaces (e.g., in restaurants). When he became self-conscious, he would diverge into sarcasm and rude humor; at times he would ridicule other patients. His psychotherapist observed that other patients felt offended and annoyed by his behavior and avoided him. He was self-centered; for instance, he did not give others space to sit in the van, or share snacks at the movie theater. He also avoided using his datebook, resulting in forgetfulness, which triggered catastrophic reactions (e.g., he became "snarky" with the therapists, blaming them for his mistakes). On one occasion, he removed his seat belt, abruptly stood up while the van was moving, and made an obscene gesture to a car that was tailgating the van. Brady had difficulty appreciating both the physical and social danger associated with such behavior.

All of these events were processed as part of his individual psychotherapy. At one juncture, Brady was suspended from the community outings until he restated his willingness to demonstrate respectful and socially acceptable behavior toward the therapists and his peers, and recommitted himself to using the necessary compensations. The relationship of his outbursts (catastrophic reactions) to self-consciousness about his physical appearance and dysarthria was also addressed as part of his individual psychotherapy, and alternative coping techniques were provided. These included working through his feelings in therapy sessions rather than projecting them onto others. Role-playing exercises were conducted in individual psychotherapy on expressing his needs in a socially acceptable manner, and "repairing" situations where he had been offensive to others. As part of his individual psychotherapy, Brady watched the movie *Pay It Forward* (Abrams et al., 2000) as an example of the benefits of giving back to his community and showing empathy rather than being judgmental. With practice and direct feedback, Brady's behavior and socialization skills improved nicely.

## REESTABLISHING FRIENDSHIPS AND PURSUING ENJOYABLE PASTIMES

Reestablishing friendships after brain injury can be a significant challenge (Charles, Butera-Prinzi, & Perlesz, 2007; Dikmen et al., 2003; Howes et al., 2005; Inzaghi et al., 2005), given the alterations in patients' personalities, cognitive status, interests, physical capabilities, accessibility, environmental constraints, commonalities, and life paths (Doig, Fleming, & Tooth, 2001). Changes in self-image and self-consciousness, including feelings of inferiority, often interfere with patients' willingness to socialize or comfort with socializing outside familiar contexts (Dikmen et al., 2003; Inzaghi et al., 2005; Kaplan De-Nour & Bauman, 1980). Younger patients in particular report abandonment by their friends, especially when the sequelae of their injuries are conspicuous or disturbing. Friendships are crucial for younger patients' maturation and self-identity (Morton & Wehman, 1995), and so feeling like a social outcast is particularly troubling. Physical limitations and the inability to drive can add to social ostracism, which results in feelings of loneliness, depression, and anxiety (see Morton & Wehman, 1995, for a review).

As part of individual psychotherapy, patients should be encouraged to explore healthy social outlets in the community. Helping patients find enjoyable relationships and leisure interests, and monitoring their involvement in these, will proactively reduce the likelihood of loneliness and social isolation. Exploration of and integration into postinjury leisure pursuits are best handled by a recreational therapist; however, a psychotherapist can also tackle this domain and can actively investigate various resources during sessions with a patient.

Positive and emotionally satisfying leisure pursuits are summarized in Figure 8.8. Community-based outlets include faith-based singles' groups; classes in patients' areas of interest at local community colleges; new hobbies and sports pursued in a group format through local parks and recreation departments; exer-

---

**Community-Based**
- Faith-based singles' groups
- Community college classes in subjects of interest to patients
- Leisure/sports groups through local parks and recreation departments
- Exercise clubs
- Cultural events
- Community support groups for patients with brain injury
- Social groups for patients with brain injury and their support networks
- Adapted sports/adventure groups
- Peer mentorship
- Work/school friendships
- Volunteer work
- Internet links (e.g., *www.meetup.com*; *www.facebook.com*)

**Home-Based**
- Crosswords, puzzles
- Handicrafts (e.g., rug hooking, knitting, embroidery, crocheting)
- Models
- Leather working
- Wood burning
- Beading
- Art projects
- Pets

**FIGURE 8.8.** Leisure pursuits.

cise clubs; community support groups for survivors of brain injury; and social groups initiated by patients and their families as extensions of groups in neurorehabilitation treatment settings. Patients can also develop new friendships through their work and school endeavors; volunteer work activities involving "giving back" to the community are psychologically fulfilling and wholesome activities as well. Peer mentorship programs (Hibbard et al., 2002) enhance patients' quality of life and feelings of empowerment. Exploration of healthy social outlets can also be conducted online; many websites (e.g., *www.meetup.com*) can now serve as social resources for patients. Other networking sites (e.g., *www.facebook.com*) can help patients both reconnect to former friends and develop new acquaintances. However, a psychotherapist should be cautious about recommending such sites if worrisome pragmatic communication problems are present. At the very least, their use may need to be monitored intermittently by family members and/or the psychotherapist. Many communities offer trips and adventures adapted for patients with brain injury (Walker, Onus, Doyle, Clare, & McCarthy, 2005), or adapted sports (e.g., horseback riding, water sports). Most communities offer periodicals advertising local concerts, art events, and other social events that can be enticing to patients. Encouraging patients to broaden their cultural interests and activities also increases their likelihood of developing new social contacts.

Often patients must shift their hobby and leisure interests away from higher-risk physical sports and toward other entertaining and productive hobbies and leisure pursuits. The psychotherapist should have access to common and diversified hobby and craft ideas, and ideally should work collaboratively with a recreational or occupational therapist in this regard. Gratifying (as well as therapeutic) activities include crosswords, puzzles, model building, leather work, wood burning, beading, art projects, and other handicrafts (e.g., rug hooking, knitting, crocheting, embroidery). Often pets provide wonderful companionship and help to alleviate loneliness, especially for patients who are more home-bound. Incidentally, pet care also provides opportunities to practice key compensations related to independence and responsibility, which will boost patients' self-confidence and psychological well-being. The resulting improvements in mood and adjustment will positively affect family and friend interactions.

## CASE STUDY

Through dialogue in individual psychotherapy, Brady gradually came to recognize the value of expanding his home- and community-based hobbies and leisure pursuits. First he adopted a kitten, which he fondly (and with a touch of humor) named "PEM" in honor of his ongoing rehabilitation. Brady enjoyed the companionship and the empowerment associated with the opportunity to take care of another being. He also became an avid fan of Sudoku, basking in the victory of solving complicated puzzles.

His psychotherapist introduced Brady to a facilitated community support group; his parents attended a similar group for family members. Several patients and families decided to begin another social group for patients and families, which met monthly on Saturdays. A local community center agreed to host this group. Interested parties agreed to share e-mail addresses, and a patient and his wife agreed to be the organizers. Each month they notified patients and families by e-mail and invited them to a social function. Events included party games, bowling, luncheons, ice cream socials, guest speakers (e.g., a local comedian who presented a humor workshop), local plays, and community sites (e.g., the zoo). Initially Brady was somewhat reluctant to participate in this group; however, his psychotherapist adopted the "Try it, you'll like it" approach. Lo and behold, over time he became friendly with some of the participants and found that he enjoyed the activities. A few months later, Brady and several group members had developed such camaraderie that they went on a cruise together.

## SUBSTANCE ABUSE AND SOCIAL ACTIVITIES

Both pre- and postinjury substance abuse can be a major impediment to reestablishing healthy recreational activities and friendships. Often the social lives of older adolescents and young adults center around parties and social gatherings with substance use or abuse (Wehman et al., 2000). Patients with traumatic brain injury also have a high prevalence of preinjury substance use disorders (Hibbard, Uysal, Kepler, Bogdany & Silver, 1998; Koponen et al., 2002; Miller, 1993; Rogers & Read, 2007; see Taylor, Kreutzer, Demm, & Meade, 2003, for a review). Maximizing postinjury neurological and functional recovery requires abstinence from alcohol and other substances (Schmidt & Heinemann, 1999); weekend social activities involving drinking or drug use should be off limits. Eventually, however, patients may drift back to these social outlets out of loneliness and desperation, or as a continuation of preinjury abuse patterns, now exacerbated by impulse control deficits (Horner et al., 2005; Langley, 1991; Schmidt & Heinemann, 1999). Postinjury mood disorders, including anxiety and depression, also predispose patients to a resurgence of substance abuse (Hibbard et al., 1998; Horner et al., 2005; Jorge et al., 2005). Lastly, reduced social and coping skills, as well as poor adaptive problem solving, predispose patients to substance abuse (Schmidt & Heinemann, 1999).

Patients who either willingly or "by default" reenter a substance-using social scene are at high risk for substance abuse, which can complicate their neurological recovery. Studies indicate that as many as 43% of patients with brain injuries can be classified as moderate to heavy drinkers (Kolakowsky-Hayner et al., 2002). Some researchers have described a "window of opportunity" in the early postinjury phases to facilitate abstinence; otherwise, patients are more likely to use substances (Bombardier, Ehde, & Kilmer, 1997; see Taylor et al., 2003, for a review). Therefore, at-risk patients should be identified and afforded relapse prevention education and treatment for substance abuse (Bombardier, Temkin, Machamer, & Dikmen, 2003; Hensold, Guercio, Grubbs, Upton, & Faw, 2006; Langley, 1991; Miller, 1993; Schmidt & Heinemann, 1999; Sparadeo, 1993; see Taylor et al., 2003, for a review), as well as introductions to healthy, diverse, and meaningful social and leisure outlets that are drug- and alcohol-free (Cox et al., 2003; see Taylor et al., 2003, for a review).

It is advisable for the individual psychotherapist to maintain a watchful eye for, and regularly inquire about, patients' postinjury substance use. Some professionals find screening tools or symptom checklists helpful, so as to ascertain the severity and extent of substance abuse (Schmidt & Heinemann, 1999; Sobell & Sobell, 2005). Patients often do not admit to substance use relapse; therefore, a trusting, nonpunitive relationship is a prerequisite for patients' willingness to make such admissions. Other therapeutic components include use of interdisciplinary services; coping skills and problem-solving training; concrete goal-directed strategies; and education about the impact of substance use on functional/independent living skills (Langley, 1991; Miller, 1993; Schmidt & Heinemann, 1999; Sparadeo, 1993). Provision of articles and educational materials to buttress recommendations for abstinence is optimal for the psychoeducational process. If need be, patients should be required to undergo random urinalysis to make sure they are abstaining, given the magnitude of the negative effects of substance abuse on recovery. Collateral input from significant others and family members can help a patient and therapist maintain factual dialogue (Sobell & Sobell, 2005). Psychoeducational and support interventions for family members are also fundamental to helping a patient achieve and maintain sobriety (Miller, 1993; Sparadeo, 1993).

The psychotherapist will need to decide how to proceed with a patient who has an active substance abuse problem, as such a patient is at risk of further injury, as well as other self-defeating behaviors. One option is to transfer treatment to a substance abuse specialist. However, to avoid abandonment or premature termination and other possible deleterious consequences, appropriate referrals must be coordinated in advance. Depending on the psychotherapist's comfort level and expertise, the patient may agree to embark on substance abuse treatment in conjunction with current psychotherapy efforts (e.g., a 12-step program, a church-related support group including a sponsor, or treatment from other substance abuse agencies) (Miller, 1993).

## DATING AND ROMANTIC RELATIONSHIPS

Initiating dating relationships after brain injury adds another level of complexity to interpersonal relationships. Many patients crave a postinjury relationship with a significant other, but struggle with how to create and then sustain a healthy, meaningful, two-way relationship (Burton, Leahy, & Volpe, 2003; Donnelly, Donnelly, & Grohman, 2005; see Morton & Wehman, 1995, for a review). Common impediments to initiating dating relationships are lowered self-esteem and changes in body image. Threats to sustaining dating relationships appear most often related to frontal lobe dysfunction and the concomitant problems in impulsivity, disinhibition, judgment, inflexibility, initiation, decision making, flat affect, and social pragmatics. Other threats include aggression, temper outbursts, and mood swings (Wood et al., 2005). Very often patients "come on too strong" and overwhelm potential mates by telephoning, texting, or e-mailing them excessively, and/or pressuring them to advance a relationship more quickly than the norm. Blunt or childlike behavior can also have a negative impact on a new relationship. Furthermore, as stated above, identifying social outlets where a patient can meet potential partners can be challenging. Patients may resort to "chat rooms" and computer dating services, which can raise some safety concerns, especially for patients with emotional and/or physical vulnerabilities.

Reestablishing a romantic relationship has its own intrinsic challenges (see Klonoff & Prigatano, 1987, for a review). Often the uninjured partner is very overwhelmed by the patient's acute neurological and functional deficiencies. The once competent and capable individual is transformed into a dependent being, at least temporarily. The personality of the injured party may also be radically altered, and he or she may seem like a stranger. Understandably but unfortunately, the patient may project his or her negative emotions onto the partner, because the partner is both familiar and accessible. A patient's inability to drive or earn an income, and other practical considerations, can further discourage a partner. When the patient's capacity for empathy and sensitivity are also affected, the partner may feel a sense of emotional emptiness. Often the partner cannot express grief for these losses, for fear of offending or distressing the patient.

Postinjury changes in sexuality can be the products of physiological, medical, reactive psychological, behavioral, and psychosocial sequelae, and they can have a major impact on self-esteem and quality of life (Ducharme, 1993; Howes, Edwards, & Benton, 2005b; Johnson, Knight, & Alderman, 2006). Changes may include sexual dysfunction and sexually intrusive or inappropriate behavior (Bezeau, Bogod, & Mateer, 2004; Johnson et al., 2006). Physiological changes may include reduced or heightened libido, cognitive inertia, and various types of sexual dysfunction affecting drive, arousal, orgasm, and ejaculation (Butler & Satz, 1988; Kreuter, Dahllof, Gudjonsson, Sullivan, & Siosteen, 1998; Sandel, Williams, Dellapietra, & Derogatis, 1996; see Schopp et al., 2006, for a review). Organically based difficulties with hormonal and neurotransmitter regulation may also have a negative impact on sexuality (Butler & Satz, 1988). The anatomical areas implicated include the orbitofrontal cortex, temporal lobes, limbic system, pituitary gland, and basal hypothalamus (Bezeau et al., 2004; Dombrowski, Petrick, & Strauss, 2000; Kreuter et al., 1998; Mills & Turnbull, 2004; Stuss & Benson, 1984).

Emotional sequelae affecting sexual interest and performance may include anxiety and depression (Butler & Satz, 1988). Psychosocial changes may include social isolation, reduced mobility (e.g., transportation), and altered interaction patterns and roles within the relationship/marriage (Butler & Satz, 1988; Dombrowski et al., 2000). Changes in self-concept and body image and a reduced sense of physical attractiveness can further inhibit patients' sexual interest. Behaviorally, patients may be perceived as excessively flirtatious, which may translate into sexual promiscuity or rejection by others.

Romantic relationships and sexuality are suitable topics to address in individual psychotherapy, as patients may place themselves in very vulnerable situations or act out because of faulty judgment and disinhibited impulses, with dire consequences (e.g., pregnancy, sexually transmitted diseases). Healthy intimate relationships are interrelated with patients' identity, self-esteem, and values (Ducharme, 1993), necessitating a holistic approach. Individual psychotherapy should explore a patient's sexual history, including the role of culture and religion (Ducharme, 1993). Techniques can include sex education; relaxation strategies; psychoeducation to improve problem solving, self-monitoring, social skills, and self-confidence; empathy training; and cognitive-behavioral techniques for anxiety-provoking social and sexual encounters (Bezeau et al., 2004; Dombrowki et al., 2000; Ducharme, 1993; Medlar, 1998; Simpson & Long, 2004). Some medications, such as antidepressants and anticonvulsants, can affect libido (Bezeau et al., 2004; Dombrowski et al., 2000). Patients are often hesitant to discuss these concerns with their treating rehabilitation physician or psychiatrist, but instead may struggle with medication compliance. The psychotherapist can function as an integral intermediary in this communication process.

Individual psychotherapy can also focus on practical advice for dating, including healthy venues for meeting prospective partners (e.g., religious social groups, interest-based classes, other social contacts) and guidelines for pacing a relationship, starting with a friendship. Faith-based reading materials can also provide guidance (e.g., Hilton, 2006). Patients should be discouraged from pursuing the "bar scene," because of the proximity to alcohol. Psychotherapy sessions can also incorporate role playing and video recording to practice anxiety-provoking situations (e.g., a first-date invitation), followed by post hoc analyses (e.g., how the invitation unfolded). The psychotherapist can discuss specific dating episodes, review e-mails, and devise a "dos and don'ts" pragmatic list specific to dating scenarios. Cueing mantras, including the "Golden Rule" ("Do unto others as you would have them do unto you"), can reinforce core relationship principles. Conjoint sessions with the partner are helpful in revealing "the other side of the story" and can facilitate psychoeducation and emotional support for both parties.

## GROUP PSYCHOTHERAPY

Group psychotherapy is an ideal setting to develop communication/social skills and discuss community reintegration after brain injury. Patient "graduates" can provide a healthy real-life perspective on these topics. The group setting can also provide firsthand practice with socially acceptable communication pragmatics, so that patients can put into action the behaviors they are studying. Applicable group discussion topics are listed in Figure 8.9. The advantage of the group format is that it gives patients multiple perspectives and sources of feedback about these complex and sensitive topics.

For example, feelings of estrangement, loneliness, and social isolation often spawn discussions about lowered self-esteem and a sense of being undesirable, like "damaged goods." As an exercise, patients rate their self-perception of postinjury problems with self-confidence on a scale from 0 (no change) to 10 (big change/ much worse). Group sharing permits venting and catharsis about these painful feelings, including infuriation, shame, and despair related to physical signs (e.g., scars, hemiparesis, ataxia) as well as to cognitive/language foibles (e.g., forgetfulness and dysarthria). Eventually, as a group exercise, patients can develop action plans to increase their social activities and reduce the likelihood of becoming "social hermits" (see Figure 8.8). In follow-up sessions, patients are held accountable by one another for following through on these intentions. Another prominent topic is understanding outsiders' avoidance reactions; often patients attribute these to insensitivity or unkindness, instead of recognizing that the aftermath of the injury often produces trepidation and sorrow in others. It is not an intentional snubbing. The more mature group members, with better self-insight, are generally

---

**Alienation, Loneliness, and Social Isolation**
- Why?
- Ways to remediate.

**Friendships**
- Changes from pre- to postinjury.
- Brain-injury-related factors affecting friendships.
- Definition of a "true friendship."
- Finding a social niche.

**Work, Love, and Play**
- Personal definitions.
- Impact of the brain injury.
- New ideas and outlets.

**Romantic Relationships**
- Perceived changes.
- Role of brain-injury-related factors.
- Empathy and the predicaments of others.
- Sexuality and intimacy.

---

**FIGURE 8.9.** Social/communication topics for group psychotherapy.

the ones who adopt this more empathic stance. They can influence patients who are experiencing hurt as a raw emotion.

Still another topic for discussion is the postinjury dissolution of friendships and romantic involvements. A psychoeducational discussion format is promoted, and patients are guided by input from the group facilitator as well as their peers to recognize their own possible negative contributions to their social alienation. The neurological correlates of these behavioral problems are also presented and discussed within the group setting (e.g., the effects of frontal lobe damage on initiation can translate into difficulty with reciprocal event planning). Likely pragmatic contributions include disinhibited comments, intrusive questions, invasion of personal space, hyperverbality, insensitivity to social cues, cognitive rigidity, and self-centered behavior. Patients have also discussed the practical consequences of their injuries for friendships, including altered interests, changed physical capabilities, and different life paths. One group compiled the components of a "true friendship," which included good listening, two-way communication, trustworthiness, commitment, sincerity, guidance, and empathy. The list provided a visual reminder of attributes group members could strive for in order to develop and enhance high-quality relationships.

A vital existential topic is consideration of the balance among work, love, and play (Prigatano, 1989). Many patients report a preinjury imbalance weighted toward work; their injuries open the door to a "second chance" (or "wake-up call"), with new and more meaningful priorities (see Chapter 9). As part of the discussion about play, patients share ideas about travel, new hobbies and outdoor activities, and other social outlets for postinjury companionship. With respect to incorporating love in their lives, patients first look up the dictionary definition and then share how their lives have included and could include both giving and receiving love. Patients also share personal outlets for, and impediments to, attaining a high postinjury quality of life and a joyful existence.

A more sensitive group psychotherapy topic relates to alterations in patients' romantic and marital relationships, including sexuality. As a group exercise, patients disclose whether or not they have experienced a relationship breakup or divorce; generally at least half the members of a group have had such experiences. Patients can then discuss the underlying reasons for disengagement and disappointment, and commiserate about painful feelings of loss. Dialogue about sexual behavior and intimacy are woven into this discussion, depending on the comfort level of the group. This topic becomes an opportunity for the facilitator to present the burdens experienced by the patients' loved ones and the ways that patients can restore their partners' interest in romance and intimacy. Specific concepts include catastrophic reactions by proxy (see Chapter 7); patients' overreliance on partners; practical stressors, including finances and transportation; personality changes, including "snarkiness"; and partners' adjusting to being with the "new" persons the patients have become. A constructive exercise is for patients to brainstorm ways to assist their significant others in their adaptation and happiness, including reiteration of the value of becoming as self-sufficient as possible (e.g., with compensations) and honing their skills as empathic and grateful individuals.

### CASE STUDY

Fifteen months after his injury, Brady was reluctant to initiate dating. He dedicated his energies to his rehabilitation and reimmersion in the community college environment. As Brady's functional and emotional status improved, however, he found himself yearning for a dating relationship. At first he considered online dating, but his psychotherapist recommended he pursue the face-to-face approach that the college environment made possible. Initially he reported considerable ineptness, and several attempts were aborted because of his self-consciousness and shyness. He then used the communication pragmatics group as a forum to practice suitable ways of introducing himself to a young lady. Helpful techniques included video recording, with a particular emphasis on active listening skills and likable humor. Brady loved popular music and took a music appreciation course; there he met a young woman with similar interests. At first, their conversations took place before and after class. Gradually, with coaching and role playing in individual psychotherapy, he worked up the courage to invite her to a concert. During their first date, Brady cautiously shared preliminary information about his traumatic brain injury. His date responded empathically to his story, and in fact had a grandmother who had suffered a stroke. Therefore, she had some understanding of the effects of brain injury on a personal level, which clearly increased her sensitivity and compassion.

As Brady navigated the early phases of the dating relationship, he made a number of errors in social judgment—at times pestering the young woman, and at other times showing some emotional volatility. Early in the relationship, Brady invited his date to attend a psychotherapy session with him, where relevant education was provided. Thereafter, both parties met periodically with his psychotherapist, particularly during times of emotional turmoil and friction. Role playing and discussions centered on enhancing his communication skills, thoughtfulness, and sensitivity to her needs. The couple had many mutual interests, which bolstered the relationship. His partner recognized and validated his talents and uniqueness, and was able to overlook and adapt to his sometimes disruptive behavior. Topics related to sexual intimacy, good judgment, and safe practices were also addressed with the couple. Brady used group psychotherapy as a good forum to discuss his growing insights and social maturation, basking in his newfound balance in work, love, and play (Prigatano, 1989). After 1 year, the romance was progressing smoothly; Brady was extremely happy and worked diligently to nurture and perpetuate the relationship.

With enhanced communication and social skills, patients are best prepared for the next phase of their psychotherapy. Chapter 9 addresses realism, adjustment, and the termination of treatment.

# Adjustment and Treatment Termination

The postinjury adjustment process consists of adaptation and assimilation (see Chapter 5). As depicted in Figure 9.1, these can be further conceptualized on three interactive and interrelated dimensions: *adaptation* (i.e., community reintegration, including the specific activities of work and school); *intrapsychic assimilation* (i.e., self-esteem, self-efficacy, mastery, and happiness); and *existential assimilation* (i.e., meaning, quality of life, self-actualization, and hope). Adjustment is an evolutionary process of transformation and transcendence grounded in realism. By *realism*, I mean the integration of accumulated internal perceptions and external life experiences to produce healthy judgments and attainable objectives for the future. This is the culmination of the awareness and acceptance process, and is depicted in Phase 6 of the PEM (see Chapter 1, Figure 1.2). This chapter discusses the three domains of the adjustment process and describes therapeutic interventions to increase realism and help patients achieve optimal outcomes. It also addresses the process of terminating psychotherapy, including suitable posttreatment resources.

## THE ADAPTATION DIMENSION

The percentages of patients after brain injury who return successfully to work and school vary, ranging from fairly meager to robust proportions (Avesani, Salvi, Rigoli, & Gambini, 2005; Klonoff et al., 2001, 2006, 2007; see Shames et al., 2007, for a review). Negative correlates of productive postinjury work and school reentry include longer periods of posttraumatic amnesia; increased injury severity,

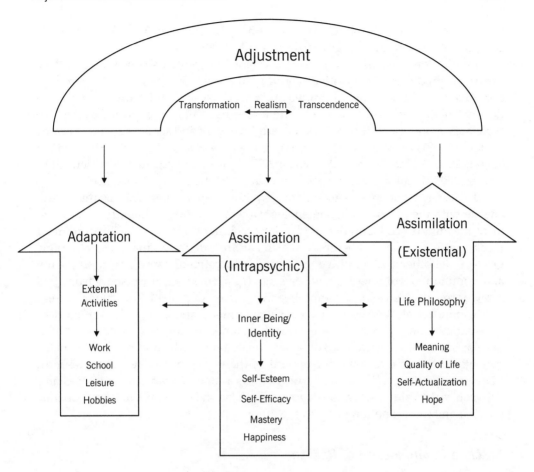

**FIGURE 9.1.** Model of adjustment.

limitations, and disability (especially disability that affects cognition, physicality, communication, and personality); a history of preexisting substance abuse; and minority group membership (Ashley, Ninomiya, Berryman, & Goodwin, 2004; Avesani et al., 2005; Cattelani, Tanzi, Lombardi, & Mazzucchi, 2002; Devitt et al., 2006; Doctor et al., 2005; Kervick & Kaemingk, 2005; Kreutzer et al., 2003; Leung & Man, 2005; Saltapidas & Ponsford, 2007; Sherer, Bergloff, High, & Nick, 1999; Sherer et al., 2007; Willemse-van Son, Ribbers, Verhagen, & Stam, 2007). Positive contributors to postinjury functionality include preinjury employment (Atchison et al., 2004; Leung & Man, 2005; Novack, Bush, Meythaler, & Canupp, 2001; Walker, Marwitz, Kreutzer, Hart, & Novack, 2006; Willemse-van Son et al., 2007); self-awareness, accurate self-appraisal, self-acceptance, and motivation (Ben-Yishay & Daniels-Zide, 2000; Kervick & Kaemingk, 2005; Klonoff et al., 2001; Mateer & Sira, 2006; Ownsworth et al., 2007; Shames et al., 2007; Wise, Ownsworth, & Fleming, 2005); better concurrent neuropsychological status (Atchison et al., 2004; Dawson et al., 2007; Sigurdardottir, Andelic, Roe, & Schanke, 2009); and younger age, male gender, higher education, non-right-hemispheric injury, and driving (Adams, Sherer, Struchen, & Nick, 2004; Dawson et al., 2007; Franulic, Carbonell, Pinto, &

Sepulveda, 2004; Goranson, Graves, Allison, & La Freniere, 2003; Klonoff et al., 2006; Kreutzer et al., 2003; Sigurdardottir et al., 2009).

In addition, various postinjury treatment interventions—including holistic treatment predicated on positive working alliances with patients and families; cognitive remediation; metacognitive and executive skills retraining; compensation instruction; and vocational rehabilitation—have all been reported as positive correlates of both early and extended postinjury work and school success (Abrams & Haffey, 1991; Avesani et al., 2005; High, Roebuck-Spencer, Sander, Struchen, & Sherer, 2006; Klonoff et al., 2001; 2006; 2007; Mateer & Sira, 2006; O'Brien, 2007; Schutz, 2007; Shames et al., 2007; Sherer et al., 2007; Turkstra & Flora, 2002).

To foster a patient's realism, the psychotherapist must first evaluate and engage with the patient's phenomenological world, and then identify and implement meaningful collaborative evidentiary techniques. If possible, I recommend incorporating a range of therapies, which can include individual psychotherapy; group psychotherapy; cognitive retraining, a vocational communication group; and community volunteer, work, or school placements. Information from this array of treatments yields a comprehensive picture of patients' functional potential (Klonoff et al., 1997). Other constructive interventions include written documentation from the work site by therapists and employers (see below). Often developing a list of work- and/or school-related strengths and difficulties helps patients adopt more realistic perceptions of their academic or career aspirations. In these ways, the psychotherapist functions as a conduit, translator, and mediator between real-world observations and feedback on the one hand, and the patients' internal ambitions and longings on the other.

## Baseline Determination of Realism

As in the awareness and acceptance process, the psychotherapist needs to establish a patient's baseline level, or entry point, of realism. Given the chronology of the process of awareness, acceptance, and realism (as depicted in the PEM), the patient may be fairly far along in psychotherapy before this can be determined. The psychotherapist's initial impressions of the patient's degree of realism are partially based on how objective evidence of the patient's capabilities and limitations compares with his or her interests and aspirations. The patient needs to have sufficient memory capacity and executive functions to be able to perform an accurate self-appraisal. Table 9.1 summarizes baseline determinants of realism after brain injury. As with the baseline determinants of acceptance listed in Table 5.1 of Chapter 5, these should be viewed as constituting a fluid continuum rather than discrete or rigid categories.

Highly realistic patients are very aware and acceptant; they are able to see the "big picture," and have identified career aspirations that closely match their neurological strengths and difficulties. These individuals temper their ambitions with real-life, objective evidence of achievements (e.g., work performance evaluations, school grades) in the context of typical external resources. They also prefer to channel their energies toward manageable and attainable goals. These patients capitalize on their strengths and effectively compensate for their deficits, so as to maximize their productivity. They recognize that success in life is not simply

**TABLE 9.1. Baseline Determinants of Realism**

| Low realism | Medium realism | High realism |
|---|---|---|
| 1. Very poor awareness and acceptance | Beginnings of awareness and acceptance | Good awareness and acceptance |
| 2. Defensive and uncomfortable demeanor with inquiry | Tentative openness and receptivity to inquiry | Open and receptive demeanor to inquiry |
| 3. Severe executive function deficits, with poor integration skills and inability to see the "big picture" | Milder executive function deficits; beginnings of integration skills and ability to see the "big picture" | More intact executive functions, with better integration skills and ability to see the "big picture" |
| 4. Poor match between neurological strengths–difficulties and career aspirations | Preliminary match between neurological strengths–difficulties and career aspirations | Good match between neurological strengths–difficulties and career aspirations |
| 5. Adamant rejection of collateral real-life data | Tentative openness to collateral real-life data | Good acceptance of collateral real-life data |
| 6. Idealism; ignoring of practicalities | Downplaying of practicalities in favor of idealistic thinking | Equal weighting of practicalities with ideals and aspirations |
| 7. Belief that anything is possible; "shooting for the stars" | Tendency to overestimate postinjury aptitudes | Belief in selecting attainable/achievable goals |
| 8. Unhealthy sense of preinjury capabilities and limitations | Satisfactory sense of preinjury capabilities and limitations | Healthy sense of preinjury capabilities and limitations |
| 9. Excessive external resources (without these, the patient fails) | External resources (necessary for the patient to achieve minimal success) | Typical external resources (facilitates the patient's success) |
| 10. Poor trust in the working alliance | Beginnings of trust and a developing working alliance | Good trust and a positive working alliance |
| 11. Unrealistic family expectations and goals | Beginnings of realistic family expectations and goals | Realistic family expectations and goals |

brought about by "mind over matter," and that all individuals (both with and without brain injury) have finite capabilities. Often these patients have had positive preinjury experiences of setting and accomplishing goals. They have also experienced periodic failures and been able to focus on making their best efforts rather than on all-or-nothing outcomes. Realistic patients are open and receptive during the inquiry phase, and they have trust in the opinions of their psychotherapists. Their family members also usually have realistic hopes for themselves and for the patients; therefore, the family environment communicates a consistent and viable set of expectations.

Patients with a medium level of baseline realism exhibit the beginnings of awareness and acceptance, with tentative receptivity to real-life data. The match between their perceived and actual neurological strengths and difficulties is "in the ballpark." These patients need external resources (e.g., tutors, job modifications) for basic accomplishments. Nonetheless, they still show a tendency to follow their dreams instead of relying on day-to-day hard evidence of abilities and limitations (e.g., their feats vs. defeats). These individuals generally had a satisfactory preinjury sense of their capabilities and limitations; now, due to executive function deficits (e.g., inability to see the "big picture") and organic unawareness, they tend to overestimate their aptitudes. However, they reveal provisional openness and receptivity during the exploratory dialogue, with the beginnings of trust and a working alliance with the psychotherapist. Their family members also demonstrate the potential to collaborate in developing realistic goals and expectations for their loved ones.

Patients with an initial unrealistic self-perception adamantly reject outside input, typically by blaming the sources of it (e.g., their work supervisors, health care professionals, and/or instructors). This unrealism emanates from poor awareness and acceptance of injury-related sequelae, and it translates into considerable discordance between aspirations and actual achievements. Upon inquiry, these patients display an uncomfortable or defensive demeanor. Generally, they also have very poor executive functions, with an inability to think on the abstract level and employ good judgment or decision making. Their mentality is that of "reaching for the stars," and they exhibit a staunch belief in infinite possibilities. They are unwilling or unable to incorporate the lessons of hard evidence (e.g., work and/or school failures). This "pie-in-the-sky" attitude precludes "down-to-earth" practicalities. These patients are initially highly suspicious of their psychotherapists, feeling that the therapists are holding them back. These patients often mirror the beliefs of their family members, who also tend to insist that "anything is possible." Because of the disparity between these patients' actual skills and the tasks they attempt, they need extraordinary external resources. The burden often falls on the shoulders of a patient's family members, who are essentially "doing the job" for the patient. Exploration of such a patient's preinjury history often reveals a similar pattern of overconfidence and underachievement.

Once a psychotherapist determines a patient's baseline level of realism, he or she has a starting point for therapeutic interventions that will either improve or reinforce the current degree and manifestations of realistic thinking, including planning for the future.

### Fostering Realism in Individual Psychotherapy

A primary component of the psychotherapy process is to foster realism as part of a patient's self-appraisal and goal setting. The psychotherapist needs to assist the patient in setting realistic vocational and training goals. Clearly, the goal of psychotherapy at this time is to generalize collaborative evidentiary techniques to the patient's world of productivity. This carries a significant degree of professional responsibility and requires empathic communication of functional recommendations. Inaccurate or incomplete data can misdirect patients, resulting in missed opportunities and shattered dreams. Therefore, although individual psychotherapy sessions are a vital sounding board for a patient's realistic decision making, the psychotherapist and patient also need data from multiple venues. This helps both parties develop a holistic overview of the patient's talents, so as to identify viable career directions.

Patients' in-session behaviors are also rich sources of information about their realism in regard to community adaptation. These include punctuality, initiation, and organization; speed of information processing, learning, and recall; auditory and written comprehension; and abstract reasoning skills. Behaviorally, the patients' emotional self-control, resiliency, motivation, self-insight, openness to feedback, and acceptance of injury-related challenges all foreshadow their interaction style and impact on outsiders (e.g., teachers, employers, and coworkers). The following discussion identifies helpful constructs or metaphors for promoting patients' realistic adaptation.

### "Raising the Bar" and Related Metaphors

As realism emerges in individual psychotherapy, it needs to be generalized to the community setting (e.g., work or school). The tolerant and supportive ambience of psychotherapy is not always replicated in the real world. The metaphor of "raising the bar" helps to prepare patients psychologically for the enhanced effort and associated angst of new, more complex challenges. However, this stage also connotes new therapeutic "windows of opportunity," as the patients in fact have shown progress in goal attainment and are now moving toward grander objectives. Comparing a patient's progress to climbing a ladder, with reference points on each "rung," can provide further graphic illustration.

### Internal Standards versus External Expectations

Often patients will protest that they are doing the best they can, based on their personal perceptions of their work performance in the context of the injury-related deficits. For example, a patient may feel that remembering only some daily assignments is acceptable, because he or she has a "good reason" for forgetfulness. Although this self-perception is legitimate in terms of the patient's internal standards, it can "miss the boat" with respect to external criteria (e.g., the objective performance standards and measures of a job, which are applicable to all employees). Part of cultivating awareness, acceptance, and ultimately realism is to help patients counterbalance their internal subjective standards of acceptable functioning with the sometimes harsher realities of work environments' objective expectations, regardless of an injury. Linking these two reference points with an arc of awareness, acceptance, and realism is a good pictorial representation of this principle.

### "The Proof Is in the Pudding" or "Show Me the Marks"

The catch phrases "The proof is in the pudding" and "Show me the marks" tell patients that despite their best intentions, actions speak louder than words. Evidence and feedback from external sources also ameliorate negative transference (or "kill the messenger") reactions from the patient, in addition to reinforcing the central life lesson that actions have consequences.

### "Plans A, B, and C"

Patients sometimes need to consider other career paths when it becomes clear that there are insurmountable obstacles to achieving their "Plan A" or first choice. Patients need ample time to reach this realization in the context of their recovery process—sometimes many months, or even up to 2 years. Patients will need to cope with the resulting feelings of loss and grief. Once they have accepted the need for a "Plan B" (or beyond), assisting them in the brainstorming process will help them determine other, more realistic avenues for their productive energies. This process helps patients diversify their thinking and "keep doors open" that otherwise they might overlook. The book *Who Moved My Cheese?* (Johnson, 1998) is an excellent resource for this process of developing realism and promoting adaptation. It reminds patients of how important it is to overcome their fears and be flexible, self-propelling, and imaginative.

## Group Psychotherapy

Group psychotherapy is a powerful venue for the process of postinjury adjustment (Klonoff, 1997). The group process allows for a vicarious experience, social persuasion, and emotional sustenance (Dixon, Thornton, & Young, 2007). Group discussions as well as structured exercises also enable beneficial peer input, self-evaluation, and concrete goal setting in regard to productive activities. Figure 9.2 summarizes pertinent group psychotherapy topics and themes for each dimension of adjustment, as well as applicable and meaningful exercises.

*Adaptation* topics include the specific struggles of patients' work and school reentry process; practical worries, including financial stressors; and the personal angst and ambivalence involved in ascertaining realistic career choices. Helpful exercises to maximize *adaptation* include encouraging the group members to realistically apportion their energies (e.g., itemizing personal work challenges and identifying realistic career paths, including specific milestones to be achieved). Another thought-provoking exercise contrasts the personal philosophies of "shooting for the stars" versus being "down to earth."

## Cognitive Retraining

As described in Chapters 3 and 5, cognitive retraining's emphasis on education, self-insight, and compensations is invaluable (Klonoff et al., 1989, 1997, 2007). Once patients select a particular academic or vocational objective, the necessary modifications and adjustments are made during cognitive retraining sessions. These include prioritizing tasks and incorporating new, relevant compensatory strategies. Practically speaking, each patient's list of strengths, difficulties, and compensations should be revised as needed to highlight those skills most germane for community-based productivity. Regular dialogue within the cognitive retrain-

**Adaptation Topics**
- How/when/where to return to work/school: What's realistic?
- Feelings about work/school failures.
- Financial stressors.
- The importance of "Plan B" (or "C, D," etc.).
- Feelings about new career directions.
- How to maximize functional recovery: The role of therapists' involvement in work/school.

**Adaptation Exercises**
- What was my preinjury work history/work ethic?
- Pros and cons of "shooting for the stars" versus being "down to earth."
- Which career path and why?
- Personal goal setting (with specific milestones), and predicted "length of stay" in treatment.
- Itemized personal challenges for work/school and how to be successful.
- Round-robin updates about work/school.

**Intrapsychic Assimilation Topics**
- Postinjury feelings of vulnerability.
- Can I be happy with my recovery?
- Expectations versus the reality of recovery.
- New feelings of mastery related to independence and work.
- "Slippage" and "flight into health."

**Intrapsychic Assimilation Exercises**
- Rating my self-confidence (and reasons for ratings).
- Describing my "pie chart" (size and components).
- My personal "progress report" and "stumbling blocks."
- What is my "personal motto"?
- Sources of pride and accomplishment (pre- vs. postinjury).
- Sources of happiness (pre- vs. postinjury).
- My year in review.
- Discussion of the short film *Boundin'* (Lasseter, Shurer, Luckey, & Gould, 2003) as an example of self-esteem.
- Discussion of the book *The Missing Piece Meets the Big O* (Silverstein, 1981) as an example of self-efficacy.

**Existential Assimilation Topics**
- Does realism mean giving up?
- How can I be emancipated?
- "To work or not to work . . . "
- Feelings about injury anniversaries.
- Uncertainty about the future.
- Was my injury a "wake-up call"?
- What will define my quality of life?
- The preciousness of life.
- What are my life goals?
- Entitlement versus giving of oneself.
- How do I maintain hope, faith, and love after my injury?

*(cont.)*

**FIGURE 9.2.** Group psychotherapy adjustment topics.

**Existential Assimilation Exercises**
- Presentations by patient "graduates":
  - "Rehab in review."
  - Hopes and plans for the future.
  - Advice to peers.
  - How does this apply to current patients?
- What would I do if I had only one more day to live?
- New Year's resolutions: Goals and aspirations.
- How has my quality of life changed since the injury?
- What am I thankful for?
- Personal choices of heroes, movies, and songs as pre- and postinjury sources of inspiration.
- Life experiences that have changed me.
- What qualities have been enhanced after injury (">100% recovery")?
- Discussion of the movies *The Pursuit of Happyness* (Alper et al., 2006) and *The Family Man* (Abraham et al., 2000), as examples of searching for meaning and self-actualization.
- Discussion of the passage "People are like teabags" (*www.catholiclinks.org/ctosipeopleareliketeabags.htm*).
- "Circle of positives."
- Personal "tool kits."
- Meaningful group projects.
- "Crystal ball" exercise: Predict my future.
- Relating the 12 gifts of the movie *The Ultimate Gift* (Eldridge et al., 2006) to personal gifts and goals.
- Personal song choices of hope and transcendence.

**Termination Topics**
- When is it enough therapy?: Criteria for termination.
- Will my recovery stop when therapy ends?
- Feelings about treatment termination and "graduation."

**Termination Exercises**
- Estimating my date for treatment termination.
- Pros and cons of treatment termination.

**FIGURE 9.2.** *(cont.)*

ing sessions, as well as during individual psychotherapy, should encompass how patients' neuropsychological, behavioral, and interpersonal status will affect their outside endeavors; generally, asterisks are placed by those abilities and compensations most likely to promote successful transitions. Whenever possible, explicit functional examples associated with work and school should be identified and noted as part of each cognitive task (Klonoff et al., 1997). Lastly, error analyses should continue regularly, so as to enhance patients' realistic grasp of specific underlying cognitive challenges that will need to be met in the work and school environments.

For patients struggling with realistic goal setting and attainment, cognitive retraining sessions are also advantageous as a training ground for potential work and school demands. For example, basic skills in mathematical computations and attention to visual detail forecast the capacity to embark on a career in bookkeeping or accounting. For students planning a return to school or college, their ability to learn and retain protocols and concepts, handle distractions in noisy environments, and master note taking are a few of the positive predictors of academic accomplishments. Patients' capacity to devise and adhere to procedural checklists is a potent indicator of their capacity for systematic and detail-oriented task completion in professional work settings. Marked discrepancies between skill sets in cognitive retraining and the required vocational/school proficiencies are "red flags" that patients have set unrealistic goals.

Improving and generalizing metacognitive skills (e.g., self-monitoring, impulse control, organization, abstraction, and "big-picture" thinking) are crucial for successful work and school adaptation (Klonoff et al., 2007). Behavioral and interpersonal variables (including distractibility, communication pragmatics, initiative, and efficiency) should also be scrutinized, measured, and integrated into cognitive retraining and psychotherapy dialogue with patients regarding realistic work and school endeavors.

### Vocational Communication Group

A vocational communication group uses didactics, group discussion, role playing, and video-recorded exercises to discuss the return to productive work. This group is best facilitated by a psychotherapist who is sensitive to the psychological issues related to self-disclosure, work readiness, and realism. The psychotherapist should consider cotreatment with a vocational counselor, occupational therapist, or speech–language pathologist knowledgeable about reintegration into work environments. Such a professional can help to remedy other work impediments, including poor interview pragmatics. Group instruction also teaches work preparatory skills and possible accommodations. One possible format is to conduct the group weekly for a sufficient period (e.g., 8–12 weeks) to enable sufficient knowledge acquisition and skill attainment.

Figure 9.3 is a purpose sheet for a vocational communication group; it lists not only the treatment purposes, but the topics covered in the group. Goals include developing interview and resumé-writing skills; understanding how the Americans with Disabilities Act (ADA; U.S. Department of Justice, 2005) affects employment opportunities; and learning and self-monitoring appropriate work behaviors. As part of the group, patients are taught how to prepare their own high-quality resumés and cover letters in specific formats, and are given practice completing job applications. Group members also receive instruction on interview skills, job development, and job search resources (see Figure 9.4). The vocational communication group also provides a potent setting for emphasizing the value of compensatory strategies in the work environment, and for encouraging patients to evaluate career decisions and the realism of their vocational paths. In order to reinforce real-life work responsibilities, group members can create in-clinic work projects (e.g., tending a small garden or fish tanks). Unresolved and emotionally laden topics can be referred to group psychotherapy for further exploration and reflection.

## Purposes

1. To become more aware of, accepting of, and realistic about the impact of our strengths and difficulties on work.
2. To acquire/improve important work-related skills (e.g., punctuality, receptivity to feedback, and follow-through).
3. To gain experience in work skills by working collaboratively on team projects.

## Goal/Outcome

1. To learn to discriminate between appropriate and inappropriate work behaviors, and to develop the ability to self-monitor/modify our behavior in work contexts.
2. To improve interviewing, resumé-writing, and job development/search skills.
3. To understand how the Americans with Disabilities Act (ADA) affects our ability to obtain and sustain gainful employment.

## Why Is This Group Important?

1. We function in the context of a professional atmosphere at work, which influences the way we communicate and interact with others.
2. The development of good work skills will assist us with seeking, obtaining, and sustaining gainful employment.

## Study Modules

- *The ADA (see above):* Learn how the ADA affects our ability to obtain and sustain gainful employment.
- *Supplemental Security Income (SSI) and Social Security Disability Insurance (SSDI):* Understand returning to work and its impact on SSI and SSDI benefits.
- *Interview Skills:* Learn how to answer interview questions and promote job skills.
- *Resumé Development:* Learn how to develop a functional and chronological resumé.
- *Job Development/Search:* Learn and understand how to find a job based on personal vocational goals.
- *Job Applications:* Learn how to complete job applications effectively.
- *Communication Pragmatics:* Understand and develop appropriate work behaviors and social/communication pragmatics.
- *Patient Concerns:* Self-assess and problem-solve issues and concerns regarding our return to work, with an emphasis on compensatory strategies.
- *Work Projects:* Work collaboratively to identify and implement in-clinic work projects, to practice important work skills and behaviors.

**This group requires active participation, role playing including video recording, and discussions.**

**FIGURE 9.3.** Vocational communication group purpose sheet.

**Sample Job Development Sources**

1. *Use Published Sources.*
   a. *O\*NET Dictionary of Occupational Titles: The Definitive Printed Reference of Occupational Information* (4th ed.) (Farr & Shatkin, 2007)
   b. *Enhanced Occupational Outlook Handbook* (7th ed.) (JIST Works, 2008)
   c. *National Trade and Professional Association of the United States* (44th ed.) (Sheridan et al., 2009)
2. *Use Career and Interest Inventories.*
   a. *Individual Employment Plan (IEP)* (Ludden & Maitlen, 2002)
   b. *Picture Interest Career Survey (PICS)* (Brady, 2007)
3. *Use the Internet.*
   a. Search online at: *www.jan.wvu.edu/index.htm*

**Sample Job Search Sources**

1. *Use Personal Contacts/Networking.*
   a. Family, friends, neighbors, teachers, and mentors
   b. Job-posting boards
2. *Make Direct Contact with Employers.*
   a. Job fairs, employer career days, cold calls
   b. Volunteer, temporary, or part-time work as a "foot in the door"
3. *Use the Internet.*
   a. Websites (e.g., *www.monster.com, www.careerbuilder.com, www.jobing.com, www.craigslist.com*)
4. *Use Job Referral Services.*
   a. State employment offices
   b. Private employment agencies

**Sample Job Topics**

1. *Interview Preparation*
   a. Work history
   b. Work interests
   c. Relevant injury-related information, including strengths and difficulties
   d. Prepare a list of potential questions for the employer
   e. Prepare a list of answers to potential questions from the employer
   f. Role-playing and video-recording exercises
2. *Interviewer Perceptions of the Interviewee*
   a. Expertise/competence
   b. Motivation
   c. Interpersonal skills
   d. Decision-making and problem-solving abilities
   e. Interest in the job or company
   f. Personality, likability, flexibility, and coachability
3. *Interviewee Goals and Expectations*
   a. Gain information about the job, employer, and organization, including health benefits
   b. Demonstrate how skills, knowledge, and abilities will fit the needs of the job and the organization

**FIGURE 9.4.** Sample job development, job search, and job interview topics.

## Observation, Liaison, and Communication Exchange

### School Reentry

It is recommended that a psychotherapist be actively involved on site at school for older teens and young adults returning to the school environment. When feasible, collaboration or cotreatment with a speech–language pathologist for the school reentry process is ideal. For patients returning to school, knowledge of the federal guidelines for provision of educational services, including the Individuals with Disabilities Education Act of 2004 (U.S. Department of Education, 2004), is mandatory in order for rehabilitation therapists to serve their patients accurately and proactively. Students attending a community college or university should be strongly encouraged to register with resource centers for students with disabilities; these centers can provide multiple advantageous accommodations (extra time for tests, note takers, etc.).

Among the most helpful precursors to the physical return to school are online or home-bound classes. These allow therapists to monitor learning styles, create and promote relevant compensatory strategies, and support patients in their academic endeavors in the comfort of a treatment environment. As patients demonstrate readiness for the classroom, the therapists can propose the necessary compensations and other measures to maximize patients' success in classroom reintegration. Provision of written educational materials about brain injury (Verburg, Borthwick, Bennett, & Rumney, 2003); attendance at individualized education program meetings; and inservices for teachers and students are all beneficial educational interventions (Klonoff, Lamb, Henderson, Reichert, et al., 2000). Other liaison mechanisms include direct observation in the classroom and provision of behavioral intervention strategies to address possible disruptive behaviors; compensatory techniques to promote academic success; and collaborative consultation with teachers, school resource personnel, and family members (Glang, Tyler, Pearson, Todis, & Morvant, 2004; Klonoff, Lamb, Henderson, Reichert, et al., 2000; Ylvisaker et al., 2001). A regular exchange of faxes, confidential e-mails, and weekly grade reports between the treating therapists and the school personnel will permit fine-tuning of clinic-based interventions.

### Study Group

In a study group, patients may spend 3–4 hours weekly working on school homework assignments. Cotreatment with a speech–language pathologist is best for the diagnostic formulation and remediation of patients' cognitive, language, and academic struggles. This group also reinforces optimal study techniques and use of compensatory strategies. Importantly, the psychotherapist monitors and addresses patients' emotional reactions to academic challenges and disappointments.

### Work Reentry

Community-based programs are designed to integrate patients directly into a naturalistic work environment. This has been termed "social role valorization" and encompasses therapies in external community settings, as well as the modification of societal attitudes toward disability (Condeluci & Gretz-Lasky, 1987). This treatment is predicated on individualized goal setting and implementation in the setting where skills are to be utilized; practical environmental manipulations to maximize performance; and a "place-and-train" approach, which includes the use of job coaches and transitional, progressive modification of supports (Oppermann, 2004; Sherer et al., 1998; Willer & Corrigan, 1994).

Psychotherapists can help coordinate job-shadowing opportunities for their patients and assist in clarifying job functions. The therapist's direct observations and evaluations of patients in prework environments (e.g., volunteer placements, work adjustment settings, or situational assessments) yield naturalistic data, which can be assimilated into psychotherapy feedback sessions and eventually applied to paid work settings. Whenever cotreatment with other therapy professionals relevant to the vocational domain is possible, this will optimize the intervention process. For example, patients returning to manual labor positions will benefit from the assessment and monitoring of work capabilities by a physical therapist, who can best assess the patients' balance, coordination, safety awareness, and so on.

The psychotherapist can also educate the patients' coworkers and employers to extend and reinforce the posttreatment training process. This advocacy can perpetuate the patients' success in the work environment, even after formal therapy concludes (Abrams & Haffey, 1991; Fraser & Shrey, 1986; Sherer et al., 1998). Barriers to sustained employment that a psychotherapist can reduce or eliminate include employers' false notions regarding disability (including unrealistic expectations of patients), and the potential for patients to have problems with professionalism, take excessive sick leave, or have difficulty meeting business productivity requirements (Giaquinto & Ring, 2007; Oppermann, 2004). To facilitate communication, employers can be asked to complete written documentation. The one-page Work Trial Rating Scale (Figure 9.5) is short and can easily be completed at regular intervals. The longer Work Skill Evaluation Form (Figure 9.6) can be used on an intermittent basis, as well as prior to therapy completion. It helps ensure that a patient has the necessary work skills and abilities. These forms represent further concrete mechanisms for promoting dialogue between the patient/worker and the employer.

## CASE STUDY

Henry was age 19 when he sustained a severe traumatic brain injury as a result of a motorcycle accident. A CT scan revealed a left frontoparietal depressed skull fracture and a left frontal parenchymal contusion. Henry was hospitalized acutely for 2 months. After limited outpatient therapies (i.e., physical therapy and speech–language therapy twice weekly for 2 months), he returned to community college. Before his injury, Henry had planned to become a business major, obtain his bachelor's degree from a local university, and then attend a prestigious business school for a master's degree. He would thus be following in the footsteps of his father, a highly successful entrepreneur. Henry had also worked successfully part-time for 2 years at a local department store, selling appliances.

After his release from therapies, Henry took two basic prerequisite classes: a remedial English class and a music appreciation class. He was unable to pay

Date: _____     Completed by: _____

Completed for: _____

**How would you rate yourself/this person in the following areas on a scale of 1 to 10 (1 is "unsatisfactory," 5 is "average," 10 is "outstanding")?**

1. Work pace/speed:                      1  2  3  4  5  6  7  8  9  10

   Comments: _____

2. Accuracy:                                 1  2  3  4  5  6  7  8  9  10

   Comments: _____

3. Focus/concentration:              1  2  3  4  5  6  7  8  9  10

   Comments: _____

4. Following directions:              1  2  3  4  5  6  7  8  9  10

   Comments: _____

5. Interactions with coworkers:     1  2  3  4  5  6  7  8  9  10

   Comments: _____

6. Endurance:                               1  2  3  4  5  6  7  8  9  10

   Comments: _____

7. Asking questions when unsure:    1  2  3  4  5  6  7  8  9  10

   Comments: _____

8. Taking feedback:                     1  2  3  4  5  6  7  8  9  10

   Comments: _____

9. Problem solving and multitasking:   1  2  3  4  5  6  7  8  9  10

   Comments: _____

10. Memory for routine:             1  2  3  4  5  6  7  8  9  10

   Comments: _____

Concerns:

**FIGURE 9.5.** Work Trial Rating Scale.

**From:** _____

**Through:** _____

**Name:** _____

**Job Classification:** _____ **Department:** _____

**Date Hired:** _____ **Evaluator:** _____

**Instructions:** Evaluate the employee on the job now being performed. Check (✓) the box above the description that most nearly expresses your overall judgment on each quality. We would appreciate comments, including recommendations for improvement to accompany each category.

| | | | | | | Consider the employee's performance since the last appraisal and show by a circle whether he/she has improved, remained consistent, or regressed in each of the qualities listed to the left. |
|---|---|---|---|---|---|---|
| **Knowledge of Work** | ☐ | ☐ | ☐ | ☐ | ☐ | **Has improved** |
| Consider knowledge of job gained through experience, general education, and specialized training. | Well informed on all phases of work. | Well-rounded job knowledge. Infrequently requires assistance. | Adequate grasp of essentials. Some assistance required. | Requires considerable assistance. | Inadequate knowledge. Requires improvement to avoid termination. | **Maintains consistency** <br><br> **Needs work** |
| COMMENTS: | | | | | | |
| **Quantity of Work** | ☐ | ☐ | ☐ | ☐ | ☐ | **Has improved** |
| Consider the volume of work produced under normal conditions. | Rapid worker. Produces exceptionally high volume. | Above-average volume. | Average volume. | Below-average volume. | Inadequate volume. Requires improvement to avoid termination. | **Maintains consistency** <br><br> **Needs work** |
| COMMENTS: | | | | | | |
| **Quality of Work** | ☐ | ☐ | ☐ | ☐ | ☐ | **Has improved** |
| Consider neatness, accuracy, and dependability of results. | Exceptional quality. Practically no mistakes. | Above-average quality. Infrequent errors. | Acceptable, seldom necessary to check work. | Often unacceptable, frequent errors. | Excessive errors or rejections. Requires improvement to avoid termination. | **Maintains consistency** <br><br> **Needs work** |
| COMMENTS: | | | | | | |

*(cont.)*

**FIGURE 9.6.** Work Skill Evaluation Form.

Adapted from East Tennessee State University (2008). Copyright 2008 by East Tennessee State University, Office of Human Resources. Adapted by permission in *Psychotherapy after Brain Injury* by Pamela S. Klonoff (Guilford Press, 2010). Permission to photocopy this figure is granted to purchasers of this book for personal use only (see copyright page for details).

| Initiative | ☐ | ☐ | ☐ | ☐ | ☐ | Has improved |
|---|---|---|---|---|---|---|
| Consider contribution of new ideas and methods; self-starting; working independently toward approved goals. | Consistently sets and works toward approved goals. | Frequently sets and works toward approved goals. | Initiates activity within normal routine. | Seldom initiates activity during normal routine. | Needs frequent direction. Requires improvement to avoid termination. | **Maintains consistency** <br><br> **Needs work** |

COMMENTS:

<br>

| Dependability/ Responsibility | ☐ | ☐ | ☐ | ☐ | ☐ | Has improved |
|---|---|---|---|---|---|---|
| Consider the degree to which employee can be relied upon to carry out duties. | Consistently fulfills all job responsibilities and duties. Totally reliable. | Can be depended upon to get the job done with little or no follow-up. Very reliable. | Assumes all responsibilities specifically assigned. Reliable. | Accepts some responsibilities, but must be cued. | Fails to accept responsibility even when specifically assigned. Requires improvement to avoid termination. | **Maintains consistency** <br><br> **Needs work** |

COMMENTS:

<br>

| Quality of Interpersonal Relationships | ☐ | ☐ | ☐ | ☐ | ☐ | Has improved |
|---|---|---|---|---|---|---|
| Consider the degree to which employee interacts and works harmoniously with the public, coworkers, and customers. | Use of exceptional tact and diplomacy. Cooperation and promotion of teamwork. | Cooperates well with others. Frequently promotes teamwork and harmony. | Adequate skills at promoting teamwork and harmony. | Has difficulty interacting with people. | Frequent conflicts with others. Requires improvement to avoid termination. | **Maintains consistency** <br><br> **Needs work** |

COMMENTS:

<br>

| Attendance | ☐ | ☐ | ☐ | ☐ | ☐ | Has improved |
|---|---|---|---|---|---|---|
| Consider appropriate requests for shifts and requests for time off. | Consistently regular in attendance. Adjusts schedule to work needs. | Regular in attendance. Frequently considers workload when requesting time off. | Generally present. Usually considers workload when requesting time off. | Frequent absences, affecting job performance. | Excessive absences. Requires improvement to avoid termination. | **Maintains consistency** <br><br> **Needs work** |

COMMENTS:

*(cont.)*

**FIGURE 9.6.** *(page 2 of 3)*

214

| Punctuality | ☐ | ☐ | ☐ | ☐ | ☐ | Has improved |
|---|---|---|---|---|---|---|
| Consider prompt attendance with regard to employee's responsibilities. | Consistently prompt. | Regularly prompt. | Seldom tardy. | Frequent tardiness. Impacts job performance. | Excessive tardiness. Requires improvement to avoid termination. | **Maintains consistency**<br><br>**Needs work** |
| COMMENTS: | | | | | | |

*(To be completed for individuals with supervisory responsibility only. Includes supervising other support employees)*

| Supervisory Abilities | ☐ | ☐ | ☐ | ☐ | ☐ | Has improved |
|---|---|---|---|---|---|---|
| Consider supervisory ability. | Exceptional ability to lead and build a team. | Exhibits good leadership skills. | Adequate supervisory abilities. | Has difficulty supervising others. | Inadequate ability to supervise. Requires improvement to maintain current supervisory responsibilities. | **Maintains consistency**<br><br>**Needs work** |
| COMMENTS: | | | | | | |

## Summary

Given what you have learned about this person while he/she has been volunteering for you, do you think that he/she will be able to return to paid employment?

Yes   Maybe   No

N/A (if already gainfully employed)

Given what you have learned about this person while he/she has been working for you, do you think that he/she will be able to sustain gainful employment indefinitely?

Yes   Maybe   No

Would you hire this person?
*(A yes response does not obligate you to consider this person for employment at this time.)*

Yes   Maybe   No

N/A (if already gainfully employed)

Additional comments:

**FIGURE 9.6.** *(page 3 of 3)*

attention in class or assimilate new information. His spelling and written formulation skills were also affected, which interfered with his ability to excel in his English class. After 6 weeks, Henry dropped out of school. At the urging of his parents and referring rehabilitation physician, he started weekly individual psychotherapy sessions and other therapies (i.e., speech–language therapy and cognitive retraining).

Henry's intake neuropsychological assessment at 6 months postinjury indicated a number of typical deficits consistent with a left frontotemporal lobe traumatic brain injury. These included moderate to severe problems with speed of information processing, attention/concentration, verbal learning and retention, and executive functions (specifically in the areas of abstract reasoning, flexible problem solving, planning, multitasking, and strategy generation). His most salient difficulty was with auditory processing and retention; his working memory scores fell in the severely impaired range. His psychological testing employed a self-report personality questionnaire (the MMPI-2; Butcher, 1990, 2005) and was suggestive of a tendency to project an unrealistically positive self-image, admit to few problems, and underreport emotional distress. His response pattern also indicated that he was socially charming and gregarious.

Henry's speech–language evaluation indicated moderate deficits in the areas of verbal abstract reasoning, spelling, auditory and reading comprehension, verbal formulation, and confrontation naming. On a positive note, Henry's communication pragmatics were unscathed; despite his challenges, he remained a very affable and outgoing person, with many retained friendships.

Henry's psychotherapist also functioned as his cognitive retraining therapist. Henry's task performance closely mirrored his neuropsychological test findings. Qualitative observations indicated problems with attention to detail, periodic "mini" catastrophic reactions, and a proclivity toward "Yeah, buts." At times he became annoyed with the regimen and slow pace of his improvements; his mantra was "Patience, patience, patience." Notably, he demonstrated relatively better procedural learning; with practice, he showed a steep learning curve. Consistent with the lateralization of his injury, his visuoperceptual and visual retention skills were also considerably stronger than his skills in the verbal domain. Behavioral observations during cognitive retraining indicated that with structure, repetition, and encouraging words, Henry's prework skills and behaviors progressed very nicely.

The initial phase of psychotherapy was spent in helping Henry develop a better appreciation of his strengths and difficulties and adopt sensible compensations. This process had its ups and downs, although Henry gradually made progress in his awareness and acceptance. His psychotherapist's initial impression of Henry's realism level was that it was low. For example, 2 months after initiating cognitive retraining and individual psychotherapy, Henry emphatically announced his unilateral decision to resume university coursework with two undergraduate business classes and one mathematics class. Secondary to his executive function deficits, he was unable to relate the challenges he was encountering in cognitive retraining and his neuropsychological deficits to the strenuous academic demands he was undertaking. Despite his prior postinjury school failures, he was steadfast in his attitude that one must "shoot for the stars" or be filled with regrets in later life. Henry was gingerly approached by his psychotherapist, as well as by his speech–language pathologist, with concerns that this plan was not realistic. In response, he became highly defensive and insulted; he declared that he would "prove to everyone" that he could resume his prior academic path, and that the therapists were underestimating and demeaning him by insinuating otherwise. An incremental game plan was mutually developed: Henry agreed that he would need at least B's in his current classes in order to consider pursuing a business degree at the university. His psychotherapist and speech–language pathologist supported him in this new undertaking by providing tutorial help and liaisoning with the resource personnel for disabled students at the university to obtain learning accommodations (e.g., extra time on tests and a note taker).

Meanwhile, Henry completed the modules in the vocational communication group, also facilitated by his psychotherapist. These included identifying and practicing the types of compensatory strategies he would need in the workplace. Ten weeks after beginning the therapeutic process, Henry returned to his part-time job on weekends at the department store. Because of his working memory and attentional difficulties, he decided that he would carry a small pocket-sized notebook at work, which he dubbed "WTR" ("Way to Remember"). Henry would continuously record customer requests and appliance code numbers, rather than attempt to retain them in his head. His sales skills were excellent; his psychotherapist observed him at work and found that his retained preaccident knowledge base, in combination with his WTR compensatory system, made him competent at work. Oral as well as written feedback on his work skills from his supervisor was highly complimentary. Positive comments included that he worked consistently, was dependable, took initiative, and worked collaboratively with others. In fact, it was the supervisor's impression that Henry was now more dedicated and enthusiastic about his job duties than had had been before his accident. Henry felt fortunate and "normal" being back at work. Three months later, he was named the top sales associate of the month and received an award.

In stark contrast, Henry's academic performance in the university was dismal. Despite his best efforts, he could not keep up with the lecture material in his business classes, nor could he retain course constructs and material between classes or on the examinations. Observations from his study group indicated that he was unable to assimilate new concepts and was having multiple catastrophic reactions. Four weeks into the term, he was failing both business classes; he had a C in the math class.

## THE INTRAPSYCHIC ASSIMILATION DIMENSION

As discussed in Chapter 4, acquired brain injury often has profound effects on an individual's sense of self and identity. As part of the intrapsychic assimilation process, patients need to reclaim self-esteem, self-efficacy, mastery, and happiness through the attainment of a productive lifestyle.

"Self-esteem" has been defined as a self-evaluative process in which an individual judges him- or herself either negatively or positively, based on personal abilities and attributes (see Vickery, Sherer, Evans, Gontkovsky, & Lee, 2008, for a review). Self-esteem has been considered a mediator of improved psychosocial functioning and facilitates adjustment to brain injury, adaptive coping, and healthy behaviors (Kendall, 2003; see Vickery et al., 2008, for a review). The recrystallization or reformulation of postinjury career expectations depends on the extent of restoration of preinjury competencies and skills, postinjury motivation to work, and environmental opportunities (Power & Hershenson, 2003). Ultimately, life satisfaction, including personal happiness, is related to reacquisition of a productive lifestyle (Corrigan et al., 2001).

"Self-efficacy" has been defined as personal belief in one's capability to organize and execute actions in striving for various attainments (Bandura, 1997; Toglia & Kirk, 2000). Self-efficacy also represents an individual's belief in his or her ability to achieve relative to personal expectations, which is a key factor in human agency (Bandura, 1997; Cicerone & Azulay, 2007). Self-discovery, in combination with increased self-efficacy and a higher internal locus of control, has been associated with better postinjury outcomes and employability (Dawson & Winocur, 2008; Lubusko, Moore, Stambrook, & Gill, 1994; Moore & Stambrook, 1995; Petrella, McColl, Krupa, & Johnston, 2005; Svendsen & Teasdale, 2006). In addition, reattainment of self-reported competency and self-esteem in the cognitive and emotional/interpersonal domains predicts better postinjury outcomes, including employment and social integration (Groswasser, Melamed, Agranov, & Keren, 1999; Sveen, Mongs, Roe, Sandvik, & Bautz-Holter, 2008).

The sense of personal mastery after brain injury is maximized when patients utilize compensatory strategies to enhance functional adjustment and ultimately achieve the necessary competencies (Ben-Yishay et al., 1985). Ben-Yishay and Lakin (1989) have postulated that through personal engagement, enhanced awareness, and systematic training in mastering "templates" of behavior, patients can improve their functioning and reacquire ego identity. Specifically, a multimodal approach to treatment, including cognitive retraining and psychotherapy, enables the therapist to address complex cognitive problems while at the same time improving patients' self-concept (Ben-Yishay & Diller, 1993).

With postinjury accomplishments comes happiness. A positive feedback loop is created: Self-esteem and mastery engender inner contentment, enthusiasm, positive affect, creativity, goodwill, and the appreciation of one's circumstances (Dalai Lama & Cutler, 1998; Miquelon & Vallerand, 2008).

## Fostering Intrapsychic Assimilation in Individual Psychotherapy

Research with neurological patients indicates that the qualities of self-reliance, recognition of improvements, determination, goal setting, and pushing one's limits all enhance self-concept (Dixon et al., 2007). Individual psychotherapy should assist patients in recognizing and embracing their postinjury assets in specific contexts both within and outside the clinic setting. This includes identifying, setting, and evaluating progress toward achieving explicit subgoals. Progression to the next challenge should be predicated on successful accomplishment of the preceding subgoals. Individual psychotherapy sessions should therefore discuss quantifiable gains in both other therapeutic areas and real-life experiences. For example, during cognitive retraining, patients can be encouraged to project their expected scores after a fixed number of task repetitions. Dialogue about the proximity (or lack of it) of their actual achievement to their projected level helps them adjust their subgoals, and thus is an excellent realism exercise. Similarly, planning for a gradual return to college coursework—beginning with easier and fewer courses, followed by an incremental increase in course number and complexity—creates a hierarchy of attainable academic goals.

Patients often begin the transition to work with a volunteer position in a protected setting. They can then build skills and confidence before entering competitive employment. In order to obtain pertinent information regarding patients' work performance, it is recommended that the psychotherapist help patients keep written notes in a central location regarding their areas of strength, difficulties, and appropriate compensations. Such notes will enable the patients to perform periodic self-appraisals of their progress and challenges. This information can be laminated and kept in the front of the datebook for easy reference. This exercise will help empower patients in deciding how, whether, and when to make the transition to a different work environment; as such, it incorporates internal locus of control, and promotes a sense of ownership and self-efficacy.

A highly effective technique for developing awareness, acceptance, and realism is to compare a patient's self-ratings on work skill evaluations with those of the monitoring therapist and the employer. Such comparisons provide wonderful "grist" for the individual psychotherapy "mill." Positive concordant ratings by all parties provide fundamental validation of the patient's skill set, and thus support the patient in feeling competent and proud. The patient's candid reactions to evaluations also reflect his or her level of acceptance and openness to feedback regarding community-based undertakings. If necessary, the psychotherapist can intervene at the level of accepting and coping with disabilities as precursors to realistic self-assessment.

In sum, any treatment plan can and often should be subdivided into meaningful and measurable subgoals. This "steppingstone" approach, with gradual and tangible progressions, builds consecutive successes and boosts patients' self-esteem. Gradually, patients develop self-recognition of errors, while building a sense of control and mastery over their performance (Sherer et al., 1998; Toglia & Kirk, 2000). The following are helpful therapeutic techniques to improve patients' intrapsychic assimilation.

### "Taming the Grandiosity," or Dealing with the "Superman Complex"

It is crucial for patients to set realistic career objectives. If patients' strivings are mismatched with their postinjury capabilities, the patients are doomed to devastating failures, which will undermine attempts to improve self-esteem and personal happiness. Bringing goals into line with capabilities has been referred to as "taming the grandiosity" (G. A. Lage, personal communication, n.d.). In order to avoid failures, regrets, and ultimately misery, patients need to modulate their aspirations to achievable levels. It is helpful to remind patients of their humanness and vulnerabilities, with the following analogy: We may sometimes have "Superman" aspirations, but we are actually all "Clark Kents." The psychotherapist needs to collaborate with patients in systematically and honestly appraising the consequences of their daily efforts. There should be synchrony among the energy investment, outcome quality, and personal fulfillment.

## *"Flight into Health" and "Slippage"*

As described in Chapter 5, when patients do not have the necessary coping skills, they may resort to minimizing and therefore underestimating the effects of their brain injuries on their functional capacities. As depicted in the Phase 6 "yellow" warning zone of the PEM, this can lead to a "flight into health." Hallmarks of this include abandoning compensatory tools and refusing to acknowledge injury-related sequelae in making daily decisions and pursuing activities. It is as if the injury no longer exists. At other times, there is a gradual process of "slippage": Patients begin to stray from the systematic use of compensations, usually in a step-wise manner. This is most noticeable when the structure and external supports of the treatment program are withdrawn. "Flight into health" and "slippage" most often occur toward the end of the treatment process or after discharge. For some patients, these are mechanisms for reframing the termination process (i.e., superficial attempts to bolster their conviction that they are ready for emancipation from the treatment environment). However, they can become dangerous if patients ignore critical warning signs and discard the teachings of psychotherapy.

## *Helping Patients Be "Comfortable in Their Own Skin"*

Patients' timidity and internal discomfort are often palpable to their supporters in the home and community. Some patients (especially those with temporal lobe damage) may become suspicious of the motives or intentions of others, and assume that they are being disrespected or demeaned. Often this assumption is an external projection of their own self-loathing. This negative cycle often contaminates the ambience of relationships, with outsiders feeling they are "walking on eggshells." Therefore, the psychotherapist needs to assist patients in recognizing their misapprehensions, while also improving their comfort with themselves. Doing so should result in improved psychological well-being and self-assurance. In general, when patients are "comfortable in their own skin," others in the environment will accord them acceptance and respect. The short film *Boundin'* (Lasseter, Shurer, Luckey, & Gould, 2003) is a wonderful therapeutic exemplar of this principle.

## *External versus Internal Self-Regulation*

Through most of the treatment process, patients' reliance on the recommendations of the psychotherapist is healthy. As treatment nears its end, however, the psychotherapist needs to assist patients in relying more on internal appraisal and ultimately self-regulation of behavior. There is an evolution of the therapist's "eye on" patients to an "eye out for" them. Intrinsic to the process of developing realism is helping patients make choices that are in their own best interest (Phase 6 of the PEM). Patients' newfound wisdom and therapeutic achievements have laid the foundation for increased self-sufficiency—of course, in the context of whatever meaningful and practical external supports are required.

*Confidence = Consistency + Competency*

After brain injury, patients' sense of adequacy and self-confidence is often shattered, perpetuating feelings of insecurity and uncertainty. The mantra "Confidence equals consistency plus competency" highlights the importance of repetition and consistency in improving skills, and ultimately in building confidence. Regular task repetition is also critical in ameliorating the disruptive effects of cognitive deficits (e.g., in memory, attention/concentration, and executive functions) on global achievements.

### Group Psychotherapy

Group psychotherapy also facilitates exploration of the intrapsychic components of adjustment. These discussions generally reach deep into the hearts of patients. Figure 9.2 lists popular *intrapsychic assimilation* topics. These include the concepts of "flight into health" and "slippage," as well as exploration of the discontent associated with plateaus in recovery. Confidence-building intrapsychic assimilation exercises include creating personalized "progress reports" and "mottos," as well as itemizing sources of happiness, pride, and accomplishment.

### CASE STUDY

Henry was initially reluctant to divulge the truth about his grades; he oscillated between avoiding and glossing over the situation. He kept the proverbial stiff upper lip, projecting a "Superman" image. He even demonstrated some "flight-into-health" behavior, proclaiming that he did not need to employ the regimented study skills he had learned in therapy. He then accused his psychotherapist of playing "Big Brother" by prying too much into his study skills and academics.

However, as the school semester unfolded, his psychotherapist observed that Henry was becoming progressively somber and socially withdrawn. These were ominous signs of internal distress, given Henry's usual happy-go-lucky demeanor. Foreshadowing his emotional capitulation, Henry participated in the "pie chart" exercise during group psychotherapy. He drew an oversized pie, symbolizing how overburdened he felt. He labeled his predominant slice as "school hassles," which were crowding out other obligations and pleasures. Then, within a few days, Henry's initial exuberance and seeming overconfidence about his intellectual capacities switched precipitously to inconsolable depression. He stated that he felt like a "fish out of water" in the university environment; he was academically overwhelmed, and anxious and insecure about his abilities. He became edgy and "snarky," and his family and therapists were "walking on eggshells." After a gentle inquiry by his psychotherapist, Henry began to weep, declaring that he was "stupid" and "incompetent." He provided a heart-wrenching example of forgetting within 2 days which small group he had been assigned to in the classroom, and being unable to recognize any of his classmates' faces. He was also unable to contribute meaningfully to classroom discussions, as he could not remember the material he had studied the prior evening. He lamented that the content on the quizzes looked like a "foreign language." He was also mortified to share his failing grades with his father, because Henry felt that he would disapprove. Soon afterward, Henry took an "all-or-nothing" approach, stopping his psychotherapist in the hallway and dogmatically announcing that he was planning to drop out of the university that afternoon. With his unrealistic goals and acute setbacks, Henry had clearly plunged into the Phase 6 "yellow" warning zone of the PEM.

His psychotherapist arranged an immediate appointment; she adopted a pragmatic, stepwise, subgoal-based approach. She agreed that it was in Henry's best interest to drop the business classes he was failing in before the looming school deadline. However, she proposed that Henry continue with the math class, as he had a satisfactory grade in that course, and the university credit could be applied to a more realistic career objective. Limited neuropsychological testing was initiated within the next week for collateral data. The specific targets were his working memory and verbal learning deficits, as almost 1 year had now passed since Henry's injury. Test results revealed no improvements since the testing several months earlier. Although this provided an important "reality check," it intensified Henry's feelings of worthlessness. His psychotherapy sessions were increased to twice weekly, and he was encouraged to continue with his psychotropic medication for his depression. He was also monitored by his psychiatrist during this time, and a conjoint meeting was soon arranged with Henry, his parents, his psychotherapist, and his psychiatrist, to discuss his mood and adjustment.

Although Henry was temporarily blinded to his strengths and capabilities, it was obvious to his treating therapists that his talents and personality made him an ideal candidate for a career in sales. His psychotherapist urged that he consider a "Plan B": attending a community college and pursuing an associate's degree in marketing or communications. The course complexity and content were considered a perfect match for a future career in sales. He also expressed eagerness to become a car salesman, which would increase his income potential. During his school and work transition, Henry shared the music and lyrics to "Working on a Dream" (Springsteen, 2009) in group psychotherapy, illustrating his enthusiastic plans. Henry later participated in the "crystal ball" exercise (see below) during group psychotherapy, seeing himself in the next 3–5 years as a successful car salesman for alternative-fuel vehicles. He received encouragement and praise for his aspirations from his fellow patients.

Henry completed his math class with a passing grade. The next semester he transferred to a local community college and undertook a 2-year degree in the field of communications. He started with three classes, and then took four for the following semesters. His grades were all A's and B's; he was genuinely happy with his new career choice. Henry was also promoted to a supervisory position at work, given his sales prowess and commitment. He was now "comfortable in his own skin," delighting in his reclaimed sense of mastery and competency. Henry was now adaptively coping (Phase 6 "green" adaptive coping zone of the PEM), as he was realistic and confident about his attainable goals. His parents were heartened and embraced Henry's new vocational direction—his "Plan B." They were highly relieved to observe his enhanced self-efficacy and renewed confidence. With encouragement from his psychotherapist to pursue other avenues for mastery and happiness, Henry also took up a new hobby: photography. This further expanded his life satisfaction. Several months later, Henry expressed gratitude to both his psychotherapist and speech–language pathologist for their patience, flexibility, and willingness to let him learn for himself. He acknowledged that he had needed to do it "my own way, and in my own time." He stated, "You've got my back," and after pondering, he restated his view of his psychotherapist as a "twin brother" (vs. the earlier "Big Brother"). This change symbolized how the working alliance was fortified and deepened.

## THE EXISTENTIAL ASSIMILATION DIMENSION

As shown in Figure 9.1, existential assimilation is the third and final component of the adjustment process. It is manifested in a patient's life philosophy, which includes meaning in life, quality of life, self-actualization, and hope. The patient undergoes an often arduous and protracted process of transformation and transcendence to attain glimmers, and then a realistic vision, of a hopeful and fulfilling future. This is a process of restoring capacities for self-agency, self-realization, human flourishing, and meaning (Jennings, 2006; Klonoff, Lamb, Henderson, Reichert, et al., 2000; Prigatano & Ben-Yishay, 1999).

"Quality of life" relates to the qualitative aspects of adjustment. It represents the subjective, "sociopersonal" aspects of existence, including physical, emotional, and material well-being; interpersonal relationships; social, community, and civic activities; recreation; and personal development and fulfillment (see Klonoff et al., 1986, for a review). Other components of quality of life include subjective well-being, a positive self-view, self-worth, and life satisfaction (Sherwin et al., 2006; Vickery, Gontkovsky, & Caroselli, 2005). Not unexpectedly, self-efficacy, especially for ameliorating cognitive deficits, is positively associated with quality of life (Cicerone & Azulay, 2007).

"Meaning in life" suggests a higher-order purpose and *raison d'être*. A vital part of the transformation and transcendence process after brain injury is defining (and often redefining) a life philosophy, including regaining identity, meaning, a sense of belonging, and hopefulness (Bay, Hagerty, Williams, Kirsch, & Gillespie, 2002; Chamberlain, 2006; Fine, 1991; Gracey et al., 2008; Haggstrom & Lund, 2008; Heller et al., 2006; Linge, 1990; Smith, 2008; Yalom, 1980). Attaining meaning can be conceptualized as finding benefit in, and making sense of, loss (Davis, Nolen-Hoeksema, & Larson, 1998). It also represents recalibration of a patient's assumptive world to accommodate life's altered course (see Corr, 2002, for a review).

Maslow (1971) described "self-actualization" as the realization of one's total potential and as the ultimate goal of all humankind (see Dhiman, 2007, for a review). The components of self-actualization or self-realization include self-acceptance, self-fulfillment, purpose in life, personal growth, positive relations with others, environmental mastery, responsibility, and autonomy (Collins, Lanham, & Sigford, 2000; Maslow, 1954, 1971; Miquelon & Vallerand, 2008). Self-actualization is also the corollary of transforming suffering into meaning and is a mechanism for personal growth (Frankl, 1984; McGrath, 2004; Paletti, 2008). Preliminary research has suggested a role for growth in the postacute phases after brain injury, including enhanced relationships with others, increased personal strength, new possibilities, greater appreciation of life, and heightened spirituality (Hawley & Joseph,

2008; Powell, Ekin-Wood, & Collin, 2007). When patients engage in productive postinjury work and/or schooling, it not only normalizes and structures their day; it puts them back into the mainstream of society and fills a social void (Johansson & Tham, 2006; Klonoff et al., 2000; Prigatano, 1989). Accomplishing these and other tangible goals can redefine life-altering events and can constitute a transformational and restorative approach (McGrath, 2004) to achieving meaning, hope, fulfillment, and quality of life (Aniskiewicz, 2007; Levack, McPherson, & McNaughton, 2004; Oppermann, 2004; Prigatano, 1991; Strom & Kosciulek, 2007).

### Fostering Existential Assimilation in Individual Psychotherapy

Psychotherapy techniques to address the existential aspects of adjustment have two objectives: (1) to reinforce compensatory strategies to ensure optimum performance across a variety of meaningful life domains; and (2) to explore higher-order values that will inspire and guide patients in their life quests. Ultimately, each patient needs to find new outlets for meaning, productivity, and humanitarianism. As portrayed in Phase 6 of the PEM, the psychotherapist must balance the two objectives in order for the patient to maintain progress toward desirable yet attainable goals. The therapy process can be likened to assisting the patient in creating a sculpture. Much like molding clay, the process can seem elusive and tentative until the patient has a firm sense of self and of how to proceed.

The psychotherapist should monitor patients' habitual use of their datebooks and other aids to compensate for memory deficits, given the positive effects of these aids on daily living, work, and quality of life (Boman et al., 2007). During individual psychotherapy sessions, patients are often invited to demonstrate the use of these compensations; this affords ongoing accountability in case of "flight into health," as well as a forum in which to initiate dialogue about specific happenings. Similarly, processing the patients' social communication skills through within-session observations, as well as inquiries about their social lives outside the sessions, allows the psychotherapist to monitor patients' social reintegration and life satisfaction (Dahlberg et al., 2006). The psychotherapist should also explore other areas relating to quality of life, including work, hobbies, and pastimes. When therapists facilitate sharing, mutual analysis, and effective problem solving, they reinforce an awareness-and-acceptance loop.

### Exploring Key Life Values

A more monumental task for the psychotherapist is assisting patients in their search for postinjury meaning and hope. Generally, this involves exploration of the patients' key life values (see Chapter 4). Ultimately, the psychotherapist can assist the patients in facing the challenges to their fundamental convictions, yet creatively reconstructing relationships and attitudes about their assumptive worlds (Corr, 2002). A number of mechanisms are helpful in this process; each is founded upon what imbues a particular patient with passion and resoluteness (i.e., what makes the patient "tick"). For example, writing a personal autobiography and imagining the future in the next 2–5 years is helpful for some patients. Sharing the autobiography in individual psychotherapy, with family members, or in group psychotherapy, can further assist such patients in articulating where they have been, where they are now, and where they aspire to go.

Sometimes patients become (understandably) mired in grief or uncertainty as they undertake this emotionally daunting journey. The psychotherapist's "shoulder to lean on" and "listening ear" often provide essential emotional support for such patients. As described elsewhere, others' soul-searching writings can help patients to recalibrate their perspectives (e.g., Bankston, 2004; Kingsley, 1987; Simon, 2002, pp. 165–166; Williams, 2004). The following is a useful metaphor for this process.

### Brain Injury as a "Wake-Up Call"

In retrospect, some patients feel that they were on the "wrong track" in life and through psychotherapy come to reframe their brain injury as a "second chance" or "wake-up call." This transforms a devastating life event into something with meaning and higher purpose (Aniskiewicz, 2007). It is as if the serendipity of survival has meaningfully altered their life course. In such cases, the psychotherapist can inquire about what the injury has done "for them" versus "to them." Often they report enrichment of sometimes underdeveloped core attributes of patience, gratitude, empathy, tolerance, and self-reflection. They also often choose to shape a new life direction, rather than return to the status quo. Interestingly, their chosen paths frequently embody existential aspirations, including helping others with life deprivations or struggles. In this way, their injuries open their eyes and their hearts.

### Group Psychotherapy

Existential topics and exercises elevate the group discussion and outlook to higher-order values and life meaning, and place brain injury into a broader life perspective (see Figure 9.2). The psychotherapist's ability to create an atmosphere that inspires self-inquiry and ingenuity plays a vital role in these discussions. Popular topics include feelings about injury anniversaries, the view of brain injury as a "wake-up call" (see above), and ways to appreciate the enhanced sense of life's preciousness. Potent group exercises include personal tabulations of enhanced humanistic qualities, things to be thankful for (especially during the end-of-year holiday season), and New Year's resolutions. The group can shift fluidly among a variety of formats, including emotional outpouring, constructive "venting," didactic education, and visits from former patients. Patients can also discuss movies—for example, *The Pursuit of Happyness* (Alper et al., & Muccino, 2006), *The Family Man* (Abraham et al., 2000), or *The Ultimate Gift* (Eldridge et al., 2006)—and review other inspirational material to reinforce the constructs of meaning, quality of life, self-actualization, and hope. One emotive group exercise is for each patient to bring in a musical choice with the lyrics, which the group sings (F. Humle, personal communication, n.d.). Following this, the individual and group explore the underlying existential messages. This bonding exercise communicates hope as patients continue their quest for belongingness, self-actualization, fulfillment, and transcendence.

Activities that unite patients and strengthen their resolve, cohesiveness, gratitude, and optimism can be incorporated into the group experience, including community service projects (e.g., serving meals at a local shelter) or creating a quilt with individualized swatches depicting patients' psychological journeys and personal mottos. A weekly "circle of positives" (P. de Visme, personal communication, February 2004); a review of patients' "tool kits" of coping and support resources; and predictions of their futures through the "crystal ball" exercise can all reinforce patients' progress and sustain the patients in their personal searches and life missions.

## CASE STUDIES

Various personal creative outlets can allow patients to adjust to new realities, yet maintain hope and optimism. For example, Laura, who sustained a traumatic brain injury, began her psychotherapy at 6 months postinjury. Prior to that time, she had sunk into deep despair and had abandoned her academic studies in interior design. After several months of twice-weekly psychotherapy, her depression lifted, and she was encouraged to reenroll in school. She carefully reentered the school in steps, first auditing classes and meeting regularly with her teachers. She enlisted her psychotherapist and speech–language pathologist to be liaisons with her instructors. This included a joint meeting wherein Laura took a leadership role in describing the effects of her brain injury. This empowered her and strengthened her resolve to complete her degree.

Laura's final course responsibility was to complete a major graduation project. Based on her recent life journey and process of self-actualization, she chose to design a recreation center for patients with acquired brain injury. She put boundless energy and devotion into the intricate details of the drawings and conceptualization, including creating the physical space in the shape of the infinity sign (see Phase 7 of the PEM in Figure 1.2). She researched and chose "healing" colors to create a warm and nurturing ambience. This project imbued her with purpose and a new, gratifying life objective. Her personal suffering was transmuted into tangible empathy and goodwill for others in similar predicaments.

Another patient, Dennis, used poetry to transcend a vanished identity and find a life purpose. Before brain injury, he had been a high-powered and accomplished hospital administrator; however, at age 62, he suffered a subarachnoid hemorrhage and was unable to return to this position. Through his psychotherapy and existential journey, Dennis rediscovered a prior love: writing. This passion had been ignored for many years because of protracted work weeks and unending work pressures. Writing became his emotional "ladder" for his progression through the stages of awareness, acceptance, and realism. The poem in Figure 9.7 depicts the transformation and transcendence process, mirrored through the story of an African parrot. Like Dennis, the parrot at first is no longer part of the (work) flock, due to his challenges. For both of them, their fate has carved a new course, and they must now find a new way to survive. Dennis's and the parrot's resourcefulness and inner talents enable them both to "meet [the] challenge" of overcoming "hindrance by happenstance"; through "reinventing" themselves, they triumph and ultimately flourish.

> This parrot hatched whiter than Antarctica's snow,
> A smashing good color for seagulls to show.
> But African parrots, contrariwise,
> Are gray with red tails and white-circled eyes.
> Worse, one wing was withered, which certainly meant
> He wouldn't be flying to places he went.
> Yet, strange as he seemed and as odd to behold,
> This parrot was crafty, his manner too bold
> To succumb to the whims of the menacing brood
> Of beasties in search of such fine feathered food.
> He instead learned to mimic the growls they convey
> To fool them and spook them and keep them away.
> Rather than surrender to his seeming sad state,
> He adjusted his life to instead compensate.
> Can we also arise to that test should it call,
> Should unforeseen hindrance by happenstance fall
> On us or on others in flocks where we live;
> And meet such a challenge, adjust and forgive,
> Reinventing ourselves, to somehow compensate
> With new talents we find in new lives we create?
> This story highlights the best lesson of all:
> Getting up is God's reason for letting us fall.
>
> —D. W. Schwesinger

**FIGURE 9.7.** Dennis's poem "The Parrot Ventriloquist."

## TERMINATION OF PSYCHOTHERAPY

Generally, termination of psychotherapy depends on a patient's knowledge acquisition, self-understanding, psychological readiness (often mirroring the process of separation and individuation), resiliency, ego strength, autonomy, and accomplishment of predetermined treatment outcomes (Joyce, Piper, Ogrodniczuk, & Klein, 2007; Quintar, 2001; Ward, 1984). Other significant considerations are the patient's prior history of loss and abandonment reactions, his or her tolerance for interpersonal conflict, and transference–countertransference reactions (Jorgensen & Thibodeau, 2007; Joyce et al., 2007; Quintar, 2001; Ward, 1984). Although the content and process of termination both need to be tailored to the individual needs of the patient, it should always include an opportunity for self-appraisal of the totality of the treatment process, a recapitulation of the lessons learned, and identification of possible unmet objectives (Joyce et al., 2007).

Relatively little has been written about the process of terminating psychotherapy after brain injury. Understandably, this population faces unique challenges regarding the "hows, whens, and whys" of treatment termination. Core considerations include the nature and extent of cognitive deficits, including a patient's capability for effective reasoning, planning, problem solving, judgment, and self-regulation. The patient should also be able to generalize the knowledge gained and techniques learned as part of the psychotherapeutic process to other life decisions and domains. To the extent that patients lack these skills and struggle to fend psychologically for themselves, the need for some form of longer-term intervention increases. This may include other formal psychotherapeutic treatment, community support groups, and/or help from family members.

Sometimes the termination process is better conceptualized as an "interruption," with the therapeutic relationship placed on hiatus until the need for further intervention emerges or is acknowledged (Joyce et al., 2007). As noted in Figure 1.2 for Phase 7 of the PEM, it can be reassuring to patients to know that the door is always open for more assistance, should the need arise. This is more likely when the injury's effects are more profound; when the patient is in the acute phases of recovery; or when new, often unexpected life-altering challenges arise down the road. Sometimes refresher sessions are needed if the patient has shown sufficient "flight into health" or "slippage" in the use of compensations to compromise productivity and quality of life. However, the reality of a managed care environment in the United States is that patients often have a predetermined number of treatment visits, which can constrain goal setting and accomplishments. In these contexts, the psychotherapist must collaborate with the patient and support system to clarify circumscribed and attainable objectives within the limits of the available resources.

## Relevant Considerations and Useful Metaphors

Figure 9.8 summarizes specific practical considerations when terminating psychotherapy after brain injury. A patient must demonstrate improved awareness, acceptance, and realism, with consistent use of compensations. Other integral elements include the patient's overall adaptation, support network, functional goal attainment, quality of life, and a meaningful existence. In essence, the patient is making the transition from Phase 6 to Phase 7 of the PEM. These criteria should be reviewed with the patient and family periodically during psychotherapy, so as to clarify the parameters of the interventions. Overall, regardless of the psychotherapeutic style or length of treatment, adequate attention to and planning for the termination process are essential for preservation of the working alliance with the current treater (and with any future treaters), for positive outcomes, and for the patient's overall emotional well-being (Joyce et al., 2007).

The following discussion describes other relevant considerations and some clinically useful metaphors for the termination process after brain injury.

### The "Long Tail of Therapy"

Patients often benefit from a tapering of psychotherapy sessions, which can be described as the "long tail of therapy." That is, the length of time between sessions is gradually increased once patients have successfully made the transition to work or school. A common schedule for the "long tail" is to move from weekly appointments to twice monthly for 1–3 months, and then monthly for 1–3 months. This eases patients and their families into the realities of a more independent existence, while at the same time providing the necessary emotional support and troubleshooting.

1. Good awareness, acceptance, and realism
   - Capacity for generalization of in-session constructs to the community
   - Capacity to function as "own therapist" (self-appraisal, judgment, and self-regulation skills)

2. Good and consistent use of compensations for deficits
   - Memory
   - Executive functions (e.g., initiation, organization, follow-through)
   - Other deficits (specify)
   - Ability to adapt/modify personalized compensations when needed

3. Psychological adaptation to the injury
   - Good communication pragmatics
   - Emotional stability
   - Sense of confidence

4. a. Working at maximum capacity (part-time or full-time)
   - Successful for a minimum of 6–8 weeks

   b. Attending school (part-time or full-time)
   - Successful for one full semester

5. Independent in transportation
   - Driving, bus, transit service

6. Support network
   - Family is "on board" and has attained knowledge and emotional support
   - Stable community supports
   - "Two-way street" in relationships

7. Good quality of life; meaningful existence
   - Work/school
   - Hobbies
   - Family life
   - Social life
   - Focusing on positives and the future
   - Sense of hope

**FIGURE 9.8.** Considerations when terminating psychotherapy after brain injury.

### "Graduation"/"Cake Day"

When patients are involved in group therapy or a program of care, holding a "graduation" ceremony not only helps define the end of the therapeutic process, but allows patients to celebrate their successes (and sometimes to acknowledge unfinished business). "Cake day" (Phase 6 of the PEM) is the culmination of their diligent efforts. In the context of group treatment, it allows for closure and the solidifying of peer relationships. Each departing patient is honored in a group setting with a cake, as well as "verbal presents" (Y. Ben-Yishay, personal communication, n.d.) from their therapists and fellow patients. The patient uses this session to discuss his or her experience of the psychotherapy and rehabilitation process. Other group participants are encouraged to share their observations and commendations about the patient's gains and to say their good-byes. This often buttresses the graduating patient's self-worth and self-assurance, and also inspires optimism in the remaining group members that their time will come.

### "Bird Out of the Nest": A Form of Therapy Is No More Therapy

Patients are often fearful about making the transition from the safety and structure of the psychotherapy relationship. They may express hesitancies, self-doubts, and sometimes profound "separation anxiety" about the future (Mander, 2000; Quintar, 2001). The metaphor of a "bird out of the nest" often helps ameliorate patients' worries and normalize the termination process; it allows them to recognize that they have "matured" to the point of readiness to "fly on their own." Providing a picture or diagram of a bird leaving the nest can be a reassuring visual reminder for patients.

### "Spreading Their Wings": Taking a Break from Psychotherapy

Sometimes patients need the opportunity to consolidate their therapeutic experiences and "spread their wings." They may therefore benefit from taking a break from the psychotherapy process. This is especially the case when patients are reacting defensively to therapeutic input because of organic unawareness, denial, and/or other neurological/characterological/emotional factors. Once they have experienced some psychological and physical distance from the therapeutic process, patients will often spontaneously reconnect with the psychotherapist and express altered views about the merits of the process.

## Group Psychotherapy

A worthwhile vehicle to prepare for the termination process is group psychotherapy. Pertinent topics and exercises are included in Figure 9.2; these include discussing general and personalized criteria for discharge, and processing patients' varied emotional reactions to ending therapy (ranging from trepidation to exultation).

## Premature Termination and Planting the Seed

As identified in the period of disintegration ("red" crisis zone) of the PEM, sometimes a patient decides to terminate the therapy process precipitously. Such a situation often results from negative reactions to the psychotherapist, intense transference reactions, triangulations, or stalemates in therapeutic interactions (Hill, Nutt-Williams, Heaton, Thompson, & Rhodes, 1996; Quintar, 2001, Ward, 1984). Also, after brain injury, patients may not recognize the need or benefit for continued treatment. Alternatively, they may be experiencing profound catastrophic reactions to confronting their deficits.

Whatever the cause of a threat to terminate treatment prematurely may be, the psychotherapist should alert the patient to his or her concerns, including the potential risks of termination (Gross, 2006). These concerns should be articulated both orally and in writing to the patient and to his or her support network, given the nature of the patient's cognitive deficits and often associated emotional instability. The psychotherapist should also be vigilant (clinically, ethically, and legally) about the destabilizing impact of unplanned treatment termination, and should provide alternative treatment interventions as necessary (Gross, 2006). When warranted, the psychotherapist should take extra steps to ensure that the patient has made a smooth transition to another treatment provider, including helping the patient set up an appointment and obtaining medical releases to forward records to ensure continuity of care. At the same time, the psychotherapist's concerns should be counterbalanced with respect for the patient's decision, should he or she insist on stopping treatment. Ideally, the psychotherapist's efforts have "planted the seed" (G. A. Lage, personal communication, n.d.) for the patient's personal growth. The psychotherapist's patience and sensitivity will preserve the working alliance, so that if the need arises, the patient will recontact the psychotherapist (Ward, 1984).

## Posttreatment Contact

### Intermittent Contact

After termination, patients sometimes appreciate the opportunity for intermittent contact with their psychotherapist. The psychotherapist must be judicious about how and when this contact is made, in order to set appropriate treatment boundaries. Acceptable formats include a prearranged follow-up appointment several months later, occasional scheduled visits to group psychotherapy, or annual holiday cards from patients (Klonoff, Lamb, Henderson, Reichert, et al., 2000; Mander, 2000; Quintar, 2001; Ward, 1984). Some rehabilitation settings schedule periodic "patient reunions," which afford a structured opportunity for patients to reunite and share their postrehabilitation stories and successes, as well as to reconnect briefly with their psychotherapist. These visits also provide a setting for the patients to reflect on life after treatment, which often has ripened into new perspectives, including attainment of meaning, productivity, and self-determination.

### Patient Aftercare Group

Aftercare support groups are a beneficial (and often an ideal) form of ongoing therapeutic and social support for patients after brain injury (Klonoff, 1997; Klonoff, Lamb, Henderson, Reichert, et al., 2000). Groups should be small enough (e.g., 12–16 patients and one to two psychotherapists), and should meet often enough (e.g., monthly) and long enough (e.g., an hour), to allow for meaningful dialogue and social familiarity. Patients can share their experiences and perturbations with colleagues who "walk in their shoes." This therapeutic setting provides opportunities for further education by the therapist(s) and peers. One suggested format for sessions is to begin by asking patients to provide introductions and status updates, especially in an open-entry group. To promote community integration, patients can identify upcoming social activities. Following this, patients can be invited to raise topics of interest or concern.

These patient discussions often cycle back through awareness, acceptance, and realism in the context of new insights and foibles that emerge as patients become further integrated into their community. Sample acceptance topics include "Why me?" and angst about using compensations for the long haul. Figure 9.9 lists common adjustment topics and exercises, grouped according to the domains of *adaptation, intrapsychic assimilation,* and *existential assimilation.* Most frequent and most poignant are patients' concerns with existential questions. These include

---

**Adaptation Topics**
- Postinjury driving and car accidents
- "To work or not to work . . .": Practical concerns.
- Financial stressors.
- New career aspirations and attainable goals.

**Adaptation Exercises**
- Round-robin updates about work/school.
- Updated itemized personal challenges for work/school and how to be successful.
- Current self-ratings of job competency (1–10; 1 = low, 10 = high), and reasons for these.

**Intrapsychic Assimilation Topics**
- "Flight into health" and "slippage" after discharge.
- Retrospective analysis of rehabilitation/psychotherapy (walk down "memory lane").
- Ways to maintain self-confidence.
- Balancing work, love, and play.

**Intrapsychic Assimilation Exercises**
- My year in review.
- Current ratings of job satisfaction (1–10; 1 = strongly dislike, 10 = love).
- Personal lists of sources of happiness (pre- vs. postinjury).

**Existential Assimilation Topics**
- Feelings about injury anniversaries.
- Is life better after the injury?
- Reciprocity in family relationships and friendships.
- What are my values/priorities now, and do I live them?
- How to overcome adversity.
- How death affects how we live.
- Is there meaning in life?
- How to enhance hope and optimism.

**Existential Assimilation Exercises**
- Objects, mementos, songs, and movies with personal meaning.
- Invent a song title that depicts your life.
- New Year's resolutions: Goals and aspirations.
- Sources of quality of life.
- "Circle of positives."
- Meaningful community service group projects.

---

**FIGURE 9.9.** Patient aftercare group topics and exercises.

how to make cosmic sense of their injuries; how to see the "silver linings" of their hardships; and how to help others struggling with life predicaments, including their families. The continued journey toward self-actualization and the quest for higher purpose and personal growth can be inspiring to fellow group members and to the psychotherapists who witness this transformation process.

A facilitating psychotherapist can take notes on an easel to track the discussions for the group. It can be helpful for the psychotherapist to transcribe the main topics and points of discussion, and then to provide these in a handout to the group at the following meeting. Provision of light snacks enhances the nurturing ambience. Concluding the group with a "circle of positives" (P. de Visme, personal communication, February 2004) borrows a comforting ritual from group psychotherapy, and also allows the group to finish on a cheerful, encouraging note. One humanitarian approach is for the psychotherapist to donate his or her time, and to charge patients only a nominal donation (e.g., $10 per session) to be used to help other patients receive rehabilitation services (this can be called a "scholarship fund"). In combination with regular community service projects, this sustains a spirit of social awareness and responsibility.

### Family Aftercare Group

The family aftercare group is an extension of the weekly family group (see Chapter 7) (Klonoff et al., 2008). Like the patient aftercare group, this group can comfortably accommodate 12–16 family members when facilitated by one or two psychotherapists. It affords extended emotional support, education, peer mentoring, and practical resources for family members. Also, similar to the patient aftercare group, it furnishes a healing social outlet for families, many of whom have developed close emotional bonds and friendships as a result of their participation in prior treatment.

Like the patient aftercare group, this group meets monthly; again, snacks and treats are supplied, to create a nurturing and relaxed atmosphere. Generally attendees share their progress and feats, as well as their disappointments, worries, fears, and even regrets. The group members often make joint efforts to identify viable solutions for colleagues facing struggles or misfortunes. When appropriate, family members may "therapeutically pressure" one another to take specific actions before the next meeting. This introduces mutual accountability, which is an outgrowth of the commitment to and compassion for each other. Common topics include patients' "flight into health" and "slippage"; patients' lingering problems with judgment, impulsivity, and safety awareness; and patients' and families' interpersonal and psychosocial challenges, especially social isolation. Without sufficient resources and support, family members may (re)lapse into emotional exhaustion or burnout. This group normalizes concerns, and is efficacious in teaching and reinforcing long-term coping techniques. Helpful adjunct interventions for family members may include joint sessions with their loved one (in family therapy or conjoint aftercare groups) to address critical concerns and issues; psychotropic medications for family members; respite care; and ongoing social activities with their peer social network.

**CASE STUDY**

Henry's individual psychotherapy visits were gradually tapered from twice weekly to once weekly and, after 1 year, to once monthly. Once he was successfully back at school and planning for a career in sales, the need for psychotherapeutic interventions waned. He was aware of his cognitive deficits and was capitalizing on his strengths. He used the necessary compensations to excel in school, including a note taker and an audio recorder. His relationship with his parents remained healthy and reciprocal. He also met a young lady through his church, and the relationship was blossoming. After 18 months, his psychological adjustment was solidifying, and Henry and his psychotherapist agreed to terminate individual psychotherapy. His support network also agreed. "Cake day" had arrived!

Henry enthusiastically attended a monthly aftercare group with a number of his fellow therapy "graduates." He also regularly participated in a social support group in the community with his parents and girlfriend. He was periodically invited to group psychotherapy by his psychotherapist; he was well liked by the "new recruits" because of his candid and entertaining ability to relate to the rigors of the psychotherapy process. He also had a "true-blue" respect and gratefulness for his substantial personal accomplishments and the maturity he had gleaned through his struggles and the psychotherapeutic process. He enjoyed the opportunity to reconnect with others still in treatment, and he felt comforted by "returning to the mother ship." In some ways, he now embraced his traumatic brain injury as a "wake-up call" to live life more purposefully. While in psychotherapy, Henry had also been introduced to the term "karma bank," as a description of how patients can express their gratitude for the treatment they have received by giving back to others. Henry began volunteering in an inpatient rehabilitation setting as a peer mentor to more acutely brain-injured patients and their families. He felt that this "closed the loop" of giving and receiving "gifts" of hope. With his evolution through Phases 4 through 7 of the PEM, Henry had matured deeply and was vibrantly reconnected to a healthy identity, loving community supports, and a meaningful existence.

Psychotherapists providing treatment interventions for patients with brain injuries and their support network encounter multiple stressors. Chapter 10 reviews techniques to avoid burnout and maintain self-care to promote professional longevity.

# Psychotherapist Self-Care
## *Managing Stress and Avoiding Burnout*

$A$ psychotherapist faces many professional hazards and stresses in treating patients with acquired brain injuries. Reasons include mismatches between the patients'/families' and the therapist's readiness and commitment to change, and elusive definitions of treatment success (McLaughlin & Carey, 1993). These patients also have intense needs stemming from the brain injuries themselves. For example, patients with executive system deficits rely on the psychotherapist for practical, daily decisions (Klonoff & Lage, 1991). Other distinct challenges emanate from the patients' interpersonal and pragmatic difficulties and from the pervasiveness and impact of their memory problems (Prigatano et al., 1986). Psychotherapists may require "thick therapeutic skins" to withstand patients' resistance and/or organic unawareness. Moreover, patients with brain injuries are prone to episodes of emotional lability or depression (Koponen et al., 2002). Those with significant temporal lobe damage can have cognitive misperceptions and distortions, as well as suspiciousness and paranoia, all of which complicate the working alliance (Prigatano et al., 1986). Lastly, family members' struggles, psychodynamics, (un)availability, and partnership (or lack of it) with the therapeutic process add a further layer of intricacy to therapy, with resulting strains on the psychotherapist. Sometimes an "adversarial alliance" ensues, and the psychotherapist may feel scapegoated by the patient and/or family (McLaughlin & Carey, 1993). Therefore, a psychotherapists must "wear many hats" in addressing the multiplicity of patients' and families' needs—functioning as a detective, trailblazer, guide, pragmatist, educator, coach, "external conscience," advocate, witness, protector, companion, and mediator.

Three constructs that potentially affect the psychotherapist and threaten the collaborative working alliance are countertransference, comorbid diagnoses, and burnout. I discuss each of these in turn.

## COUNTERTRANSFERENCE

"Countertransference" refers to a psychotherapist's feelings and attitudes toward a patient. These arise because specific qualities of the patient are perceived through the lens of the psychotherapist's past significant relationships, which have affected the psychotherapist's personality and development (Lewis, 1999; Sandler, Dare, & Holder, 1973). Countertransference is a valuable source of therapeutic information to supplement the psychotherapist's insights, interpretations, and interventions (Clarkson & Nuttall, 2000; Dieckmann, 1991; Gabbard, 2001; Guy & Brady, 2001; Swift & Wonderlich, 1993). However, it does represent a distortion, and it can be beneficial or detrimental, depending on the psychothcrapist's insight, skill, and integrity (Clarkson & Nuttall, 2000).

A psychotherapist may experience countertransference toward multiple aspects of a patient with brain injury, including the actual deficits, the patient's attitude toward his or her deficits, and/or the patient's transference (Lewis, 1999). Countertransference problems result when a psychotherapist has inaccurate perceptions of a brain-injured patient (Pepping, 1993). Sometimes the patient may consciously or unconsciously press the psychotherapist's professional "hot buttons." A patient's noncompliance with treatment recommendations may also induce feelings of helplessness or "My psychotherapeutic hands are tied" in the therapist.

Figure 10.1 lists "professional beacons" for dealing with countertransference—that is, guidelines for self-monitoring countertransference reactions to patients with brain injury. Countertransference feelings become problematic when they are out of a psychotherapist's awareness, chronic, counterproductive to the therapeu-

---

- Differentiate between helpful and deleterious countertransference reactions through awareness, self-scrutiny, supervision/mentoring, and a professional support group.
- Be vigilant about "Achilles' heel" countertransference liabilities.
- Monitor warning signs:
  - Inappropriate or excessive self-disclosure.
  - Impasses or stalemates.
  - Treatment failures and abrupt terminations.
  - Angry outbursts toward patients.
  - Postponing or avoiding termination for the psychotherapist's needs rather than the patient's.
  - Sexual liaisons.

**FIGURE 10.1.** Professional beacons for dealing with countertransference.

tic process, or distressing (Clarkson & Nuttall, 2000; Sandler et al., 1973). Clearly, the psychotherapist needs to differentiate between countertransference reactions that are helpful and empathetically responsive to the patient's unmet needs, and those that are potentially harmful and due to the psychotherapist's unresolved longings (Guy & Brady, 2001).

To maintain effectiveness and ethical standards of practice, psychotherapists must be aware of, acknowledge, and address both their positive and negative reactions to their patients (Dieckmann, 1991; Gans, 1983; Groves, 1978; Gunther, 1994; Kraemer, 1958; Sandler et al., 1973). Psychotherapists need to be prepared to be "disturbed" by their "disturbing" patients (Rothstein, 1999). Conversely, fears of countertransference may inhibit creative responses to patients' needs (Strozier, 2001), and so these fears should also be examined.

The psychotherapist's introspective process extends to his or her perceptions of the patient's progress in psychotherapy; therefore, the psychotherapist must be willing to examine his or her own contributions to the therapy and to remove any inner barriers (Kohut, 1984a; Newman, 2002). The ultimate gauge is the best interest of the patient (Ward, 1984). Moreover, the psychotherapist needs to be vigilant about whatever his or her personal "Achilles' heel" of countertransference overreactions or distortions may be. One warning sign is inappropriate or excessive self-disclosure—that is, the sharing of personal information that benefits the psychotherapist more than the patient (Barglow, 2005; Yalom, 2002). Other unrecognized countertransference reactions can result in impasses or stalemates, treatment failures, abrupt unilateral terminations, angry outbursts toward patients, unnecessary postponement of termination, and sexual liaisons (Hill et al., 1996; Swift & Wonderlich, 1993; Ward, 1984). Self-scrutiny, external supervision, and a psychotherapist support group are potent ways to combat the professional hazards caused by unmonitored countertransference (Teitelbaum, 1991; Yalom, 2002).

## COMORBID DIAGNOSES

Patients with acquired brain injury may also have comorbid diagnoses (Gagnon, Bouchard, & Rainville, 2006), including substance use disorders, attention-deficit/hyperactivity disorder, and learning disabilities, as well as other preexisting Axis I and Axis II diagnoses. Some patients demonstrate conscious exaggeration of symptoms (i.e., malingering). Psychotherapists therefore need well-honed differential diagnostic skills, as well as treatment techniques spanning a wide range of diagnostic categories (Gagnon et al., 2006; Klonoff & Dawson, 2004; Prigatano et al., 1986).

The psychotherapist must be realistic about characterological problems and their potential for negative impact on treatment outcome. When patients' cognitive capacities are compromised, they may be more treatment-compliant initially. However, as their neuropsychological status improves and as reactive emotional difficulties are ameliorated (e.g., depression), characterological symptoms increasingly emerge. These may include the refusal to follow rules; refusal to complete datebook and homework assignments; lack of empathy and consideration of others' needs; arrogant, disrespectful, and "snarky" interactions; distrust and argumentative behavior; dishonest and manipulative conduct; poor work skills; and impulsive, risk-taking, and dangerous behavior. Other patients demonstrate helplessness and neediness; overstatement of problem areas; and/or overt noncompliance with gainful work recommendations. In a group treatment or milieu environment, patients with any of these symptoms may attempt to undermine the therapists' authority and generally contaminate the collaborative, harmony-based ambience. Similar characterological and compliance problems are also often encountered with their family members.

The likelihood of relapse for patients with substance use disorders is substantial after brain injury (MacMillan et al., 2002)—in part due to the addictive process itself, and in part to the compromised judgment and impulse control resulting from the organic brain damage (see Chapter 8). Most worrisome can be the possibility of assault or violence toward the psychotherapist. Research indicates that this possibility is most heightened in a neurological patient with a preexisting history of violence and/or substance abuse (Miller, 1998).

Figure 10.2 summarizes professional beacons for treating patients with comorbid diagnoses. Patients should be screened early for such diagnoses. Careful diagnostic formulation is essential in determining the relative contributions of neurological injury, psychiatric factors, and conscious effort to each patient's symptom picture. I strongly recommend that current symptom severity, course, and chronicity be determined by a combination of the following: (1) acute neurological/neuroradiographic correlates; (2) a detailed intake interview exploring pre- and postinjury psychiatric and functional status; (3) collateral interviews and objective psychosocial data; and (4) neuropsychological test performance (with quantitative and qualitative observations, symptom validity, and personality questionnaires). This comprehensive evaluation is required to ascertain the appropriate diagnoses and to promote optimal treatment planning (Babin & Gross, 2002; Klonoff & Dawson, 2004; Klonoff & Lamb, 1998; Lynch, 2004).

---

- Conduct early screening and careful diagnostic formulations, including assessment of the patient's motivation.
- Limit/monitor size of caseload.
- Set clear treatment rules and expectations.
- Seek cotreatment with specialists, involvement in a multidisciplinary team, and supervisory relationships whenever possible.
- If necessary, postpone treatment until any litigation is resolved.
- Assess and modify treatment plans as necessary for a patient at risk for aggressiveness.
- Consider psychotropic medication.
- Consider placing a highly resistant/noncompliant patient on probationary status.
- Consider judicious termination when all other possibilities have been exhausted.

---

**FIGURE 10.2.** Professional beacons for treating patients with comorbid diagnoses.

To the extent possible, psychotherapists may need to limit the size of their caseloads of patients with severe comorbid diagnoses, or be prepared for the complexity and demands of treating these populations. Such a patient's motivation for psychotherapy should be explored and assessed as early as possible and monitored throughout the treatment process, to avoid unwarranted expenditure of a psychotherapist's emotional energies and a misuse of funding resources. When noncompliant patients are involved in litigation, it is sometimes necessary to postpone psychotherapy until the litigation is resolved (Klonoff & Lamb, 1998).

Making and enforcing clear treatment rules are most efficacious for managing problem behaviors in patients with Axis II disorders. Such rules also protect the psychotherapist from attempts at deception and manipulation. Cotreatment with specialists in Axis II diagnoses and/or substance use disorders (e.g., psychiatrists, psychologists), or involvement in a multidisciplinary treatment team, also provides necessary professional and collegial resources (Warriner & Velikonja, 2006).

If a patient is at risk for aggression, the treatment environment can be modified to reduce conditions that could provoke or agitate the patient or escalate violent behavior. For example, sessions can be shorter; the treatment approach can be supportive or behavioral rather than insight-oriented; and the patient can be excluded from group psychotherapy (Alpert & Spillmann, 1997; Bruns & Disorbio, 2000; Klonoff et al., 1993). Sometimes it is also necessary to transfer the patient to a self-contained, specialized treatment unit that is better equipped to address severe behavioral problems (Alpert & Spillmann, 1997; Manchester, Hodgkinson, & Casey, 1997). At a minimum, the psychotherapist should carefully monitor the patient's disposition during psychotherapeutic discussions, and be sensible and pragmatic about the limits and efficacy of his or her interventions.

Adjunct psychopharmacological interventions can provide symptom relief. For example, SSRIs can be prescribed for irritability, emotional lability, agitation, and aggression (Klonoff et al., 1993; Vaishnavi et al., 2009; Warriner & Velikonja, 2006), which can result from the organic effects of brain injury, in combination with the preexisting personality problems. Supervisory relationships for clinicians immersed in these complex diagnoses are also warranted and strongly urged.

As discussed in Chapter 5, a psychotherapist may place a highly resistant and noncompliant patient on probation, with specific requirements for continued psychotherapy clearly delineated. Proper documentation and communication with relevant parties (the patient, family, referring physician, funding sources, etc.) are also necessary. This holds the patient accountable for his or her earnest commitment to psychotherapy.

If the patient does not demonstrate the necessary investment or therapeutic gains after the steps described above have been taken, the psychotherapist may decide to discontinue treatment. To avoid abandonment, the patient and family must then be provided with other applicable treatment resources (Vasquez, Bingham, & Barnett, 2008). There should be clear protocols in place for treating patients at risk for self-harm (or harm to others) and/or substance abuse (see Chapters 4 and 8). This should include arrangement with accessible, competent outside resources, such as psychiatrists and psychiatric inpatient facilities.

## BURNOUT

Without careful self-monitoring, a psychotherapist treating patients with brain injuries may unwittingly succumb to "compassion fatigue," emotional exhaustion, or "burnout" (Miller, 1998). Burnout is a process, not an endpoint (see Emerson & Markos, 1996, for a review). Precursors of burnout include an overwhelming sense of responsibility, overinvolvement, or overcommitment; excessive idealism; and unrealistic self-expectations (Emerson & Markos, 1996; Sapienza & Bugental, 2000). Burnout is manifested in the working alliance by clinician underinvolvement (see Emerson & Markos, 1996, for a review). Other warning signs include feelings of emotional depletion, depression, and worthlessness; disorganization and chaos; numbness or depersonalization; alienation, detachment, or even hatred toward patients; and a sense of futility about the effectiveness of the therapist's work (Emerson & Markos, 1996; Gans, 1983; Madhavilatha, 2008; McCarthy & Frieze, 1999; Pais, 2002; Sapienza & Bugental, 2000).

Other antecedents of burnout in the psychotherapist are problems in personal and work environments. For example, any taxing personal problem can negatively affect work performance by sapping and diverting the psychotherapist's psychic energies and emotional resources. "System failures" at work can include a lack of administrative support, bottom-line pressures, or personnel problems. The maze of insurance and reimbursement, and the fragmentation of health care delivery among physicians and other treaters, can have a negative impact not only on patients but ultimately on the psychotherapist (who feels responsible for safeguarding the patients' emotional well-being).

## AVOIDING BURNOUT: THE PSYCHOTHERAPIST'S "SURVIVAL KIT"

In keeping with psychologists' ethical principles, they have a professional obligation to be aware of the potential effect of their physical and mental health on those they help (American Psychological Association, 2002, Principle A) and engage in self-care (American Psychological Association Practice Organization, 2009). Many different strategies are available to help a psychotherapist avoid or reduce burnout, as listed in Figure 10.3 and discussed in the remainder of this chapter. These techniques are designed to preserve the psychotherapist's sense of enjoyment, fulfillment, renewal, and self-efficacy in work, as well as to promote personal growth (Norcross & Guy, 2005, 2007). Pais (2002, p. 109) has aptly described this process as remembering to "place the oxygen mask on yourself first."

### Personal Attributes and Coping Style

Professional burnout is diminished in the empathic psychotherapist (Linley & Joseph, 2007). The psychotherapist must be heedful of counterhostility, coldness, emotional distance, inflexibility, rejection, complacency, and scornfulness as markers of burnout (Holmqvist & Armelius, 2006; Strupp, 1980). Good antidotes to these include the capacity to laugh at him- or herself and to recognize innocent

**Personal Attributes and Coping Styles**
- Empathy
- Mindfulness
- Sense of humor
- Problem-solving ability
- Ability to compromise
- Capacity to "know thyself"
- Realism

**Division of Labor**

**Adjusting Expectations**
- Prepare to be unpopular
- Avoid power struggles and "pick your battles"
- Aspire to fairness
- Focus on process versus outcome
  - "Things take time" ("TTT")
  - "Plant the seed"

**Self-Examination, Supervision/Mentorship, and Personal Therapy**

**Professional Development**
- Research
- Professional organizations
- Community groups
- Scientific conferences

**System Supports and Professional Camaraderie**
- Institutional leadership that promotes professional growth
- Staff social events and recognition
- Community projects

**Balance between Work and Personal Life**
- Family life
- Friendships
- Hobbies/other leisure activities
- Regular exercise
- Proper nutrition
- Good sleep hygiene
- Small indulgences (e.g., chocolate)
- Vacations

**Creativity, Vision, and Hope**
- "Vicarious resilience"
- Adjunct psychotherapy treatment techniques
  - Art
  - Music
  - Literature
  - Movies
- Inspirational resources
  - Songs, literature, movies (see Figure 10.4)
  - Patient alumni visits to group psychotherapy
  - Yearly graduations/reunions and projects
  - "Imaginative conviction"

**FIGURE 10.3.** Avoiding burnout: The psychotherapist's survival kit.

humor in clinical vignettes. This not only refreshes the psychotherapist, but also engenders levity and a healthy therapeutic outlet and perspective (Norcross & Guy, 2005, 2007; Scholl & Ragan, 2003). Research suggests that therapists who utilize a problem-solving coping style, including "taking one step at a time" and the capacity to compromise, cope better with the inherent demands of working with patients with acquired brain injury (McLaughlin & Erdman, 1992).

Given the intensity and nature of the work, the psychotherapist who heeds the adage "Know thyself" will be mindful of his or her work capacities and limitations, and acknowledge the inability to cure every patient (Norcross & Guy, 2005). This type of mindfulness includes not practicing outside his or her areas of expertise and comfort zones. "Therapeutic ambitiousness" can be detrimental if it overtaxes a patient and sets unattainable expectations (Gans, 1983). The psychotherapist's ability to set realistic parameters and explicit time frames facilitates self-care, and preserves long-term therapeutic effectiveness and personal well-being (Pais, 2002; Prigatano et al., 1986).

## Division of Labor

In situations where psychotherapists work as part of an interdisciplinary treatment team, or with other clinicians, they have the opportunity of sharing responsibilities through cotreatment with other professionals. As thorny treatment issues arise, the psychotherapists can assume alternate roles (e.g., the "good cop/ bad cop"). This allows each clinician to trade off taking a more confrontive role with taking a supportive role.

Every clinician has preferences and areas of expertise; however, psychotherapists must also be wary of "overspecialization" (Yalom, 2002). Seeing too many patients of the same types can lead to burnout. A mix of patients in the caseload preserves the psychotherapist's psychic energies and zeal.

## Adjusting Expectations

Working with brain-injured patients can be difficult in some predictable ways. Expecting and preparing for these difficulties will minimize their impact. The following are some typical examples.

### Prepare to Be Unpopular

Psychotherapists treating patients with acquired brain injuries are frequently the bearers of bad news. They share information about the often devastating consequences of brain injury with patients who (due to organic unawareness and/or other factors) cannot fathom the complexities of their condition, and with family members who often cannot digest or tolerate the stark realities. Psychotherapists must also perform the taxing and sometimes worrisome task of therapeutically confronting patients (Norcross & Guy, 2005). Psychotherapists should therefore not expect to feel appreciated, affirmed, or popular, especially until trusting working alliances are fortified. Patients and families may use therapists as scapegoats

(McLaughlin & Carey, 1993) or want to "kill the messenger." Therapists can neutralize the patients' and families' hostilities by recognizing the behavior for what it is—the need to vent in a setting where they feel understood and safe.

## Avoid Power Struggles and "Pick Your Battles"

The psychotherapist must be attentive to the covert development of an imbalance in the collaboration process. The patient may lag in his or her commitment and investment; however, the psychotherapist must be careful about "picking battles." Sometimes, despite the psychotherapist's best intentions, the process backfires: The harder the psychotherapist pushes, the, more the patient may resist and push back. This results in ultimatums and a power struggle (Pepping, 1993). The impetus for change must emanate partially from the patient, not just the psychotherapist. At this juncture, the psychotherapist can fall prey to taking the patient's rebuffs personally. Instead, the therapist should conduct a self-appraisal and ask, "Do I want the therapy more than the patient does?" (R. Wienecke, personal communication, n.d.). If a skewed or one-sided alliance has developed, it should be explored with the patient and resolved through the psychotherapist's supervisory relationship and/or self-examination.

## Aspire to Fairness

Dedication can be a finite resource for psychotherapists. There are long-term unhealthy consequences when relationships are unbalanced. Psychotherapists can enhance their professional longevity by aspiring to be fair to themselves, as well as to their professional colleagues and patients. Fairness includes the system within which therapists work; it involves the expectations for workload (relative to those of others in the department), reimbursement and the compensation package, "on-call" schedules, vacations, and the like. There should also be fairness in the collaborative relationship with the patient and family. When there is too much of an imbalance for too long between the psychotherapist's and the patient's efforts, the psychotherapist can feel exploited, exhausted, and depleted. The book *The Giving Tree* (Silverstein, 1964) eloquently illustrates the insidiously destructive impact of unbalanced relationships. Therefore, a helpful internal signal is the psychotherapist's gut feeling about the fairness of his or her professional and clinical relationships. It is essential to set appropriate boundaries, with professional expectations and limitations (Norcross & Guy, 2005, 2007).

## Focus on Process versus Outcome

Despite everyone's best efforts, the desired outcome for a patient cannot always be achieved. For their own psychological well-being and that of their patients, psychotherapists should focus their energies on the therapeutic journey rather than the destination; that is, they should nurture the working alliance, regardless of the treatment outcome or endpoint.

Like patients, psychotherapists sometimes lapse into wanting instant results. But recovery after brain injury takes considerable time. It behooves a psychotherapist to remember that patients deserve the opportunity to test the validity of treatment recommendations in their own way. The recovery and adjustment process often spans months or years, even after the psychotherapy process ends. A mantra that is as useful for psychotherapists as it is for patients is "Things take time," or just "TTT" (Hein, 2004). When the psychotherapist demonstrates an attitude of patience, humility, and flexibility, the working alliance is solidified and often strengthened (allowing future interventions, if and when needed).

Related to this is the sustaining idea that the benefits of psychotherapy after brain injury do not always emerge during the treatment. It can be enough to "plant the seed" (G. A. Lage, personal communication, n.d.) that bears fruit only later (see Chapter 9). This idea helps the psychotherapist to take a step back and respect the right of patients to make their own decisions (Melamed & Szor, 1999). By affording patients the "dignity of risk" in their life choices (M. Pepping, personal communication, n.d.; see Chapter 7), the psychotherapist also avoids the pitfall of becoming too dogmatic and/or taking things personally.

### Self-Examination, Supervision/Mentorship, and Personal Therapy

An introspective and reflective psychotherapist can utilize his or her skills to self-monitor burnout and enhance self-understanding (Danieli, 2005; Miller, 1998; Sapienza & Bugental, 2000; Skovholt, Grier, & Hanson, 2001). Self-nourishment and self-compassion are vital for "keeping our [psychotherapy] instruments finely tuned" (Sapienza & Bugental, 2000, p. 458).

Additional techniques for avoiding burnout and recalibrating the psychotherapist's perspective include processing emotional reactions and angst in team meetings and staff retreats, during clinical supervision, or through personal therapy (Baldwin et al., 2007; Danieli, 2005; Gans, 1983; Gottesfeld & Lieberman, 1979; Gunther, 1994; Judd & Wilson, 2005; Linley & Joseph, 2007; Miller, 1998; Norcross, 2005; Norcross & Guy, 2005, 2007; Pais, 2002; Prigatano et al., 1986; Yalom, 2002). All these outlets encourage group exchange, self-expression, and clarity of thinking. Supervision or a formal mentorship furnishes sponsorship and role modeling as well (Norcross & Guy, 2005, 2007; Payne & Huffman, 2005). Mentorship further combats burnout by normalizing the psychotherapist's need for guidance; providing comfort in the demanding work world; and facilitating the transmission of virtues, values, and the ethics of our profession (Allen, Day, & Lentz, 2005; Dearing, Maddux, & Tangney, 2005; Warren, 2005).

"Psychological debriefing," which encourages ventilation, catharsis, and education, should be accessible to all psychotherapists and other neurorehabilitation staff to allay their fears and woes (Miller, 1998). This becomes particularly crucial when countertransference reactions are negatively affecting the working alliance, or when the psychotherapist is disappointed in the outcome of therapeutic interventions. The "detoxification" process (Gunther, 1994) of sharing feelings with other therapists allows for peer support and informal mentoring. Personal therapy has been shown to revitalize the therapist, as well as to facilitate empathy, tolerance, warmth, and insight (Norcross, 2005).

## Professional Development

Psychotherapists who strive to expand and diversify their professional knowledge and interests through conferences, workshops, and courses usually find renewal and new meaning in their work (Pepping, 1993). This can take the form of doing research, exploring new theories, and learning new treatment techniques, as well as becoming involved in professional organizations or community groups (Prigatano et al., 1986; Skovholt et al., 2001). Attendance at scientific conferences and association with other dedicated and like-minded professionals furthers professional development as it rejuvenates psychotherapists. Innovative research can generate enthusiasm and allow for professional collaboration, especially when it tests the efficacy of clinical interventions.

## System Supports and Professional Camaraderie

A work atmosphere that promotes professionalism, growth, and resource reconstitution helps avert burnout. This "professional greenhouse" should include perceptive leadership and support at the clinical and institutional levels, as well as peer and mentor tutelage (Gans, 1983; Gottesfeld & Lieberman, 1979; Miller, 1998; Norcross & Guy, 2005, 2007; Skovholt et al., 2001).

When the psychotherapist is part of a treatment cohort, periodic social events also build rapport, mutual bonding, and keenness for the work. Examples include celebrations of birthdays; breakfast and "happy hour" get-togethers; and recognition of personal accomplishments, such as promotions or parenthood. Community projects that exemplify and enhance the treatment team's social awareness and commitment to community service are other excellent professional and team-building opportunities.

## Balance between Work Life and Personal Life

Finding a balance between work demands and replenishing personal pursuits is key for the emotional health of psychotherapists. Self-care should be practiced in the physical, spiritual, emotional, and social domains (Norcross & Guy, 2007; Pais, 2002; Skovholt et al., 2001). Restorative "decompression" and stress reduction options include family life, friendships, and hobbies/other leisure activities, as well as physical fitness, proper nutrition, and good sleep hygiene (Danieli, 2005; Judd & Wilson, 2005; Madhavilatha, 2008; Miller, 1998; Norcross & Guy, 2005, 2007; Pais, 2002; Skovholt et al., 2001). Small innocuous indulgences (e.g., chocolate) can offer a momentary respite in a hectic and often stressful schedule. Regular (even if short) vacations are also integral to preserving psychotherapists' freshness for their work and reinforce balanced self-care (Norcross & Guy, 2005, 2007).

## Creativity, Vision, and Hope

Witnessing traumatic loss in patients and families can also shatter a psychotherapist's assumptive world, especially when he or she is inclined to believe that life should be fair and that undeserving people should not have tragedies befall them.

A remedy for this is "vicarious resilience," or the positive influence on the psychotherapist of patients' coping with adversity (Hernandez, Gangsei, & Engstrom, 2007). Witnessing and reflecting on patients' healing capacity through empathic engagement can transform the psychotherapist's view of hope and commitment (Hernandez et al., 2007), and strengthen his or her own courage and resolve (Aniskiewicz, 2007).

Psychotherapists can also enhance the intrinsic rewards of their work by incorporating creativity into the "art" of psychotherapy. Art, music, literature, and movie analysis are just a few practices that can assist the psychotherapist in connecting creatively and meaningfully with his or her patients. These media speak to patients with different voices that can reinforce therapeutic messages. Using artistic works in this way creates a positive feedback loop, whereby psychotherapists also feel energized in their efforts.

Inspirational readings and other resources can motivate not only patients, but psychotherapists. I encourage psychotherapists to identify works in various media that inspire them and sustain their dedication to their efforts; I personally derive solace from Figure 2.3, which is a visual reminder of the healing power of the working alliance and collaborative process. Such reminders become especially meaningful during the inevitable periods of disenchantment and sorrow that we as psychotherapists experience as part of our toils. Figure 10.4 lists some examples of literature, movies, and music I have found to anchor, recalibrate, and rekindle my (and hopefully others') psychic energies by affirming universal values and existential realities.

A critical component of the psychotherapist's sustenance is the ability to maintain an attitude of hopefulness about the future (Judd & Wilson, 2005; Klonoff, 1997; Newman, 2002; Prigatano et al., 1986). This transcends the preoccupation with "right now" and promotes patience. Various treatment practices can contribute to this positive outlook, including visits to group psychotherapy by former patients who have achieved contentment and quality of life. Similarly, celebrating patients' progress with a yearly graduation or other rites of passage renews a sense of purpose and signifies the psychotherapist's "fruits of his or her labor."

As a counterpart to the patient's "dignity of risk" (M. Pepping, personal communication, n.d.), the psychotherapist who employs "imaginative conviction"—encompassing zeal, hopefulness, creativity, and pluck—internalizes and resonates with a passion to propel his or her treatment interventions and efforts to the highest realm possible. Ideally, this passion is transmitted to, and reverberates within, the psychotherapist's colleagues, patients, and families.

**Professional Angst**

- Songs
  "Everybody Hurts" (Berry, Buck, Mills, & Stipe, 1992)
  "Stuck in a Moment You Can't Get Out Of" (Clayton, Evans, Hewson, & Mullen, 2000)
  "Nobody's Perfect" (Gerrard & Nevil, 2007)
  "These Hard Times" (Rinehart, Rinehart, Bolt, & Stillwell, 2009b)

- Literature
  *Man's Search for Meaning* (Frankl, 1984)

- Movies
  *Million Dollar Baby* (Eastwood et al., 2004)

**The Working Alliance**

- Songs
  "You'll Never Walk Alone" (Rodgers & Hammerstein, 1956/2001)
  "Help!" (Lennon & McCartney, 1965a)
  "We Can Work It Out" (Lennon & McCartney, 1965b)
  "Fix You" (Martin, Buckland, Berryman, & Champion, 2005)
  "Say" (Mayer, 2007)
  "Lay 'Em Down" (Rinehart, Rinehart, Bolt, & Stillwell, 2009a)

- Literature
  "The Love That Is Enough: Countertransference and the Ego Processes of Staff Members in a Therapeutic Milieu" (Bettelheim, 1975)

- Movies
  *The Karate Kid* (Weintraub et al., 1984)
  *Good Will Hunting* (Armstrong et al., 1997)
  *The Sixth Sense* (Kennedy, Marshall, Mendel, Mercer, & Shyamalan, 1999)

**Professional Camaraderie/Empathy**

- Songs
  "You've Got a Friend" (King, 1971)
  "Valerie" (Winwood, 1982)
  "On the Turning Away" (Gilmour & Moore, 1987)
  "If Everyone Cared" (Adair, Kroeger, Kroeger, & Peake, 2005)

- Literature
  *Tuesdays with Morrie* (Albom, 1997)
  *The Five People You Meet in Heaven* (Albom, 2003)
  "The Friend Who Just Stands By" (Williams, 2004)

- Movies/Short Films
  *The Doctor* (Feldman et al., 1991)
  *Crash* (Cheadle et al., 2004)
  *Boundin'* (Lasseter, Shurer, Luckey, & Gould, 2003)

**Acceptance, Coping, and Resiliency**

- Songs
  "Revolution" (Lennon, 1968/2002)
  "Don't Worry, Be Happy" (McFerrin, 1988)
  "Times like These" (Johnson, 2003)
  "Little Wonders" (Tomas, 2007)
  "Shiver" (Rudd, 2008)

*(cont.)*

**FIGURE 10.4.** Inspirational songs, literature, and movies for the psychotherapist.

- Literature
  *Daily Motivator* (Marsten, n.d.)
  "Attitude" (Swindoll, n.d.)
- Movies/Short Films
  *Defiance* (Balciunaite et al., 2008)
  *Up* (Con et al., 2009)
  *Partly Cloudy* (Reher & Sohn, 2009)

**Hope, Inspiration, and Transcendence**
- Songs
  "We Shall Overcome" (Carawan, Carawan, & Tindley, n.d./2006)
  "Ooh Child" (Vincent, 1972)
  "Pass It On" (Marley, 1973)
  "Israel Kamakawiwo'ole's Somewhere over the Rainbow" (Arlen, Harburg, Thiele, Weiss, & Kamakawiwo'ole," 1993)
  "Optimistic" (Greenwood, Yorke, Greenwood, O'Brien, & Selway, 2000)
  "Better Way" (Harper, 2006)
- Literature
  *The Last Lecture* (Pausch & Zaslow, 2008)
- Movies
  *Rocky* (Chartoff, Kirkwood, Winkler, & Avildsen, 1976)
  *E. T.: The Extra-Terrestrial* (Kennedy, Spielberg, Mathison, & Spielberg, 1982)
  *Pay It Forward* (Abrams et al., 2000)
  *Freedom Writers* (DeVito et al., 2007)

**FIGURE 10.4.** *(cont.)*

# References

Abraham, M., Bernstein, A., Bliss, T. A., Davis, A. Z., Freitag, J. M., Levine, J., et al. (Producers), & Ratner, B. (Director). (2000). *The family man* [Motion picture]. United States: Universal Studios.

Abrams, P., Carson, P., Levy, R., McLaglen, M., Reuther, S., Treisman, J. (Producers), & Leder, M. (Director). (2000). *Pay it forward* [Motion picture]. United States: Warner Bros. Entertainment.

Abrams, D. L., & Haffey, W. J. (1991). Blueprint for success in vocational restoration: The work re-entry program. In B. T. McMahon & L. R. Shaw (Eds.), *Work worth doing: Advances in brain injury rehabilitation* (pp. 221–244). Orlando, FL: Deutsch.

Ackerman, S. J., & Hilsenroth, M. J. (2001). A review of therapist characteristics and techniques negatively impacting the therapeutic alliance. *Psychotherapy, 38*(2), 171–185.

Ackerman, S. J., & Hilsenroth, M. J. (2003). A review of therapist characteristics and techniques positively impacting the therapeutic alliance. *Clinical Psychology Review, 23*(1), 1–33.

Adair, D., Kroeger, M., Kroeger, C., & Peake, R. (2005). If everyone cared [Recorded by Nickelback]. On *All the right reasons* [CD]. New York: Roadrunner Records.

Adams, R. A., Sherer, M., Struchen, M. A., & Nick, T. G. (2004). Post-acute brain injury rehabilitation for patients with stroke. *Brain Injury, 18*(8), 811–823.

Aesop. (1984). *The tortoise and the hare*. New York: Holiday House Books.

Albom, M. (1997). *Tuesdays with Morrie*. New York: Random House.

Albom, M. (2003). *The five people you meet in heaven*. New York: Hyperion.

Allen, T., Day, R., & Lentz, E. (2005). The role of interpersonal comfort in mentoring relationships. *Journal of Career Development, 31*(3), 155–169.

Alper, D., Black, T., Blumenthal, J., Clayman, M., D'Esposito, L., Gardner, L., et al. (Producers), & Muccino, G. (Director). (2006). *The pursuit of happyness* [Motion picture]. United States: Columbia Pictures Industries.

Alpert, J. E., & Spillmann, M. K. (1997). Psychotherapeutic approaches to aggressive and violent patients. *Psychiatric Clinics of North America, 20*(2), 453–472.

American Psychiatric Association. (2000). *Diagnostic and statistical manual of mental disorders* (fourth ed., text rev.). Washington, DC: Author.

American Psychological Association. (2002). *Ethical principles of psychologists and code of conduct.* Retrieved July 26, 2009, from *www.apa.org/ethics/code2002.html#principle_a.*

American Psychological Association Practice Organization. (2009, Spring–Summer). An action plan for self-care. *Good Practice*, pp. 16–17.

American Speech–Language–Hearing Association. (1997–2005). *Pragmatics, socially speaking.* Retrieved April 1, 2008, from *www.asha.org/public/speech/development/pragmatics. htm.*

Anderson, M. I., Parmenter, T. R., & Mok, M. (2002). The relationship between neurobehavioural problems of severe traumatic brain injury (TBI), family functioning and the psychological well-being of the spouse/caregiver: Path model analysis. *Brain Injury, 16*(9), 743–757.

Andrews, S. S., Gerhart, K. A., & Hosack, K. R. (2004). Therapeutic recreation in traumatic brain injury rehabilitation. In M. J. Ashley (Ed.), *Traumatic brain injury: Rehabilitative treatment and case management* (pp. 539–557). Boca Raton, FL: CRC Press.

Aniskiewicz, A. S. (2007). *Psychotherapy for neuropsychological challenges.* Lanham, MD: Jason Aronson.

Anka, P., Revaux, J., Thibault, G., & Frankois, C. (1969). My way [Recorded by F. Sinatra]. On *My way* [Album]. Burbank, CA: Reprise Records.

Anson, K., & Ponsford, J. (2006a). Who benefits?: Outcome following a coping skills group intervention for traumatically brain injured individuals. *Brain Injury, 20*(1), 1–13.

Anson, K., & Ponsford, J. (2006b). Evaluation of a coping skills group following traumatic brain injury. *Brain Injury, 20*(2), 167–178.

Anson, K., & Ponsford, J. (2006c). Coping and emotional adjustment following traumatic brain injury. *Journal of Head Trauma Rehabilitation, 21*(3), 248–259.

Arlen, H., Harburg, E., Thiele, B., Weiss, G., & Kamakawiwo'ole, I. (1993). Israel Kamakawiwo'ole's Somewhere over the rainbow [Recorded by I. Kamakawiwo'ole]. On *Facing future* [CD]. Honolulu, HI: Mountain Apple.

Armstrong, S., Bender, L., Gordon, J., Moore, C., Mosier, S., Smith, K., et al. (Producers), & Van Sant, G. (Director). (1997). *Good will hunting* [Motion picture]. United States: Miramax Films.

Armstrong, L., with Jenkins, S. (2000). *It's not about the bike: My journey back to life.* New York: Putnam.

Ashley, M. J., Ninomiya, J., Jr., Berryman, A., & Goodwin, K. (2004). Vocational rehabilitation. In M. J. Ashley (Ed.), *Traumatic brain injury: Rehabilitative treatment and case management* (pp. 509–537). Boca Raton, FL: CRC Press.

Atchison, T. B., Sander, A. M., Struchen, M. A., High, W. M. Jr., Roebuck, T. M., Contant, C. F., et al. (2004). Relationship between neuropsychological test performance and productivity at 1-year following traumatic brain injury. *Clinical Neuropsychologist, 18*(2), 249–265.

Avesani, R., Salvi, L., Rigoli, G., & Gambini, M. G. (2005). Reintegration after severe brain injury: A retrospective study. *Brain Injury, 19*(11), 933–939.

Babin, P. R., & Gross, P. (2002). Traumatic brain injury when symptoms don't add up: Conversion and malingering in the rehabilitation setting. *Journal of Rehabilitation, 68*(2), 4–13.

Bachelor, A., Laverdiere, O., Gamache, D., & Bordeleau, V. (2007). Clients' collaboration in therapy: Self-perceptions and relationships with client psychological functioning, interpersonal relations, and motivation. *Psychotherapy: Theory, Research, Practice, Training, 44*(2), 175–192.

Baker, H. S., & Baker, M. N. (1987). Heinz Kohut's self psychology: An overview. *American Journal of Psychiatry, 144*(1), 1–9.

Balciunaite, E., Boden, A., Brugge, P. J., Frohman, C., Herskokvitz, M., Katz, A., et al. (Producers), & Zwick, E. (Director). (2008). *Defiance* [Motion picture]. United States: Paramount Vantage.

Baldwin, S. A., Wampold, B. E., & Imel, Z. E. (2007). Untangling the alliance–outcome correlation: Exploring the relative importance of therapist and patient variability in the alliance. *Journal of Consulting and Clinical Psychology, 75*(6), 842–852.

Balk, D. E. (2004). Recovery following bereavement: An examination of the concept. *Death Studies, 28*(4), 361–374.

Balkis, M., & Duru, E. (2007). The evaluation of the major characteristics and aspects of the procrastination in the framework of psychological counseling and guidance. *Educational Sciences: Theory and Practice, 7*(1), 376–385.

Bandura, A. (1997). *Self-efficacy: The exercise of control.* New York: Freeman.

Bankston, L. (2004). *The mayonnaise jar and 2 cups of coffee.* Retrieved October 19, 2008, from *www.ecst.csuchico.edu/~renner/csci330/Activities/priorities.html*

Barco, P. B., Crosson, B., Bolesta, M. M., Werts, D., & Stout, R. (1991). Training awareness and compensation in post-acute head injury rehabilitation. In J. S. Kreutzer & P. H. Wehman (Eds.), *Cognitive rehabilitation for persons with traumatic brain injury: A functional approach* (pp. 129–146). Baltimore: Brookes.

Barglow, P. (2005). Self-disclosure in psychotherapy. *American Journal of Psychotherapy, 59*(2), 83–99.

Barnathan, M. (Producer), & Columbus, C. (Director). (1998). *Stepmom* [Motion picture]. United States: Columbia Pictures Industries.

Barrie, J. M. (1985). *Peter Pan..* New York: Bantam Classics. (Original work published 1904)

Bay, E., Hagerty, B. M., Williams, R. A., Kirsh, N., & Gillespie, B. (2002). Chronic stress, sense of belonging, and depression among survivors of traumatic brain injury. *Journal of Nursing Scholarship, 34*(3), 221–226.

Beck, J. S. (2005). *Cognitive therapy for challenging problems.* New York: Guilford Press.

Becker, M. E., & Vakil, E. (1993). Behavioral psychotherapy of the frontal-lobe-injured patient in an outpatient setting. *Brain Injury, 7*(6), 515–523.

Ben-Yishay, Y. (1996). Reflections on the evolution of the therapeutic milieu concept. *Neuropsychological Rehabilitation, 6*(4), 327–343.

Ben-Yishay, Y., & Daniels-Zide, E. (2000). Diller Lecture. Examined lives: Outcomes after holistic rehabilitation. *Rehabilitation Psychology, 45*(2), 112–129.

Ben-Yishay, Y., & Diller, L. (1993). Cognitive remediation in traumatic brain injury: Update and issues. *Archives of Physical Medicine and Rehabilitation, 74*(2), 204–213.

Ben-Yishay, Y., & Lakin, P. (1989). Structured group treatment for brain-injury survivors. In D. W. Ellis & A.-L. Christensen (Eds.), *Neuropsychological treatment after brain injury* (pp. 271–295). Boston: Kluwer Academic.

Ben-Yishay, Y., Rattok, J., Lakin, P., Piasetsky, E. B., Ross, B., Silver, S., et al. (1985). Neuropsychologic rehabilitation: Quest for a holistic approach. *Seminars in Neurology, 5*(3), 252–259.

Berry, B., Buck, P., Mills, M., & Stipe, M. (1992). Everybody hurts [Recorded by R.E.M.]. On *Automatic for the people* [CD]. New York: Warner Bros./WEA.

Bettelheim, B. (1975). The love that is enough: Countertransference and the ego processes of staff members in a therapeutic milieu. In P. Giovacchini (Ed.), *Tactics and techniques in psychoanalytic therapy* (Vol. 2, pp. 251–278). New York: Aronson.

Beutler, L. E., Moleiro, C., & Talebi, H. (2002). Resistance in psychotherapy: What conclusions are supported by research. *Journal of Clinical Psychology/In Session, 58*(2), 207–217.

Bezeau, S. C., Bogod, N. M., & Mateer, C. A. (2004). Sexually intrusive behaviour following brain injury: Approaches to assessment and rehabilitation. *Brain Injury, 18*(3), 299–313.

Bisiach, E., & Geminiani, G. (1991). Anosognosia related to hemiplegia and hemianopia. In G.P. Prigatano & D.L. Schacter (Eds.), *Awareness of deficit after brain injury: Clinical and theoretical issues* (pp. 17–39). New York: Oxford University Press.

Bivona, U., Ciurli, P., Barba, C., Onder, G., Azicnuda, E., Silvestro, D., et al. (2008). Executive function and metacognitive self-awareness after severe traumatic brain injury. *Journal of the International Neuropsychological Society, 14*, 862–868.

Blais, M. C., & Boisvert, J.-M. (2007). Psychological adjustment and marital satisfaction following head injury: Which critical personal characteristics should both partners develop? *Brain Injury, 21*(4), 357–372.

Boman, I., Tham, K., Granqvist, A., Bartfai, A., & Hemmingsson, H. (2007). Using electronic aids to daily living after acquired brain injury: A study of the learning process and the usability. *Disability and Rehabilitation: Assistive Technology, 2*(1), 23–33.

Bombardier, C. H., Ehde, D., & Kilmer, J. (1997). Readiness to change alcohol drinking habits after traumatic brain injury. *Archives of Physical Medicine and Rehabilitation, 78*(6), 592–596.

Bombardier, C. H., Temkin, N. R., Machamer, J., & Dikmen, S. S. (2003). The natural history of drinking and alcohol-related problems after traumatic brain injury. *Archives of Physical Medicine and Rehabilitation, 84*(2), 185–191.

Bordin, E. S. (1979). The generalizability of the psychoanalytic concept of the working alliance. *Psychotherapy: Theory, Research, and Practice, 16*(3), 252–260.

Borgaro, S., Caples, H., & Prigatano, G. P. (2003). Non-pharmacological management of psychiatric disturbances after traumatic brain injury. *International Review of Psychiatry, 15*(4), 371–379.

Bowen, C. (2007). Family therapy and neuro-rehabilitation: Forging a link. *International Journal of Therapy and Rehabilitation, 14*(8), 344–349.

Boyle, G. J., & Haines, S. (2002). Severe traumatic brain injury: Some effects on family caregivers. *Psychological Reports, 90*(2), 415–425.

Bradbury, C. L., Christensen, B. K., Lau, M. A., Ruttan, L. A., Arundine, A. L., & Green, R. E. (2008). The efficacy of cognitive behavior therapy in the treatment of emotional distress after acquired brain injury. *Archives of Physical Medicine and Rehabilitation, 89*(Suppl. 2), S61–S68.

Bradley, S. S., & Bentley, K. J. (2003). The psychology of the psychopharmacology triangle: The client, the clinicians, and the medication. *Psychiatric Medication Issues for Social Workers, Counselors and Psychologists, 1*(4), 29–50.

Brady, R. P. (2007). *Picture Interest Career Survey (PICS)*. Indianapolis, IN: JIST Works.

Braverman, S. E., Spector, J., Wardern, D. L., Wilson, B. C., Ellis, T. E., Bamdad, M. J., et al. (1999). A multidisciplinary TBI inpatient rehabilitation programme for active duty service members as part of a randomized clinical trial. *Brain Injury, 13*(6), 405–415.

Brenner, L. A., Homaifar, B. Y., & Schultheis, M. T. (2008). Driving, aging, and traumatic brain injury: Integrating findings from the literature. *Rehabilitation Psychology, 53*(1), 18–27.

Brouwer, W. H., Withaar, F. K., Tant, M. L. M., & van Zomeren, A. H. (2002). Attention and driving in traumatic brain injury: A question of coping with time-pressure. *Journal of Head Trauma Rehabilitation, 17*(1), 1–15.

Brown, D., Lyons, E., & Rose, D. (2006). Recovery from brain injury: Finding the missing bits of the puzzle. *Brain Injury, 20*(9), 937–946.

Bruns, D., & Disorbio, J. M. (2000). Violent ideation in physical rehabilitation patients. *Pain Medicine, 1*(2), 190–191.

Burridge, A. C., Huw Williams, W., Yates, P. J., Harris, A., & Ward, C. (2007). Spousal relationship satisfaction following acquired brain injury: The role of insight and socioemotional skill. *Neuropsychological Rehabilitation, 17*(1), 95–105.

Burton, L. A., Leahy, D. M., & Volpe, B. (2003). Traumatic brain injury brief outcome interview. *Applied Neuropsychology, 10*(3), 145–152.

Butcher, J. N. (1990). *The MMPI-2 in psychological treatment.* New York: Oxford University Press.

Butcher, J. N. (2005). *Minnesota Multiphasic Personality Inventory–2: The Minnesota Report, Adult Clinical System—Revised* (4th Edition). Minneapolis, MN: NCS/Pearson.

Butcher, J. N., & Williams, C. L. (2000). *Essentials of MMPI-2 and MMPI-A interpretation* (2nd ed.). Minneapolis: University of Minnesota Press.

Butler, R. W., & Satz, P. (1988). Individual psychotherapy with head-injured adults: Clinical notes for the practitioner. *Professional Psychology: Research and Practice, 19*(5), 536–541.

Carawan, G., Carawan, C., & Tindley, C. (2006). We shall overcome [Recorded by B. Springsteen]. On *We shall overcome: The Seeger sessions* [CD]. New York: Sony Records. (Original work n.d.)

Cattelani, R., Tanzi, F., Lombardi, F., & Mazzucchi, A. (2002). Competitive re-employment after severe traumatic brain injury: Clinical, cognitive and behavioural predictive variables. *Brain Injury, 16*(1), 51–64.

Chamberlain, D. J. (2006). The experience of surviving traumatic brain injury. *Journal of Advanced Nursing, 54*(4), 407–417.

Channon, S., & Watts, M. (2003). Pragmatic language interpretation after closed head injury: Relationship to executive functioning. *Cognitive Neuropsychiatry, 8*(4), 243–260.

Charles, N., Butera-Prinzi, F., & Perlesz, A. (2007). Families living with acquired brain injury: A multiple family group experience. *NeuroRehabilitation, 22*, 61–76.

Chartoff, R., Kirkwood, G., Winkler, I. (Producers), & Avildsen, J. (Director). (1976). *Rocky* [Motion picture]. United States: United Artists.

Cheadle, D., Danbury, B., Finn, S., Grasic, M., Haggis, P., Harris, M., et al. (Producers), & Haggis, P. (Director). (2004). *Crash* [Motion picture]. United States: Lions Gate Films.

Chen, L.-C. (1997). Grief as a transcendent function and teacher of spiritual growth. *Pastoral Psychology, 46*(2), 79–84.

Cheng, S. K. W., & Man, D. W. K. (2006). Management of impaired self-awareness in persons with traumatic brain injury. *Brain Injury, 20*(6), 621–628.

Christensen, A.-L., Pinner, E. M., Moller Pedersen, P., Teasdale, T. W., & Trexler, L. E. (1992). Psychosocial outcome following individualized neuropsychological rehabilitation of brain damage. *Acta Neurologica Scandinavica, 85*, 32–38.

Churchill, F., Harline, L., & Smith, J. (2001). Heigh-ho [The dwarf chorus]. On *Walt Disney's Snow White and the seven dwarfs: Classic soundtrack series* [CD]. Burbank, CA: Walt Disney Records. (Original work released 1937)

Cicerone, K. D. (1989). Psychotherapeutic interventions with traumatically brain-injured patients. *Rehabilitation Psychology, 34*, 105–114.

Cicerone, K. D., & Azulay, J. (2007). Perceived self-efficacy and life satisfaction after traumatic brain injury. *Journal of Head Trauma Rehabilitation, 22*(5), 257–266.

Cicerone, K. D., Levin, H., Malec, J., Stuss, D., & Whyte, J. (2006). Cognitive rehabilitation interventions for executive function: Moving from bench to bedside in patients with traumatic brain injury. *Journal of Cognitive Neuroscience, 18*(7), 1212–1222.

Cicerone, K. D., Mott, T., Azulay, J., Sharlow-Galella, M. A., Ellmo, W. J., Paradise, S., et al. (2008). A randomized controlled trial of holistic neuropsychologic rehabilitation after traumatic brain injury. *Archives of Physical Medicine and Rehabilitation, 89*, 2239–2249.

Clarkson, P., & Nuttall, J. (2000). Working with countertransference. *Psychodynamic Counselling, 6*(3), 359–379.

Clayton, A., Evans, D., Hewson, P., & Mullen L. (2000). Stuck in a moment you can't get out of [Recorded by U2]. On *All that you can't leave behind* [CD]. Santa Monica, CA: Interscope Records.

Coelho, C. A., Youse, K. M., & Le, K. N. (2002). Conversational discourse in closed-head-injured and non-brain-injured adults. *Aphasiology, 16*(4–6), 659–672.

Coetzer, R. (2006). *Traumatic brain injury rehabilitation: A psychotherapeutic approach to loss and grief.* New York: Nova Science.

Coetzer, R. (2007). Psychotherapy following traumatic brain injury: Integrating theory and practice. *Journal of Head Trauma Rehabilitation, 22*(1), 39–47.

Collins, R., Lanham, R. A., Jr., & Sigford, B. J. (2000). Reliability and validity of the Wisconsin HSS Quality of Life Inventory in traumatic brain injury. *Journal of Head Trauma Rehabilitation, 15*(5), 1139–1148.

Con, L., Lasseter, J., Rivera, J., Stanton, A. (Producers), & Docter, P., Peterson, B. (Directors). (2009). *Up* [Motion picture]. United States: Walt Disney Pictures & Pixar Animation Studios.

Condeluci, A., Cooperman, S., & Seif, B. A. (1987). Independent living: Settings and supports. In M. Ylvisaker & E. M. R. Gobble (Eds.), *Community re-entry for head injured adults* (pp. 301–347). Boston: Little, Brown.

Condeluci, A., & Gretz-Lasky, S. (1987). Social role valorization: A model for community reentry. *Journal of Head Trauma Rehabilitation, 2*, 49–56.

Conti, B., Connors, C., & Robbins, A. (1976). Gonna fly now (Rocky's theme) [Recorded by B. Conti, D. E. Little, & N. Pigford]. On *Rocky soundtrack* [Album]. Los Angeles: Capitol Records.

Corkery, S., & Fairweather, M. (2009). The impact of executive function impairments on communication. In M. Oddy, & A. Worthington (Eds.), *The rehabilitation of executive disorders: A guide to theory and practice* (pp. 153–173). New York: Oxford University Press.

Corr, C. A. (2002). Coping with challenges to assumptive worlds. In J. Kauffman (Ed.), *Loss of the assumptive world: A theory of traumatic loss* (pp. 127–138). New York: Brunner-Routledge.

Corrigan, P. W., & Bach, P. A. (2005). Behavioral treatment. In J. M. Silver, T. W. McAllister, & S. C. Yudofsky (Eds.), *Textbook of traumatic brain injury* (pp. 661–678). Washington, DC: American Psychiatric Publishing.

Corrigan, J. D., Bogner, J. A., Mysiw, J. W., Clinchot, D., & Fugate, L. (2001). Life satisfaction after traumatic brain injury. *Journal of Head Trauma Rehabilitation, 16*(6), 543–555.

Cowan, R. (Producer), & Winkler, I. (Director). (2001). *Life as a house* [Motion picture]. United States: New Line Cinema.

Cox, W. M., Heinemann, A. W., Miranti, S. V., Schmidt, M., Klinger, E., & Blount, J. (2003). Outcomes of systematic motivational counseling for substance use following traumatic brain injury. *Journal of Addictive Diseases, 22*(1), 93–110.

Crimmins, C. (2000). *Where is the Mango Princess?: A journey back from brain injury.* New York: Vintage Books.

Critchley, H. D. (2005). Neural mechanisms of autonomic, affective, and cognitive integration. *Journal of Comparative Neurology, 493*(1), 154–166.

Culbertson, W. C., & Zillmer, E. A. (2005). *Tower of London: Drexel University* (2nd ed.). North Tonawanda, NY: Multi-Health Systems.

Cummings, L. (2007). Pragmatics and adult language disorders: Past achievements and future directions. *Seminars in Speech and Language, 28*(2), 96–110.

Curran, C. A., Ponsford, J. L., & Crowe, S. (2000). Coping strategies and emotional outcome following traumatic brain injury: A comparison with orthopedic patients. *Journal of Head Trauma Rehabilitation, 15*(6), 1256–1274.

Curtiss, G., Klemz, S., & Vanderploeg, R. D. (2000). Acute impact of severe traumatic brain injury on family structure and coping responses. *Journal of Head Trauma Rehabilitation, 15*(5), 1113–1122.

Cusack, J., Loh, G., Niederhoffer, G., Lundberg, D. T., Rattray, C. (Producers), & Strouse, J. C. (Director). (2007). *Grace is gone* [Motion picture]. United States: The Weinstein Company.

Dahlberg, C. A., Cusick, C. P., Hawley, L. A., Newman, J. K., Morey, C. E., Harrison-Felix, C.

L., et al. (2007). Treatment efficacy of social communication skills training after traumatic brain injury: A randomized treatment and deferred treatment controlled trial. *Archives of Physical Medicine and Rehabilitation, 88*(12), 1561–1573.

Dahlberg, C., Hawley, L., Morey, C., Newman, J., Cusick, C. P., & Harrison-Felix, C. (2006). Social communication skills in persons with post-acute traumatic brain injury: Three perspectives. *Brain Injury, 20*(4), 425–435.

Dalai Lama, & Cutler, H. C. (1998). *The art of happiness: A handbook for living.* New York: Riverhead Books.

Danieli, Y. (2005). Guide: Some principles of self care. *Journal of Aggression, Maltreatment and Trauma, 10*(1–2), 663–665.

Davis, C. G., Nolen-Hoeksema, S., & Larson, J. (1998). Making sense of loss and benefiting from the experience: Two construals of meaning. *Journal of Personality and Social Psychology, 75*(2), 561–574.

Davis, J. R., Gemeinhardt, M., Gan, C., Anstey, K., & Gargaro, J. (2003). Crisis and its assessment after brain injury. *Brain Injury, 17*(5), 359–376.

Dawson, D. R., Schwartz, M. L., Winocur, G., & Stuss, D. T. (2007). Return to productivity following traumatic brain injury: Cognitive, psychological, physical, spiritual, and environmental correlates. *Disability and Rehabilitation, 29*(4), 301–313.

Dawson, D. R., & Winocur, G. (2008). Psychosocial considerations in cognitive rehabilitation. In D. T. Stuss, G. Winocur, & I. H. Robertson (Eds.), *Cognitive neurorehabilitation: Evidence and application* (2nd ed., pp. 232–249). New York: Cambridge University Press.

Dearing, R. L., Maddux, J. E., & Tangney, J. P. (2005). Predictors of psychological help seeking in clinical and counseling psychology graduate students. *Professional Psychology: Research and Practice, 36*(3), 323–329.

Degeneffe, C. E. (2001). Family caregiving and traumatic brain injury. *Health & Social Work, 26*(4), 257–268.

Delis, D. C., Kramer, J. H., Kaplan, E., & Ober, B. A. (2000). *California Verbal Learning Test— Second Edition, Adult Version.* San Antonio, TX: Psychological Corporation/Harcourt Brace Jovanovich.

Delmonico, R. L., Hanley-Peterson, P., & Englander, J. (1998). Group psychotherapy for persons with traumatic brain injury: Management of frustration and substance abuse. *Journal of Head Trauma Rehabilitation, 13*(6), 10–22.

Demark, J., & Gemeinhardt, M. (2002). Anger and its management for survivors of acquired brain injury. *Brain Injury, 16*(2), 91–108.

DeVito, D., Durning, T., Glick-Franzheinn, J., Levine, D., Morales, N., Shamberg, M., et al. (Producers), & La Gravenese, R. (Director). (2007). *Freedom writers* [Motion picture]. United States: Paramount Pictures.

Devitt, R., Colantonio, A., Dawson, D., Teare, G., Ratcliff, G., & Chase, S. (2006). Prediction of long-term occupational performance outcomes for adults after moderate to severe traumatic brain injury. *Disability and Rehabilitation, 28*(9), 547–559.

Dhiman, S. (2007). Personal mastery: Our quest for self-actualization, meaning, and highest purpose. *Interbeing, 1*(1), 25–35.

Dieckmann, H. (1991). *Methods in analytical psychology: An introduction.* Wilmette, IL: Chiron.

Dikmen, S. S., Machamer, J. E., Powell, J. M., & Temkin, N. R. (2003). Outcome 3 to 5 years after moderate to severe traumatic brain injury. *Archives of Physical Medicine and Rehabilitation, 84*, 1449–1457.

Dixon, G., Thornton, E. W., & Young, C. A. (2007). Perceptions of self-efficacy and rehabilitation among neurologically disabled adults. *Clinical Rehabilitation, 21*(3), 230–240.

Doctor, J. N., Castro, J., Temkin, N. R., Fraser, R. T., Machamer, J. E., & Dikmen, S. S. (2005). Workers' risk of unemployment after traumatic brain injury: A normed comparison. *Journal of the International Neuropsychological Society, 11*, 747–752.

Doig, E., Fleming, J., & Tooth, L. (2001). Patterns of community integration 2–5 years post-discharge from brain injury rehabilitation. *Brain Injury, 15*(9), 747–762.

Dombrowski, L. K., Petrick, J. D., & Strauss, D. (2000). Rehabilitation treatment of sexuality issues due to acquired brain injury. *Rehabilitation Psychology, 45*(3), 299–309.

Donnelly, J. P., Donnelly, K., & Grohman, K. K. (2005). A multi-perspective concept mapping study of problems associated with traumatic brain injury. *Brain Injury, 19*(13), 1077–1085.

Douglas, H. (2007). Brain injury experience: From black and white to color. *Barrow Quarterly, 23*(3), 13–65.

Douglas, J. M., & Spellacy, F. J. (2000). Correlates of depression in adults with severe traumatic brain injury and their carers. *Brain Injury, 14*(1), 71–88.

Ducharme, S. H. (1993). Beyond the management of sexual problems: Creating a therapeutic environment for addressing sexuality issues. In C. J. Durgin, N. D. Schmidt, & L. J. Fryer (Eds.), *Staff development and clinical intervention in brain injury rehabilitation* (pp. 211–228). Gaithersburg, MD: Aspen.

Dumont, C., Gervais, M., Fougeyrollas, P., & Bertrand, R. (2004). Toward an explanatory model of social participation for adults with traumatic brain injury. *Journal of Head Trauma Rehabilitation, 19*(6), 431–444.

East Tennessee State University (2008). *Classified personnel performance review form.* Retrieved November 4, 2008, from *www.etsu.edu/HUMANRES/forms/staffeval.pdf*

Eastwood, C., Haggis, P., Lorenz, R., Lucchesi, G., Moresco, R., Rosenberg, T., et al. (Producers), & Eastwood, C. (Director). (2004). *Million dollar baby* [Motion picture]. United States: Warner Bros. Entertainment.

Eldridge, R., Brooks, P., Fithian, S., Landsberd, C., Ross, D., Shepherd, J., et al. (Producers), & Sajbel, M. O. (Director). (2006). *The ultimate gift* [Motion picture]. United States: 20th Century Fox Home Entertainment.

Emerson, S., & Markos, P. A. (1996). Signs and symptoms of the impaired counselor. *Journal of Humanistic Education and Development, 34*(3), 108–117.

Ergh, T. C., Hanks, R. A., Rapport, L. J., & Coleman, R. D. (2003). Social support moderates caregiver life satisfaction following traumatic brain injury. *Journal of Clinical and Experimental Neuropsychology, 25*(8), 1090–1101.

Erickson, R. C. (1995). A review and critique of the process approach in neuropsychological assessment. *Neuropsychology Review, 5*(4), 223–243.

Ewing, M. (Producer), & Segal, P. (Director). (2004). *50 first dates* [Motion picture]. United States: Sony/Columbia Pictures.

Eysenck, H. J. (2006). *The biological basis of personality.* New Brunswick, NJ: Transaction. (Original work published 1967)

Fann, J. R., Jones, A. L., Dikmen, S. S., Temkin, N. R., Esselman, P. C., & Bombardier, C. H. (2009). Depression treatment preferences after traumatic brain injury. *Journal of Head Trauma Rehabilitation, 24*(4), 272–278.

Farr, J. M. & Shatkin, L. (2007). *O*NET dictionary of occupational titles: The definitive printed reference of occupational information* (4th ed.). Indianapolis, IN: JIST Works.

Felde, A. B., Westermeyer, J., & Thuras, P. (2006). Co-morbid traumatic brain injury and substance use disorder: Childhood predictors and adult correlates. *Brain Injury, 20*(1), 41–49.

Feldman, E., Glick, M., Ziskin, L. (Producers), & Haines, R. (Director). (1991). *The doctor* [Motion picture]. United States: Touchstone Pictures.

Filley, C. M. (2008). Neuroanatomy for the neuropsychologist. In J. E. Morgan & J. H. Ricker (Eds.), *Textbook of clinical neuropsychology* (pp. 61–82). New York: Taylor & Francis Group.

Fine, S. B. (1991). Resilience and human adaptability: Who rises above adversity? 1990 Eleanor Clarke Slagle Lecture. *American Journal of Occupational Therapy, 45*(6), 493–503.

Fischer, S., Trexler, L. E., & Gauggel, S. (2004). Awareness of activity limitations and prediction of performance in patients with brain injuries and orthopedic disorders. *Journal of the International Neuropsychological Society, 10,* 190–199.

Flashman, L. A., Amador, X., & McAllister, T. W. (2005). Awareness of deficits. In J. M. Silver, T. W. McAllister, & S. C. Yudofsky (Eds.), *Textbook of traumatic brain injury* (pp. 353–367). Washington, DC: American Psychiatric Publishing.

Fleming, J. M., & Ownsworth, T. (2006). A review of awareness interventions in brain injury rehabilitation. *Neuropsychological Rehabilitation, 16*(4), 474–500.

Fleming, J. M., Strong, J., & Ashton, R. (1996). Self-awareness of deficits in adults with traumatic brain injury: How best to measure? *Brain Injury, 10*(1), 1–15.

Fleminger, S., Oliver, D. L., Williams, W. H., & Evans, J. (2003). The neuropsychiatry of depression after brain injury. *Neuropsychological Rehabilitation, 13*(1–2), 65–87.

Florian, V., & Katz, S. (1991). The other victims of traumatic brain injury: Consequences for family members. *Neuropsychology, 5*(4), 267–279.

Fluharty, G., & Priddy, D. (1993). Methods of increasing client acceptance of a memory book. *Brian Injury, 7*(1), 85–88.

Forman, A. C. M., Vesey, P. A., & Lincoln, N. B. (2006). Effectiveness of an adjustment group for brain injury patients: A pilot evaluation. *International Journal of Therapy and Rehabilitation, 13*(5), 223–228.

Forssmann-Falck, R., & Christian, F. M. (1989). The use of group therapy as a treatment modality for behavioral change following brain injury. *Psychiatric Medicine, 7*(1), 43–50.

Forssmann-Falck, R., Christian, F. M., & O'Shanick, G. (1989). Group therapy with moderately neurologically damaged patients. *Health and Social Work, 14*(4), 235–243.

Frankl, V. E. (1984). *Man's search for meaning* (3rd ed.). New York: Simon & Schuster.

Franulic, A., Carbonell, C. G., Pinto, P., & Sepulveda, I. (2004). Psychosocial adjustment and employment outcome 2, 5 and 10 years after TBI. *Brain Injury, 18*(2), 119–129.

Fraser, R. T., & Shrey, D. F. (1986). Perceived barriers to job placement revisited: Towards practical solutions. *Journal of Rehabilitation, 52*(4), 26–30.

Freed, P. (2002). Meeting of the minds: Ego reintegration after traumatic brain injury. *Bulletin of the Menninger Clinic, 66*(1), 61–78.

Freeman, A., Pretzer, J., Fleming, B., & Simon, K. M. (2004). *Clinical applications of cognitive therapy* (2nd ed.). New York: Kluwer Academic/Plenum.

Friedland, D., & Miller, N. (1998). Conversation analysis of communication breakdown after closed head injury. *Brain Injury, 12*(1), 1–14.

Friendly, D. T., Saraf, P., Turtletaub, M. (Producers), & Dayton, J., Faris, V. (Directors). (2006). *Little Miss Sunshine* [Motion picture]. United States: Fox Searchlight Pictures.

Gabbard, G. O. (2001). A contemporary psychoanalytic model of countertransference. *Journal of Clinical Psychology/In Session, 57*(8), 983–991.

Gagnon, J., Bouchard, M. A., & Rainville, C. (2006). Differential diagnosis between borderline personality disorder and organic personality disorder following traumatic brain injury. *Bulletin of the Menninger Clinic, 70*(1), 1–28.

Galski, T., Ehle, H. T., McDonald, M. A., & Mackevich, J. (2000). Evaluating fitness to drive after cerebral injury: Basic issues and recommendations for medical and legal communities. *Journal of Head Trauma Rehabilitation, 15*(3), 895–908.

Galski, T., Tompkins, C., & Johnston, M. V. (1998). Competence in discourse as a measure of social integration and quality of life in persons with traumatic brain injury. *Brain Injury, 12*(9), 769–782.

Gan, C., Campbell, K. A., Gemeinhardt, M., & McFadden, G. T. (2006). Predictors of family system functioning after brain injury. *Brain Injury, 20*(6), 587–600.

Gan, C., & Schuller, R. (2002). Family system outcome following acquired brain injury: Clinical and research perspectives. *Brain Injury, 16*(4), 311–322.

Gans, J. S. (1983). Hate in the rehabilitation setting. *Archives of Physical Medicine and Rehabilitation, 64,* 176–179.

Genevro, J. L., Marshall, T., & Miller, T. (2004). Chapter 2: Themes in research on bereavement and grief. *Death Studies, 28*(6), 498–505.

Gerrard, M., & Nevil, R. (2007). Nobody's perfect [Recorded by Miley Cyrus]. On *Hannah Montana 2: Meet Miley Cyrus* [CD]. Burbank, CA: Walt Disney Records.

Ghaffar, O., & Feinstein, A. (2008). Mood, affect and motivation in rehabilitation. In D. T. Stuss, G. Winocur, & I. H. Robertson (Eds.), *Cognitive neurorehabilitation: Evidence and application* (2nd ed. pp. 205–217). New York: Cambridge University Press.

Giaquinto, S., & Ring, H. (2007). Return to work in selected disabilities. *Disability and Rehabilitation, 29*(17), 1313–1316.

Giles, G. M., & Manchester, D. (2006). Two approaches to behavior disorder after traumatic brain injury. *Journal of Head Trauma Rehabilitation, 21*(2), 168–178.

Gilliand, B. E., & James, R. K. (1988). *Crisis intervention strategies*. Belmont, CA: Brooks/ Cole.

Gilmour, D., & Moore, A. (1987). On the turning away [Recorded by Pink Floyd]. On *A momentary lapse of reason* [Album]. Los Angeles: Capitol Records.

Gladsjo, J. A., Heaton, R. K., Palmer, B. W., Taylor, M. J., & Jeste, D. V. (1999). Use of oral reading to estimate premorbid intellectual and neuropsychological functioning. *Journal of the International Neuropsychological Society, 5*(3), 247–254.

Glang, A., Tyler, J., Pearson, S., Todis, B., & Morvant, M. (2004). Improving educational services for students with TBI through statewide consulting teams. *NeuroRehabilitation, 19*(3), 219–231.

Gleckman, A. D., & Brill, S. (1995). The impact of brain injury on family functioning: Implications for subacute rehabilitation programmes. *Brain Injury, 9*(4), 385–393.

Gleser, J., & Brown, P. (1988). Judo principles and practices: Applications to conflict-solving strategies in psychotherapy. *American Journal of Psychotherapy, 42*(3), 437–447.

God will save me. (n.d.). Retrieved February 28, 2009, from *www.pennyparker2.com/saveme. html*

Godfrey, H. P. D., & Shum, D. (2000). Executive functioning and the application of social skills following traumatic brain injury. *Aphasiology, 14*(4), 433–444.

Goldberg, E., & Barr, W. (1991). Three possible mechanisms of unawareness of deficit. In G. P. Prigatano & D. L. Schacter (Eds.), *Awareness of deficit after brain injury: Clinical and theoretical issues* (pp. 152–175). New York: Oxford University Press.

Goldstein, K. (1952). The effect of brain damage on the personality. *Psychiatry, 15*(3), 245–260.

Goldstein, K. (1954). The concept of transference in treatment of organic and functional nervous disease. *Acta Psychotherapeutica Psychosomatica et Orthopaedagogica, 2*(3–4), 334–353.

Goodglass, H., & Kaplan, E. (2000). *Boston Naming Test*. Philadelphia: Lippincott Williams & Wilkins.

Goranson, T. E., Graves, R. E., Allison, D., & La Freniere, R. (2003). Community integration following multidisciplinary rehabilitation for traumatic brain injury. *Brain Injury, 17*(9), 759–774.

Gordon, W. A., Cantor, J., Ashman, T., & Brown, M. (2006). Treatment of post-TBI executive dysfunction: Application of theory to clinical practice. *Journal of Head Trauma Rehabilitation, 21*(2), 156–167.

Gosling, J., & Oddy, M. (1999). Rearranged marriages: Marital relationships after head injury. *Brain Injury, 13*(10), 785–796.

Gottesfeld, M. L., & Lieberman, F. (1979). The pathological therapist. *Social Casework: The Journal of Contemporary Social Work*, 387–393.

Gouick, J., & Gentleman, D. (2004). The emotional and behavioural consequences of traumatic brain injury. *Trauma, 6*(4), 285–292.

Goverover, Y. (2004). Categorization, deductive reasoning, and self-awareness: Association with everyday competence in persons with acute brain injury. *Journal of Clinical and Experimental Neuropsychology, 26*(6), 737–749.

Gracey, F., Palmer, S., Rous, B., Psaila, K., Shaw, K., O'Dell, J., et al. (2008). "Feeling part of things": Personal construction of self after brain injury. *Neuropsychological Rehabilitation, 18*(5–6), 627–650.

Graham, J. R. (2006). *MMPI-2: Assessing personality and psychopathology* (4th ed.). New York: Oxford University Press.

Green, J. L. (2007). *Technology for communication and cognitive treatment: The clinician's guide.* Potomac, MD: Innovative Speech Therapy.

Greenwood, C., Yorke, T., Greenwood, J., O'Brien, E., & Selway, P. (2000). Optimistic [Recorded by Radiohead]. On *Kid A* [CD]. Los Angeles: Capitol Records.

Gregory, B. M., (2007, December). *Cognitive behavioral treatment.* Paper presented at a continuing education course sponsored by PESI Health Care, Phoenix, AZ.

Gross, B. (2006). When enough is enough. *Annals of the American Psychotherapy Association, 9*(2), 37–40.

Groswasser, Z., Melamed, S., Agranov, E., & Keren, O. (1999). Return to work as an integrative outcome measure following traumatic brain injury. *Neuropsychological Rehabilitation, 9*(3–4), 493–504.

Groth-Marnat, G. (2003). *Handbook of psychological assessment* (4th ed.). New York: Wiley.

Groves, J. E. (1978). Taking care of the hateful patient. *New England Journal of Medicine, 298,* 883–887.

Gunther, M. S. (1994). Countertransference issues in staff caregivers who work to rehabilitate catastrophic-injury survivors. *American Journal of Psychotherapy, 48*(2), 208–220.

Gutman, S. A. (1999). Alleviating gender role strain in adult men with traumatic brain injury: An evaluation of a set of guidelines for occupational therapy. *American Journal of Occupational Therapy, 53*(1), 101–110.

Gutman, S. A., & Napier-Klemic, J. (1996). The experience of head injury on the impairment of gender identity and gender role. *American Journal of Occupational Therapy, 50*(7), 535–544.

Guy, J. D., & Brady, J. L. (2001). Identifying the faces in the mirror: Untangling transference and countertransference in self psychology. *Journal of Clinical Psychology/In Session, 57*(8), 993–997.

Haggstrom, A., & Lund, M. L. (2008). The complexity of participation in daily life: A qualitative study of the experiences of persons with acquired brain injury. *Journal of Rehabilitation Medicine, 40*(2), 89–95.

Hallett, J. D., Zasler, N. D., Maurer, P., & Cash, S. (1994). Role change after traumatic brain injury in adults. *American Journal of Occupational Therapy, 48*(3), 241–246.

Hanks, R. A., Rapport, L. J., & Vangel, S. (2007). Caregiving appraisal after traumatic brain injury: The effects of functional status, coping style, social support and family functioning. *NeuroRehabilitation, 22,* 43–52.

Harper, B. (2006). Better way. On *Both sides of the gun* [CD]. New York: Virgin Records America.

Harris, J. K. J., Godfrey, H. P. D., Partridge, F. M., & Knight, R. G. (2001). Caregiver depression following traumatic brain injury (TBI): A consequence of adverse effects on family members? *Brain Injury, 15*(3), 223–238.

Hart, T., Buchhofer, R., & Vaccaro, M. (2004). Portable electronic devices as memory and organizational aids after traumatic brain injury: A consumer survey study. *Journal of Head Trauma Rehabilitation, 19*(5), 351–365.

Hart, T., Hanks, R., Bogner, J. A., Millis, S., & Esselman, P. (2007). Blame attribution in intentional and unintentional traumatic brain injury: Longitudinal changes and impact on subjective well-being. *Rehabilitation Psychology, 52*(2), 152–161.

Hart, T., Millis, S., Novack, T., Englander, J., Fidler-Sheppard, R., & Bell, K. R. (2003). The relationship between neuropsychologic function and level of caregiver supervision at 1-year after traumatic brain injury. *Archives of Physical Medicine and Rehabilitation, 84,* 221–230.

Hart, T., Sherer, M., Whyte, J., Polansky, M., & Novack, T. A. (2004). Awareness of behavioral, cognitive, and physical deficits in acute traumatic brain injury. *Archives of Physical Medicine and Rehabilitation, 85,* 1450–1456.

Hartman, J. J. (1971). The case conference as a reflection of unconscious patient–therapist interaction. *Contemporary Psychoanalysis, 8,* 1–17.

Hartman-Maeir, A., Soroker, N., Oman, S. D., & Katz, N. (2003). Awareness of disabilities in stroke rehabilitation: A clinical trial. *Disability and Rehabilitation, 25*(1), 35–44.

Hawley, C. A., & Stephen, J. (2008). Predictors of positive growth after traumatic brain injury: A longitudinal study. *Brain Injury, 22*(5), 427–435.

Hayes, S. C., Strosahl, K. D., & Wilson, K. G. (1999). *Acceptance and commitment therapy: An experiential approach to behavior change.* New York: Guilford Press.

Heaton, R. K. (2003). *Wisconsin Card Sorting Test* (Computer version, 4th research ed.). Lutz, FL: Psychological Assessment Resources.

Heaton, R. K., Grant, I., & Matthews, C. G. (2004). *Revised comprehensive norms for an expanded Halstead–Reitan Battery (Computer version).* Lutz, FL: Psychological Assessment Resources.

Heaton, R., Miller, W., Taylor, M., & Grant, I. (2004). *Revised comprehensive norms for an expanded Halstead–Reitan Battery: Demographically adjusted neuropsychological norms for African American and Caucasian adults.* Lutz, FL: Psychological Assessment Resources.

Hein, P. (2004). T. T. T. In *Piet Hein—poems: Classic poetry series.* Retrieved from *www.poemhunter.com/i/ebooks/pdf/piet_hein_2004_9.pdf*

Heller, W., Levin, R. L., Mukherjee, D., & Reis, J. P. (2006). Characters in contexts: Identity and personality processes that influence individual and family adjustment to brain injury. *Journal of Rehabilitation, 72*(2), 44–49.

Hensold, T. C., Guercio, J. M., Grubbs, E. E., Upton, J. C., & Faw, G. (2006). A personal intervention substance abuse treatment approach: Substance abuse treatment in a least restrictive residential model. *Brain Injury, 20*(4), 369–381.

Hernandez, P., Gangsei, D., & Engstrom, D. (2007). Vicarious resilience: A new concept in work with those who survive trauma. *Family Process, 46*(2), 229–241.

Hibbard, M. R., Bogdany, J., Uysal, S., Kepler, K., Silver, J. M., Gordon, W. A., et al. (2000). Axis II psychopathology in individuals with traumatic brain injury. *Brain Injury, 14*(1), 45–61.

Hibbard, M. R., Cantor, J., Charatz, H., Rosenthal, R., Ashman, T., Gundersen, N., et al. (2002). Peer support in the community: Initial findings of a mentoring program for individuals with traumatic brain injury and their families. *Journal of Head Trauma Rehabilitation, 17*(2), 112–131.

Hibbard, M. R., Uysal, S., Kepler, K., Bogdany, J., & Silver, J. (1998). Axis I psychopathology in individuals with traumatic brain injury. *Journal of Head Trauma Rehabilitation, 13*(4), 24–39.

High, W. M., Jr., Roebuck-Spencer, T., Sander, A. M., Struchen, M. A., & Sherer, M. (2006). Early versus later admission to postacute rehabilitation: Impact on functional outcome after traumatic brain injury. *Archives of Physical Medicine and Rehabilitation, 87,* 334–342.

Hill, N. (1994). *Napoleon Hill's keys to success: The 17 principles of personal achievement.* New York: Dutton.

Hill, C. E., Nutt-Williams, E., Heaton, K. J., Thompson, B. J., & Rhodes, R. H. (1996). Therapist retrospective recall impasses in long-term psychotherapy: A qualitative analysis. *Journal of Counseling Psychology, 43*(2), 207–217.

Hilton, J., III. (2006). *I lost my phone number, can I have yours?: Pick-up lines that don't work, scriptural advice that does!* Salt Lake City, UT: Deseret Book.

Hinkebein, J. H., & Stucky, R. C. (2007). Coping with traumatic brain injury: Existential challenges and managing hope. In E. Martz, H. Livneh, & B. A. Wright (Eds.), *Coping with chronic illness and disability: Theoretical, empirical, and clinical aspects* (pp. 389–409). New York: Springer.

Hiott, D. W., & Labbate, L. (2002). Anxiety disorders associated with traumatic brain injuries. *NeuroRehabilitation, 17*(4), 345–355.

Hiscock, M., & Hiscock, C. K. (1989). Refining the forced-choice method for the detection of malingering. *Journal of Clinical and Experimental Neuropsychology, 11,* 967–974.

Hobson, R. P., & Kapur, R. (2005). Working in the transference: Clinical and research perspectives. *Psychology and Psychotherapy: Theory, Research and Practice, 78*(3), 275–293.

Holland, D., & Shigaki, C. L. (1998). Educating families and caretakers of traumatically brain injured patients in the new health care environment: A three phase model and bibliography. *Brain Injury, 12*(12), 993–1009.

Holmqvist, R., & Armelius, B. (2006). Sources of psychiatric staff members' feelings towards patients and treatment outcome. *Psychology and Psychotherapy: Theory, Research and Practice, 79,* 571–584.

Hoofien, D., Gilboa, A., Vakil, E., & Barak, O. (2004). Unawareness of cognitive deficits and daily functioning among persons with traumatic brain injuries. *Journal of Clinical and Experimental Neuropsychology, 26*(2), 278–290.

Horner, M. D., Ferguson, P. L., Selassie, A. W., Labbate, L. A., Kniele, K., & Corrigan, J. D. (2005). Patterns of alcohol use 1 year after traumatic brain injury: A population-based, epidemiological study. *Journal of the International Neuropsychological Society, 11*(3), 322–330.

Horvath, A. O., & Luborsky, L. (1993). The role of the therapeutic alliance in psychotherapy. *Journal of Consulting and Clinical Psychology, 61*(4), 561–573.

House, A. (2003). Psychiatry in neurological rehabilitation. In R. J. Greenwood, M. P. Barnes, T. M. McMillan, & C. D. Ward (Eds.), *Handbook of neurological rehabilitation* (2nd ed., pp. 433–442). New York: Psychology Press.

Howes, H., Benton, D., & Edwards, S. (2005). Women's experience of brain injury: An interpretative phenomenological analysis. *Psychology and Health, 20*(1), 129–142.

Howes, H., Edwards, S., & Benton, D. (2005a). Female body image following acquired brain injury. *Brain Injury, 19*(6), 403–415.

Howes, H., Edwards, S., & Benton, D. (2005b). Male body image following acquired brain injury. *Brain Injury, 19*(2), 135–147.

Inman, T., Vickery, C., Berry, D., Lamb, D., Edwards, C., & Smith, G. (1998). The Letter Memory Test. *Psychological Assessment, 10,* 128–139.

Inzaghi, M. G., De Tanti, A., & Sozzi, M. (2005). The effects of traumatic brain injury on patients and their families: A follow up study. *Europa Medicophysica, 41,* 265–273.

Jackson, H., & Manchester, D. (2001). Towards the development of brain injury specialists. *NeuroRehabilitation, 16*(1), 27–40.

Jemmer, P. (2006). Beliefs, values and the vacuum of choice. *European Journal of Clinical Hypnosis, 6*(4), 16–21.

Jennings, B. (2006). The ordeal of reminding. *Hastings Center Report, 36*(2), 29–37.

JIST Works. (2008). *Enhanced occupational outlook handbook* (7th ed). Indianapolis IN: Author.

Johansson, U., & Tham, K. (2006). The meaning of work after acquired brain injury. *American Journal of Occupational Therapy, 60*(1), 60–69.

Johnson, J. (2003). Times like these. On *On and on* [CD]. Universal City, CA: UMVD Labels.

Johnson, S. (1998). *Who moved my cheese?: An a-mazing way to deal with change in your work and in your life.* New York: Putnam.

Johnson, C., Knight, C., & Alderman, N. (2006). Challenges associated with the definition and assessment of inappropriate sexual behavior amongst individuals with an acquired neurological impairment. *Brain Injury, 20*(7), 687–693.

Jorge, R. E., & Robinson, R. G. (2003). Mood disorders following traumatic brain injury. *International Review of Psychiatry, 15*(4), 317–327.

Jorge, R. E., Starkstein, S. E., Arndt, S., Moser, D., Crespo-Facorro, B., & Robinson, R. G. (2005). Alcohol misuse and mood disorders following traumatic brain injury. *Archives of General Psychiatry, 62*(7), 742–749.

Jorgensen, R. S., & Thibodeau, R. (2007). Defensive avoidance of disapproval: The relationship of a defensive style to physical and mental health. *Harvard Review of Psychiatry, 15*(1), 9–17.

Jourard, S. M. (1971). *The transparent self.* New York: Van Nostrand Reinhold.

Joyce, A. S., Piper, W. E., Ogrodniczuk, J. S., & Klein, R. H. (2007). *Termination in psychotherapy: A psychodynamic model of processes and outcomes.* Washington, DC: American Psychological Association.

Judd, D., & Wilson, S. L. (2005). Psychotherapy with brain injury survivors: An investigation of the challenges encountered by clinicians and their modifications to therapeutic practice. *Brain Injury, 19*(6), 437–449.

Jureidini, J. (1988). Psychotherapeutic implications of severe physical disability. *American Journal of Psychotherapy, 42*(2), 297–307.

Kant, R., Duffy, J. D., & Pivovarnik, A. (1998). Prevalence of apathy following head injury. *Brain Injury, 12*(1), 87–92.

Kaplan De-Nour, A., & Bauman, A. (1980). Psychiatric treatment in severe brain injury: A case report. *General Hospital Psychiatry, 2*(1), 23–34.

Karg, R. S., & Wiens, A. N. (2005). Improving diagnostic and clinical interviewing. In G. P. Koocher, J. C. Norcross, & S. S. Hill III (Eds.), *Psychologists' desk reference* (2nd ed., pp. 11–14). New York: Oxford University Press.

Karlovits, T., & McColl, M. A. (1999). Coping with community reintegration after severe brain injury: A description of stresses and coping strategies. *Brain Injury, 13*(11), 845–861.

Kauffman, J. (2002). Introduction. In J. Kauffman (Ed.), *Loss of the assumptive world: A theory of traumatic loss* (pp. 1–9). New York: Brunner-Routledge.

Kendall, E. (2003). Predicting vocational adjustment following traumatic brain injury: A test of a psychosocial theory. *Journal of Vocational Rehabilitation, 19*(1), 31–45.

Kennedy, K., Marshall, F., Mendel, B., Mercer, S. (Producers), & Shyamalan, M. (Director). (1999). *The sixth sense* [Motion picture]. United States: Buena Vista Motion Pictures.

Kennedy, K., Spielberg, S., Mathison, M. (Producers), & Spielberg, S. (Director). (1982). *E. T.: The extra-terrestrial* [Motion picture]. United States: Universal Studios.

Kerner, E. A., & Fitzpatrick, M. R. (2007). Integrating writing into psychotherapy practice: A matrix of change processes and structural dimensions. *Psychotherapy: Theory, Research, Practice, Training, 44*(3), 333–346.

Kervick, R. B., & Kaemingk, K. L. (2005). Cognitive appraisal accuracy moderates the relationship between injury severity and psychosocial outcomes in traumatic brain injury. *Brain Injury, 19*(11), 881–889.

Kesler, S. R., Adams, H. F., Blasey, C. M., & Bigler, E. D. (2003). Premorbid intellectual functioning, education, and brain size in traumatic brain injury: An investigation of the cognitive reserve hypothesis. *Applied Neuropsychology, 10*(3), 153–162.

Kim, S. C., Kim, S., & Boren, D. (2008). The quality of therapeutic alliance between patient and provider predicts general satisfaction. *Military Medicine, 173*(1), 85–90.

King, C. (1971). You've got a friend [Recorded by J. Taylor]. On *Mud Slide Slim and the blue horizon* [Album]. Burbank, CA: Warner Bros. Records.

Kingsley, E. P. (1987). Welcome to Holland. Retrieved November 13, 2008, from *users.erols. com/jmatts/welcome%20to%20holland.html*

Klonoff, P. S. (1997). Individual and group psychotherapy in milieu-oriented neurorehabilitation. *Applied Neuropsychology, 4*(2), 107–118.

Klonoff, P. S. (2004, November). *Neuropsychological rehabilitation with adults using the milieu
approach at B.N.I.* Paper presented at Academy of Multidisciplinary Neurotraumatol-
ogy Conference, Phoenix, AZ.

Klonoff, P. S. (2005). The art and science of milieu-oriented neurorehabilitation. *Barrow
Quarterly, 21*(2), 14–21.

Klonoff, P. S., & Dawson, L. K. (2004). Commentary—Neuropsychological evaluation of
patients with traumatic brain injury: Polarization versus holistic integration. *Archives
of Clinical Neuropsychology, 19*, 1095–1101.

Klonoff, P. S., Koberstein, E. J., Talley, M. C., & Dawson, L. K. (2008). A family experiential
model of recovery after brain injury. *Bulletin of the Menninger Clinic, 72*(2), 109–129.

Klonoff, P. S., & Lage, G. A. (1991). Narcissistic injury in patients with traumatic brain
injury. *Journal of Head Trauma Rehabilitation, 6*(4), 11–21.

Klonoff, P. S., & Lage, G. A. (1995). Suicide in patients with traumatic brain injury: Risk and
prevention. *Journal of Head Trauma Rehabilitation, 10*(6), 16–24.

Klonoff, P. S., Lage, G. A., & Chiapello, D. A. (1993). Varieties of the catastrophic reaction
to brain injury: A self psychology perspective. *Bulletin of the Menninger Clinic, 57*(2),
227–241.

Klonoff, P. S., & Lamb, D. G. (1998). Mild head injury, significant impairment on neuropsychological test scores, and psychiatric disability. *The Clinical Neuropsychologist, 12*(1),
31–42.

Klonoff, P. S., Lamb, D. G., Chiapello, D. A., Kime, S. K., Shepherd, J., & Cunningham, M.
(1997). Cognitive retraining in a milieu-oriented outpatient rehabilitation program. In
M. E. Maruish & J. A. Moses (Eds.), *Clinical neuropsychology: Theoretical foundations for
practitioners* (pp. 219–236). Mahwah, NJ: Erlbaum.

Klonoff, P. S., Lamb, D. G., & Henderson, S. W. (2001). Outcomes from milieu-based neurorehabilitation at up to 11 years post-discharge. *Brain Injury, 15*(5), 413–428.

Klonoff, P. S., Lamb, D., Henderson, S., Dawson, L., Lutton, J., Grady, J., et al. (2003). Neu-
ropsychological rehabilitation in the community. In M. P. Barnes & H. Radermacher
(Eds.), *Community rehabilitation in neurology* (pp. 212–236). Cambridge, UK: Cambridge
University Press.

Klonoff, P. S., Lamb, D. G., Henderson, S. W., Reichert, M. V., & Tully, S. L. (2000). Milieu-
based neurorehabilitation at the Adult Day Hospital for Neurological Rehabilitation.
In A.-L. Christensen & B. P. Uzzell (Eds.), *International handbook of neuropsychological
rehabilitation* (pp. 195–213). New York: Kluwer Academic/Plenum.

Klonoff, P. S., Lamb, D. G., Henderson, S. W., & Shepherd, J. (1998). Outcome assessment
after milieu-oriented rehabilitation: New considerations. *Archives of Physical Medicine
and Rehabilitation, 79*, 684–690.

Klonoff, P. S., O'Brien, K. P., Prigatano, G. P., Chiapello, D. A., & Cunningham, M. (1989).
Cognitive retraining after traumatic brain injury and its role in facilitating awareness.
*Journal of Head Trauma Rehabilitation, 4*(3), 37–45.

Klonoff, P. S., & Prigatano, G. P. (1987). Reactions of family members and clinical intervention after traumatic brain injury. In M. Ylvisaker & E. M. R. Gobble (Ed.), *Community
re-entry for head injured adults* (pp. 381–402). Boston: Little, Brown.

Klonoff, P. S., Sheperd, J. C., O'Brien, K. P., Chiapello, D. A., & Hodak, J. A. (1990). Rehabilitation and outcome of right-hemisphere stroke patients: Challenges to traditional
diagnostic and treatment methods. *Neuropsychology, 4*, 147–163.

Klonoff, P. S., Snow, W. G., & Costa, L. D. (1986). Quality of life in patients 2 to 4 years after
closed head injury. *Neurosurgery, 19*(5), 735–743.

Klonoff, P. S., Talley, M. C., Dawson, L. K., Myles, S. M., Watt, L. M., Gehrels, J., et al. (2007).
The relationship of cognitive retraining to neurological patients' work and school status. *Brain Injury, 21*(11), 1097–1107.

Klonoff, P. S., Watt, L. M., Dawson, L. K., Henderson, S. W., Gehrels, J., & Voreis Wethe, J. (2006). Psychosocial outcomes 1–7 years after comprehensive milieu-oriented neurorehabilitation: The role of pre-injury status. *Brain Injury, 20*(6), 601–612.

Kohut, H. S. (1972). Thoughts on narcissism and narcissistic rage. *Psychoanalytic Study of the Child, 27,* 360–400.

Kohut, H. S. (1984a). The role of empathy in psychoanalytic cure. In A. Goldberg & P. Stepansky (Eds.), *How does analysis cure?* (pp. 172–191). Chicago: University of Chicago Press.

Kohut, H. S. (1984b). A reexamination of castration anxiety. In A. Goldberg & P. Stepansky (Eds.), *How does analysis cure?* (pp. 13–33). Chicago: University of Chicago Press.

Kolakowsky-Hayner, S. A., Gourley, E. V., III., Kreutzer, J. S., Marwitz, J. H., Meade, M. A., & Cifu, D. X. (2002). Post-injury substance abuse among persons with brain injury and persons with spinal cord injury. *Brain Injury, 16*(7), 583–592.

Koponen, S., Taiminen, T., Portin, R., Himanen, L., Isoniemi, H., Heinonen, H., et al. (2002). Axis I and II psychiatric disorders after traumatic brain injury: A 30-year follow-up study. *American Journal of Psychiatry, 159*(8), 1315–1321.

Kortte, K. B., Hill-Briggs, F., & Wegener, S. T. (2005). Psychotherapy with cognitively impaired adults. In G. P. Koocher, J. C. Norcross, & S. S. Hill III (Eds.), *Psychologists' desk reference* (2nd ed., pp. 342–346). New York: Oxford University Press.

Kortte, K. B., & Wegener, S. T. (2004). Denial of illness in medical rehabilitation populations: Theory, research, and definition. *Rehabilitation Psychology, 49*(3), 187–199.

Kortte, K. B., Wegener, S. T., & Chwalisz, K. (2003). Anosognosia and denial: Their relationship to coping and depression in acquired brain injury. *Rehabilitation Psychology, 48*(3), 131–136.

Kraemer, W. P. (1958). The dangers of unrecognized counter-transference. *Journal of Analytical Psychology, 3*(1), 29–41.

Kreuter, M., Dahllof, A. G., Gudjonsson, G., Sullivan, M., & Siosteen, A. (1998). Sexual adjustment and its predictors after traumatic brain injury. *Brain Injury, 12*(5), 349–368.

Kreutzer, J. S., Kolakowsky-Hayner, S. A., Demm, S. R., & Meade, M. A. (2002). A structured approach to family intervention after brain injury. *Journal of Head Trauma Rehabilitation, 17*(4), 349–367.

Kreutzer, J. S., Marwitz, J. H., Hsu, N., Williams, K., & Riddick, A. (2007). Marital stability after brain injury: An investigation and analysis. *NeuroRehabilitation, 22*(1), 53–59.

Kreutzer, J. S., Marwitz, J. H., & Kepler, K. (1992). Traumatic brain injury: Family response and outcome. *Archives of Physical Medicine and Rehabilitation, 73,* 771–778.

Kreutzer, J. S., Marwitz, J. H., Walker, W., Sander, A., Sherer, M., Bogner, J., et al. (2003). Moderating factors in return to work and job stability after traumatic brain injury. *Journal of Head Trauma Rehabilitation, 18*(2), 128–138.

Kuipers, P., & Lancaster, A. (2000). Developing a suicide prevention strategy based on the perspectives of people with brain injuries. *Journal of Head Trauma Rehabilitation, 15*(6), 1275–1284.

Kushner, H. (1981). *When bad things happen to good people.* New York: Schocken Books.

Lamb, W. (1998). *I know this much is true.* New York: Regan Books.

Landa-Gonzalez, B. (2001). Multicontextual occupational therapy intervention: A case study of traumatic brain injury. *Occupational Therapy International, 8*(1), 49–62.

Langenbahn, D. M., Sherr, R. L., Simon, D., & Hanig, B. (1999). Group psychotherapy. In K. G. Langer, L. Laatsch, & L. Lewis (Eds.), *Psychotherapeutic interventions for adults with brain injury or stroke: A clinician's treatment resource* (pp. 167–189). Madison, CT: Psychosocial Press.

Langer, K. G. (1994). Depression and denial in psychotherapy of persons with disabilities. *American Journal of Psychotherapy, 48*(2), 181–194.

Langer, K. G. (1999). Awareness and denial in psychotherapy. In K. G. Langer, L. Laatsch,

& L. Lewis (Eds.), *Psychotherapeutic interventions for adults with brain injury or stroke: A clinician's treatment resource* (pp. 75–96). Madison, CT: Psychosocial Press.

Langley, M. J. (1991). Preventing post-injury alcohol-related problems: A behavioral approach. In B. T. McMahon & L. R. Shaw (Eds.), *Work worth doing: Advances in brain injury rehabilitation* (pp. 251–275). Orlando, FL: Deutsch.

Laroi, F. (2003). The family systems approach to treating families of persons with brain injury: A potential collaboration between family therapist and brain injury professional. *Brain Injury, 17*(2), 175–187.

Lasseter, J., Shurer, O. (Producers), & Luckey, B., Gould, R. (Directors). (2003). *Boundin'* [Short motion picture]. United States: Pixar Animation Studios.

Lassiter, J., Mordaunt, W., Smith, W., Tadross, M., Zee, T. (Producers), & Tennant, A. (Director). (2005). *Hitch* [Motion picture]. United States: Columbia Pictures.

Lee, H., Kim, S.-W., Kim, J.-M., Shin, I.-S., Yang, S.-J., & Yoon, J.-S. (2005). Comparing effects of methylphenidate, Sertraline and placebo on neuropsychiatric sequelae in patients with traumatic brain injury. *Human Psychopharmacology: Clinical and Experimental, 20*, 97–104.

Lefebvre, H., Pelchat, D., Swaine, B., Gelinas, I., & Levert, M. J. (2005). The experiences of individuals with a traumatic brain injury, families, physicians and health professionals regarding care provided throughout the continuum. *Brain Injury, 19*(8), 585–597.

Lennon, J. (2002). Revolution [Recorded by Grandaddy]. On *I Am Sam—Music from and inspired by the motion picture soundtrack* [CD]. New York: V2 North America. (Original work recorded 1968)

Lennon, J., & McCartney, P. (1965a). Help! [Recorded by The Beatles]. On *Help!* [Album]. London: EMI Group.

Lennon, J., & McCartney, P. (1965b). We can work it out [Recorded by The Beatles]. On *Day tripper/We can work it out* [Single record]. London: EMI Group.

Leon-Carrion, J., De Serdio-Arias, M. L., Cabezas, F. M., Dominguez Roldan, J. M., Dominguez-Morales, R., Barroso y Martins, J. M., et al. (2001). Neurobehavioural and cognitive profile of traumatic brain injury patients at risk for depression and suicide. *Brain Injury, 15*(2), 175–181.

LeRoy, M. (Producer), & Fleming, V. (Director). (1939). *The wizard of Oz* [Motion picture]. United States: Metro-Goldwyn-Mayer.

Leung, K. L., & Man, D. W. K. (2005). Prediction of vocational outcome of people with brain injury after rehabilitation: A discriminant analysis. *Work, 25*, 333–340.

Levack, W., McPherson, K., & McNaughton, H. (2004). Success in the workplace following traumatic brain injury: Are we evaluating what is most important? *Disability and Rehabilitation, 26*(5), 290–298.

Lewis, L. (1991). Role of psychological factors in disordered awareness. In G. P. Prigatano & D. L. Schacter (Eds.), *Awareness of deficit after brain injury: Clinical and theoretical issues* (pp. 223–239). New York: Oxford University Press.

Lewis, L. (1999). Transference and countertransference in psychotherapy with adults having traumatic brain injury. In K.G. Langer, L. Laatsch, & L. Lewis (Eds.), *Psychotherapeutic interventions for adults with brain injury or stroke: A clinician's treatment resource* (pp. 113–127). Madison, CT: Psychosocial Press.

Lewis, L., & Rosenberg, S. J. (1990). Psychoanalytic psychotherapy with brain injured adult psychiatric patients. *Journal of Nervous and Mental Disease, 178*(2), 69–77.

Lezak, M. (1978). Living with the characterologically altered brain injured patient. *Journal of Clinical Psychiatry, 39*, 592–598.

Lezak, M. D., Howieson, D. B., Loring, D. W., Hannay, H. J., & Fischer, J. S. (2004). *Neuropsychological assessment* (4th ed.). New York: Oxford University Press.

Linden, A., Boschian, K., Eker, C., Schalen, W., & Nordstrom, C.-H. (2005). Assessment of motor and process skills reflects brain-injured patients' ability to resume independent living better than neuropsychological tests. *Acta Neurologica Scandinavica, 111*, 48–53.

Linge, F. R. (1990). Faith, hope, and love: Nontraditional therapy in recovery from serious head injury. A personal account. *Canadian Journal of Psychology, 44*(2), 116–129.

Linley, P. A., & Joseph, S. (2007). Therapy work and therapists' positive and negative well-being. *Journal of Social and Clinical Psychology, 26*(3), 385–403.

Lomas, P. (1993). *The psychotherapy of everyday life.* New Brunswick, NJ: Transaction.

Lombard, L. A., & Zafonte, R. D. (2005). Agitation after traumatic brain injury: Considerations and treatment options. *American Journal of Physical Medicine and Rehabilitation, 84*(10), 797–812.

Luborsky, L. (1976). Helping alliances in psychotherapy. In J. L. Claghorn (Ed.), *Successful psychotherapy* (pp. 92–116). New York: Brunner/Mazel.

Lubusko, A. A., Moore, A. D., Stambrook, M., & Gill, D. D. (1994). Cognitive beliefs following severe traumatic brain injury: Association with post-injury employment status. *Brain Injury, 8*(1), 65–70.

Ludden, L. L., & Maitlen, B. (2002). *Individual employment plan (IEP).* Indianapolis, IN: JIST.

Lundqvist, A., & Alinder, J. (2007). Driving after brain injury: Self-awareness and coping at the tactical level of control. *Brain Injury, 21*(11), 1109–1117.

Lundqvist, A., Alinder, J., & Rönnberg, J. (2008). Factors influencing driving 10 years after brain injury. *Brain Injury, 22*(4), 295–304.

Lynch, W. J. (2004). Determination of effort level, exaggeration, and malingering in neurocognitive assessment. *Journal of Head Trauma Rehabilitation, 19*(3), 277–283.

Machamer, J., Temkin, N., & Dikmen, S. (2002). Significant other burden and factors related to it in traumatic brain injury. *Journal of Clinical and Experimental Neuropsychology, 24*(4), 420–433.

MacMillan, P. J., Hart, R. P., Martelli, M. F., & Zasler, N. D. (2002). Pre-injury status and adaptation following traumatic brain injury. *Brain Injury, 16*(1), 41–49.

Madhavilatha, M. (2008). What makes the counselor effective? *ICFAI Journal of Soft Skills, 2*(2), 47–51.

Mainio, A., Kyllonen, T., Viilo, K., Hakko, H., Sarkioja, T., & Rasanen, P. (2007). Traumatic brain injury, psychiatric disorders and suicide: A population-based study of suicide victims during the years 1988–2004 in northern Finland. *Brain Injury, 21*(8), 851–855.

Malec, J. F., Testa, J. A., Rush, B. K., Brown, A. W., & Moessner, A. M. (2007). Self-assessment of impairment, impaired self-awareness, and depression after traumatic brain injury. *Journal of Head Trauma Rehabilitation, 22*(3), 156–166.

Mammi, P., Zaccaria, B., & Franceschini, M. (2006). Early rehabilitative treatment in patients with traumatic brain injuries: Outcome at one-year follow-up. *Europa Medicophysica, 42*, 17–22.

Man, D. W. K. (2001). A preliminary study to investigate the empowerment factors of survivors who have experienced brain damage in rehabilitation. *Brain Injury, 15*(11), 961–973.

Man, D. W. K. (2002). Family caregivers' reactions and coping for persons with brain injury. *Brain Injury, 16*(12), 1025–1037.

Manchester, D., Hodgkinson, A., & Casey, T. (1997). Prolonged, severe behavioural disturbance following traumatic brain injury: What can be done? *Brain Injury, 11*(8), 605–618.

Mander, G. (2000). Beginnings, endings and outcome: A comparison of methods and goals. *Psychodynamic Counselling, 6*(3), 301–317.

Markey, P., & Redford, R. (Producers), & Redford, R. (Director). (1998). *The horse whisperer* [Motion picture]. United States: Touchstone Pictures.

Marley, B. (1973). Pass it on [Recorded by B. Marley & the Wailers]. On *Burnin* [Album]. Kingston, Jamaica: Island/Tuff Gong Productions.

Marsten, R. S. (n.d.). *Daily motivator*. Retrieved September 2, 2008, from *greatday.com/motivate/index.html*

Martelli, M. F., Nicholson, K., & Zasler, N. D. (2008). Skill reacquisition after acquired brain injury: A holistic habit retraining model of neurorehabilitation. *NeuroRehabilitation, 23*(2), 115–126.

Martin, C., Buckland, J., Berryman, G., & Champion, W. (2005). Fix you [Recorded by Coldplay]. On *X&Y* [CD]. Los Angeles: Capitol Records.

Maslow, A. H. (1954). *Motivation and personality*. New York: Harper.

Maslow, A. H. (1971). *The farther reaches of human nature*. New York: Viking Press.

Mateer, C. A. (2005). Fundamentals of cognitive rehabilitation. In P. W. Halligan, & D. T. Wade (Eds.), *The effectiveness of rehabilitation for cognitive deficits* (pp. 21–29). New York: Oxford University Press.

Mateer, C. A., & Sira, C. S. (2006). Cognitive and emotional consequences of TBI: Intervention strategies for vocational rehabilitation. *NeuroRehabilitation, 21*(4), 315–326.

Mateer, C. A., & Sira, C. S. (2008). Practical rehabilitation strategies in the context of clinical neuropsychology feedback. In J. E. Morgan & J. H. Ricker (Eds.), *Textbook of clinical neuropsychology* (pp. 996–1007). New York: Taylor & Francis.

Mateer, C. A., Sira, C. S., & O'Connell, M. E. (2005). Putting Humpty Dumpty together again. *Journal of Head Trauma Rehabilitation, 20*(1), 62–75.

Mathiesen, B. B., & Weinryb, R. M. (2004). Unstable identity and prefrontal injury. *Cognitive Neuropsychiatry, 9*(4), 249–266.

Matthews, L. T., & Marwit, S. J. (2006). Meaning reconstruction in the context of religious coping: Rebuilding the shattered assumptive world. *Omega: Journal of Death and Dying, 53*(1–2), 87–104.

Mauss-Clum, N., & Ryan, M. (1981). Brain injury and the family. *Journal of Neurosurgical Nursing, 13*(4), 165–169.

May, R. (1977). *The meaning of anxiety* (rev. ed.). New York: Norton.

Mayer, J. (2007). Say. On *Continuum* [CD]. New York: Sony Records.

Mazaux, J.-M., Masson, F., Levin, H. S., Alaoui, P., Maurette, P., & Barat, M. (1997). Long-term neuropsychological outcome and loss of social autonomy after traumatic brain injury. *Archives of Physical Medicine and Rehabilitation, 78*, 1316–1320.

McAllister, T. W. (2005). Mild brain injury and the postconcussion syndrome. In J. M. Silver, T. W. McAllister, & S. C. Yudofsky (Eds.), *Textbook of traumatic brain injury* (pp. 279–308). Washington, DC: American Psychiatric Publishing.

McCarthy, W. C., & Frieze, I. H. (1999). Negative aspects of therapy: Client perceptions of therapists' social influence, burnout, and quality of care. *Journal of Social Issues, 55*(1), 33–50.

McColl, M. A., Bickenbach, J., Johnston, J., Nishihama, S., Schumaker, M., Smith, K., et al. (2000a). Spiritual issues associated with traumatic-onset disability. *Disability and Rehabilitation, 22*(12), 555–564.

McColl, M. A., Bickenbach, J., Johnston, J., Nishihama, S., Schumaker, M., Smith, K., et al. (2000b). Changes in spiritual beliefs after traumatic disability. *Archives of Physical Medicine and Rehabilitation, 81*, 817–823.

McCrea, M. A. (2007). *Mild traumatic brain injury and postconcussion syndrome: The new evidence base for diagnosis and treatment*. New York: Oxford University Press.

McDonald, B. C., Flashman, L. A., & Saykin, A. J. (2002). Executive dysfunction following traumatic brain injury: Neural substrates and treatment strategies. *NeuroRehabilitation, 17*, 333–344.

McFerrin, B. (1988). Don't worry, be happy. On *Simple pleasures* [CD]. Los Angeles: EMI-Manhattan.

McGlynn, S. M., & Schacter, D. L. (1989). Unawareness of deficits in neuropsychological syndromes. *Journal of Clinical and Experimental Neuropsychology, 11*(2), 143–205.

McGrath, J. C. (2004). Beyond restoration to transformation: Positive outcomes in the rehabilitation of acquired brain injury. *Clinical Rehabilitation, 18*(7), 767–775.

McGrath, J. C., & Linley, P. A. (2006). Post-traumatic growth in acquired brain injury: A preliminary small scale study. *Brain Injury, 20*(7), 767–773.

McLaughlin, A. M., & Carey, J. L. (1993). The adversarial alliance: Developing therapeutic relationships between families and the team in brain injury rehabilitation. *Brain Injury, 7*(1), 45–51.

McLaughlin, A. M., & Erdman, J. (1992). Rehabilitation staff stress as it relates to patient acuity and diagnosis. *Brain Injury, 6*(1), 59–64.

McPherson, K. M., Pentland, B., & McNaughton, H. K. (2000). Brain injury: The perceived health of carers. *Disability and Rehabilitation, 22*(15), 683–689.

Medlar, T. (1998). The sexuality education program of the Massachusetts Statewide Head Injury Program. *Sexuality and Disability, 16*(1), 11–19.

Melamed, Y., & Szor, H. (1999). The therapist and the patient: Coping with noncompliance. *Comprehensive Psychiatry, 40*(5), 391–395.

Messer, S. B. (2002). A psychodynamic perspective on resistance in psychotherapy: Vive la resistance. *Journal of Clinical Psychology/In Session, 58*(2), 157–163.

Metzgar, E. D. (Producer & Director). (2008). *Life. Support. Music.* [Motion picture]. United States: Merigold Moving Pictures.

Meyers, J. E., & Meyers, K. R. (1995). *Rey Complex Figure Test and Recognition Trial: Professional manual.* Lutz, FL: Psychological Assessment Resources.

Middelkamp, W., Moulaert, V. R. M. P., Verbunt, J. A., van Heugten, C. M., Bakx, W. G., & Wade, D. T. (2007). Life after survival: Long-term daily life functioning and quality of life of patients with hypoxic brain injury as a result of a cardiac arrest. *Clinical Rehabilitation, 21*, 425–431.

Middleton, W., Raphael, B., Martinek, N., & Misso, V. (1993). Pathological grief reactions. In M. S. Stroebe, W. Stroebe, & R. O. Hansson (Eds.) *Handbook of bereavement: Theory, research and intervention* (pp. 44–61). Cambridge, UK: Cambridge University Press.

Miller, L. (1991, March–April). Psychotherapy of the brain-injured patient: Principles and practices. *Cognitive Rehabilitation*, pp. 24–30.

Miller, L. (1993). *Psychotherapy of the brain-injured patient: Reclaiming the shattered self.* New York: Norton.

Miller, L. (1998). *Shocks to the system: Psychotherapy of traumatic disability syndromes.* New York: Norton.

Miller, L. (1999). A history of psychotherapy with patients with brain injury. In K.G. Langer, L. Laatsch, & L. Lewis (Eds.), *Psychotherapeutic interventions for adults with brain injury or stroke: A clinician's treatment resource* (pp. 27–43). Madison, CT: Psychosocial Press.

Millis, S. R. (2008). Assessment of incomplete effort and malingering in the neuropsychological examination. In J. E. Morgan & J. H. Ricker (Eds.), *Textbook of clinical neuropsychology* (pp. 891–904). New York: Taylor & Francis.

Millon, T. (2005). *Millon Clinical Multiaxial Inventory–III.* Minneapolis, MN: NCS/Pearson.

Mills, B., & Turnbull, G. (2004). Broken hearts and mending bodies: The impact of trauma on intimacy. *Sexual and Relationship Therapy, 19*(3), 265–289.

Mintz, M. C., Van Horn, K. R., & Levine, M. J. (1995). Developmental models of social cognition in assessing the role of family stress in relatives' predictions following traumatic brain injury. *Brain Injury, 9*(2), 173–186.

Miquelon, P., & Vallerand, R. J. (2008). Goal motives, well-being, and physical health: An integrative model. *Canadian Psychology, 49*(3), 241–249.

Moore, A. D., & Stambrook, M. (1995). Cognitive moderators of outcome following traumatic brain injury: A conceptual model and implications for rehabilitation. *Brain Injury, 9*(2), 109–130.

Morris, K. C. (2001). Psychological distress in carers of head injured individuals: The provision of written information. *Brain Injury, 15*(3), 239–254.

Morton, M. V., & Wehman, P. (1995). Psychosocial and emotional sequelae of individuals with traumatic brain injury: A literature review and recommendations. *Brain Injury, 9*(1), 81–92.

Mukerjee, D., Reis, J. P., & Heller, W. (2003). Women living with traumatic brain injury: Social isolation, emotional functioning and implications for psychotherapy. *Women and Therapy, 26*(1–2), 3–26.

Murphy, F. C., Nimmo-Smith, I., & Lawrence, A. D. (2003). Functional neuroanatomy of emotions: A meta-analysis. *Cognitive, Affective, and Behavioral Neuroscience, 3*(3), 207–233.

Myles, S. M. (2004). Understanding and treating loss of sense of self following brain injury: A behavior analytic approach. *International Journal of Psychology and Psychological Therapy, 4*(3), 487–504.

Myles, S. M. (2007, February). *Changes to sense-of-self post-brain injury: Research and treatment.* Paper presented at the 35th Annual Meeting of the International Neuropsychological Society (Continuing Education Program), Portland, OR.

Mynatt, S., & Cunningham, P. (2007). Unraveling anxiety and depression. *Nurse Practitioner, 32*(8), 28–37.

Newman, C. F. (2002). A cognitive perspective on resistance in psychotherapy. *Journal of Clinical Psychology/In Session, 58*(2), 165–174.

Niemeier, J., Kennedy, R., McKinley, W., & Cifu, D. (2004). The Loss Inventory: Preliminary reliability and validity data for a new measure of emotional and cognitive responses to disability. *Disability and Rehabilitation, 26*(10), 614–623.

Nochi, M. (1998). "Loss of self" in the narratives of people with traumatic brain injuries: A qualitative analysis. *Social Science and Medicine, 46*(7), 869–878.

Noé, E., Ferri, J., Caballero, M. C., Villodre, R., Sanchez, A., & Chirivella, J. (2005). Self-awareness after brain injury: Predictors and rehabilitation. *Journal of Neurology, 252*, 168–175.

Norcross, J. C. (2005). The psychotherapist's own psychotherapy: Educating and developing psychologists. *American Psychologist, 60*(8), 840–853.

Norcross, J. C., & Guy, J. D., Jr. (2005). Therapist self-care checklist. In G. P. Koocher, J. C. Norcross, & S. S. Hill III (Eds.), *Psychologists' desk reference* (2nd ed., pp. 677–682). New York: Oxford University Press.

Norcross, J. C., & Guy, J. D., Jr. (2007). *Leaving it at the office: A guide to psychotherapist self-care.* New York: Guilford Press.

Novack, T. A., Alderson, A. L., Bush, B. A., Meythaler, J. M., & Canupp, K. (2000). Cognitive and functional recovery at 6 and 12 months post-TBI. *Brain Injury, 14*(11), 987–996.

Novack, T. A., Bush, B. A., Meythaler, J. D., & Canupp, K. (2001). Outcome after traumatic brain injury: Pathway analysis of contributions from premorbid, injury severity, and recovery variables. *Archives of Physical Medicine and Rehabilitation, 82*, 300–305.

O'Brien, L. (2007). Achieving a successful and sustainable return to the workforce after ABI: A client-centered approach. *Brain Injury, 21*(5), 465–478.

O'Callaghan, C., Powell, T., & Oyebode, J. (2006). An exploration of the experience of gaining awareness of deficit in people who have suffered brain injury. *Neuropsychological Rehabilitation, 16*(5), 579–593.

Oddy, M. (2003). Psychosocial consequences of brain injury. In R. J. Greenwood, M. P. Barnes, T. M. McMillan, & C. D. Ward (Eds.), *Handbook of neurological rehabilitation* (2nd ed., pp. 453–462). New York: Psychology Press.

Ondrasik, J. (2000). Superman (It's not easy) [Recorded by Five for Fighting]. On *America town* [CD]. New York: Sony Records.

Oppermann, J. D. (2004). Interpreting the meaning individuals ascribe to returning to work after traumatic brain injury: A qualitative approach. *Brain Injury, 18*(9), 941–955.

Orlinsky, D. E., & Howard, K. I. (1995). Unity and diversity among psychotherapies: A comparative perspective. In B. Bongar & L. E. Beutler (Eds.), *Comprehensive textbook of psychotherapy: Theory and practice* (pp. 3–23). New York: Oxford University Press.

Ownsworth, T., Fleming, J., Strong, J., Radel, M., Chan, W., & Clare, L. (2007). Awareness typologies, long-term emotional adjustment and psychosocial outcomes following acquired brain injury. *Neuropsychological Rehabilitation, 17*(2), 129–150.

Ownsworth, T. L., & McFarland, K. (2004). Investigation of psychological and neuropsychological factors associated with clinical outcome following a group rehabilitation programme. *Neuropsychological Rehabilitation, 14*(5), 535–562.

Ownsworth, T. L., McFarland, K., & Young, R. M. (2002). The investigation of factors underlying deficits in self-awareness and self-regulation. *Brain Injury, 16*(4), 291–309.

Padrone, F. J. (1999). Psychotherapeutic issues in treating family members. In K. G. Langer, L. Laatsch, & L. Lewis (Eds.), *Psychotherapeutic interventions for adults with brain injury or stroke: A clinician's treatment resource* (pp. 191–209). Madison, CT: Psychosocial Press.

Pagulayan, K. F., Temkin, N. R., Machamer, J. E., & Dikmen, S. S. (2007). The measurement and magnitude of awareness difficulties after traumatic brain injury: A longitudinal study. *Journal of the International Neuropsychological Society, 13*, 561–570.

Pais, S. (2002). "Remember to place the oxygen mask on yourself first . . . " *Journal of Clinical Activities, Assignments and Handouts in Psychotherapy Practice, 2*(4), 109–115.

Paletti, R. (2008). Recovery in context: Bereavement, culture, and the transformation of the therapeutic self. *Death Studies, 32*(1), 17–26.

Palmer, S., & Glass, T. A. (2003). Family function and stroke recovery: A review. *Rehabilitation Psychology, 48*(4), 255–265.

Pausch, R., & Zaslow, J. (2008). *The last lecture.* New York: Hyperion.

Payne, S. C., & Huffman, A. H. (2005). A longitudinal examination of the influence of mentoring on organizational commitment and turnover. *Academy of Management Journal, 48*(1), 158–168.

Pearlin, L. I., Mullan, J. T., Semple, S. J., & Skaff, M. M. (1990). Caregiving and the stress process: An overview of concepts and their measures. *The Gerontologist, 30*(5), 583–594.

Pepping, M. (1993). Transference and countertransference issues in brain injury rehabilitation: Implications for staff training. In C. J. Durgin, N. D. Schmidt, & L. J. Fryer (Eds.), *Staff development and clinical intervention in brain injury rehabilitation* (pp. 87–103). Gaithersburg, MD: Aspen.

Perlesz, A., Kinsella, G., & Crowe, S. (2000). Psychological distress and family satisfaction following traumatic brain injury: Injured individuals and their primary, secondary, and tertiary carers. *Journal of Head Trauma Rehabilitation, 15*(3), 909–929.

Persel, C. S., & Persel, C. H. (2004). The use of applied behavior analysis in traumatic brain injury rehabilitation. In M. J. Ashley (Ed.), *Traumatic brain injury: Rehabilitative treatment and case management* (pp. 403–453). Boca Raton, FL: CRC Press.

Persinger, M. A. (1993). Personality changes following brain injury as a grief response to the loss of sense of self: Phenomenological themes as indices of local lability and neurocognitive structuring as psychotherapy. *Psychological Reports, 72*, 1059–1068.

Petrella, L., McColl, M. A., Krupa, T., & Johnston, J. (2005). Returning to productive activities: Perspectives of individuals with long-standing acquired brain injuries. *Brain Injury, 19*(9), 643–655.

Pierce, C. A., & Hanks, R. A. (2006). Life satisfaction after traumatic brain injury and the World Health Organization model of disability. *American Journal of Physical Medicine and Rehabilitation, 85*(11), 889–898.

Pies, R. (2008). The anatomy of sorrow: A spiritual, phenomenological, and neurological perspective. *Philosophy, Ethics, and Humanities in Medicine, 3*, 1–8.

Piolino, P., Desgranges, B., Manning, L., North, P., Jokic, C., & Eustache, F. (2007). Autobiographical memory, the sense of recollection and executive functions after severe traumatic brain injury. *Cortex, 43*(2), 176–195.

Piper, W. (1986). *The easy-to-read little engine that could.* New York: Platt & Munk.

Ponsford, J., Olver, J., Ponsford, M., & Nelms, R. (2003). Long-term adjustment of families following traumatic brain injury where comprehensive rehabilitation has been provided. *Brain Injury, 17*(6), 453–468.

Porteus, S. D. (1965). *Porteus Maze Test: Fifty years' application.* Palo Alto, CA: Pacific Books.

Powell, T., Ekin-Wood, A., & Collin, C. (2007). Post-traumatic growth after head injury: A long-term follow-up. *Brain Injury, 21*(1), 31–38.

Power, P. W., & Hershenson, D. B. (2003). Work adjustment and readjustment of persons with mid-career onset traumatic brain injury. *Brain Injury, 17*(12), 1021–1034.

Prigatano, G. P. (1989). Work, love, and play after brain injury. *Bulletin of the Menninger Clinic, 53*(5), 414–431.

Prigatano, G. P. (1991). Disordered mind, wounded soul: The emerging role of psychotherapy in rehabilitation after brain injury. *Journal of Head Trauma Rehabilitation, 6*(4), 1–10.

Prigatano, G. P. (1999). *Principles of neuropsychological rehabilitation.* New York: Oxford University Press.

Prigatano, G. P. (2005a). Disturbances of self-awareness and rehabilitation of patients with traumatic brain injury: A 20-year perspective. *Journal of Head Trauma Rehabilitation, 20*(1), 19–29.

Prigatano, G. P. (2005b). Impaired self-awareness after moderately severe to severe traumatic brain injury. *Acta Neurochirurgica,* Suppl. 93, 39–42.

Prigatano, G. P. (2008a). Neuropsychological rehabilitation and psychodynamic psychotherapy. In J. E. Morgan & J. H. Ricker (Eds.), *Textbook of clinical neuropsychology* (pp. 985–995). New York: Taylor & Francis.

Prigatano, G. P. (2008b). Anosognosia and the process and outcome of neurorehabilitation. In D. T. Stuss, G. Winocur, & I. H. Robertson (Eds.), *Cognitive neurorehabilitation: Evidence and application* (2nd ed., pp. 218–231). New York: Cambridge University Press.

Prigatano, G. P., & Ben-Yishay, Y. (1999). Psychotherapy and psychotherapeutic interventions in brain injury rehabilitation. In M. Rosenthal, E. R. Griffith, J. S. Kreutzer, & B. Pentland (Eds.), *Rehabilitation of the adult and child with traumatic brain injury* (3rd ed., pp. 271–283). Philadelphia: Davis.

Prigatano, G. P., Fordyce, D. J., Zeiner, H. K., Roueche, J. R., Pepping, M., & Wood, B. C. (1986). *Neuropsychological rehabilitation after brain injury.* Baltimore: Johns Hopkins University Press.

Prigatano, G. P., & Klonoff, P. S. (1988). Psychotherapy and neuropsychological assessment after brain injury. *Journal of Head Trauma Rehabilitation, 3*(1), 45–56.

Prigatano, G. P., & Klonoff, P. S. (1998). A clinician's rating scale for evaluating impaired self-awareness and denial of disability after brain injury. *The Clinical Neuropsychologist, 12*(1), 56–67.

Prigatano, G. P., & Schacter, D. L. (Eds.). (1991). *Awareness of deficit after brain injury: Clinical and theoretical issues.* New York: Oxford University Press.

Quintar, B. (2001). Termination phase. *Journal of Psychotherapy in Independent Practice, 2*(3), 43–60.

Rawn, M. L. (1991). The working alliance: Current concepts and controversies. *The Psychoanalytic Review, 78*(3), 379–389.

Redding, O. (1967). Respect [Recorded by A. Franklin]. On *I never loved a man the way I love you* [Album]. New York: Atlantic Records. (Original work released 1965)

Reher, K. (Producer), & Sohn, P. (Director). (2009). *Partly cloudy* [Short motion picture]. United States: Pixar Animation Studios.

Riley, G. A., Brennan, A. J., & Powell, T. (2004). Threat appraisal and avoidance after traumatic brain injury: Why and how often are activities avoided? *Brain Injury, 18*(9), 871–888.

Rinehart, B., Rinehart, B., Bolt, S., & Stillwell, J. (2009a). Lay 'em down [Recorded by Need to Breathe]. On *The outsiders* [CD]. New York: Atlantic Records.

Rinehart, B., Rinehart, B., Bolt, S., & Stillwell, J. (2009b). These hard times [Recorded by Need to Breathe]. On *The outsiders* [CD]. New York: Atlantic Records.

Rodgers, R., & Hammerstein, O. (2001). You'll never walk alone [Recorded by S. Jones]. On *Carousel soundtrack* [CD]. New York: Angel Records. (Original work released 1956)

Rogers, R. (2005). Assessment of malingering on psychological measures. In G. P. Koocher, J. C. Norcross, & S. S. Hill III (Eds.), *Psychologists' desk reference* (2nd ed., pp. 67–71). New York: Oxford University Press.

Rogers, J. M., & Read, C. A. (2007). Psychiatric comorbidity following traumatic brain injury. *Brain Injury, 21*(13–14), 1321–1333.

Roter, D. L., Cole, K. A., Kern, D. E., Barker, L. R., & Grayson, M. (1990). An evaluation of residency training in interviewing skills and the psychosocial domain of medical practice. *Journal of General Internal Medicine, 5,* 347–354.

Rothstein, A. (1999). Some implications of the analyst feeling disturbed while working with disturbed patients. *Psychoanalytic Quarterly, 68*(4), 541–558.

Rothwell, N. A., LaVigna, G. W., & Willis, T. J. (1999). A non-aversive rehabilitation approach for people with severe behavioural problems resulting from brain injury. *Brain Injury, 13*(7), 521–533.

Rotondi, A. J., Sinkule, J., Balzer, K., Harris, J., & Moldovan, R. (2007). A qualitative needs assessment of persons who have experienced traumatic brain injury and their primary family caregivers. *Journal of Head Trauma Rehabilitation, 22*(1), 14–25.

Rudd, X. (2008). Shiver. On *Dark shades of blue* [CD]. Los Angeles: Anti.

Rudin, S. (Producer), & Dey, T. (Director). (2006). *Failure to launch* [Motion picture]. United States: Paramount Pictures.

Ruff, R. M. (1996). *Ruff Figural Fluency Test administration manual.* Lutz, FL: Psychological Assessment Resources.

Saltapidas, H., & Ponsford, J. (2007). The influence of cultural background on motivation for and participation in rehabilitation and outcome following traumatic brain injury. *Journal of Head Trauma Rehabilitation, 22*(2), 132–139.

Sandel, M. E., Williams, K. S., Dellapietra, L., & Derogatis, L. R. (1996). Sexual functioning following traumatic brain injury. *Brain Injury, 10*(10), 719–728.

Sander, A. M., Caroselli, J. S., High, W. M., Jr., Becker, C., Neese, L., & Scheibel, R. (2002). Relationship of family functioning to progress in a post-acute rehabilitation programme following traumatic brain injury. *Brain Injury, 16*(8), 649–657.

Sander, A. M., Sherer, M., Malec, J. F., High, W. M., Jr., Thompson, R. N., Moessner, A. M., et al. (2003). Preinjury emotional and family functioning in caregivers of persons with traumatic brain injury. *Archives of Physical Medicine and Rehabilitation, 84,* 197–203.

Sandler, J., Dare, C., & Holder, A. (1973). *The patient and the analyst: The basis of the psychoanalytic process.* New York: International Universities Press.

Sapienza, B. G., & Bugental, J. F. T. (2000). Keeping our instruments finely tuned: An existential–humanistic perspective. *Professional Psychology: Research and Practice, 31*(4), 458–460.

Satz, P. (1993). Brain reserve capacity on symptom onset after brain injury: A formulation and review of evidence for threshold theory. *Neuropsychology, 7,* 273–295.

Schanke, A.-K., & Sundet, K. (2000). Comprehensive driving assessment: Neuropsychological testing and on-road evaluation of brain injured patients. *Scandinavian Journal of Psychology, 41,* 113–121.

Schmidt, M. F., & Heinemann, A. W. (1999). Substance abuse interventions for people with brain injury. In K. G. Langer, L. Laatsch, & L. Lewis (Eds.), *Psychotherapeutic interventions for adults with brain injury or stroke: A clinician's treatment resource* (pp. 211–238). Madison, CT: Psychosocial Press.

Scholl, J. C., & Ragan, S. L. (2003). The use of humor in promoting positive provider–patient interactions in a hospital rehabilitation unit. *Health Communication, 15*(3), 319–330.

Schönberger, M., Humle, F., & Teasdale, T. W. (2006a). The development of the therapeutic working alliance, patients' awareness and their compliance during the process of brain injury rehabilitation. *Brain Injury, 20*(4), 445–454.

Schönberger, M., Humle, F., & Teasdale, T. W. (2006b). Subjective outcome of brain injury rehabilitation in relation to the therapeutic working alliance, client compliance and awareness. *Brain Injury, 20*(12), 1271–1282.

Schönberger, M., Humle, F., Zeeman, P., & Teasdale, T. (2006). Working alliance and patient compliance in brain injury rehabilitation and their relation to psychosocial outcome. *Neuropsychological Rehabilitation, 16*(3), 298–314.

Schopp, L. H., Good, G. E., Barker, K. B., Mazurek, M. O., & Hathaway, S. L. (2006). Masculine role adherence and outcomes among men with traumatic brain injury. *Brain Injury, 20*(11), 1155–1162.

Schultheis, M. T., Matheis, R. J., Nead, R., & DeLuca, J. (2002). Driving behaviors following brain injury: Self-report and motor vehicle records. *Journal of Head Trauma Rehabilitation, 17*(1), 38–47.

Schutz, L. E. (2007). Models of exceptional adaptation in recovery after traumatic brain injury: A case series. *Journal of Head Trauma Rehabilitation, 22*(1), 48–55.

Schwaber, E. A. (1979). *Narcissism, self psychology, and the listening perspective.* Paper presented at a staff psychiatry conference, Mt. Auburn Hospital, Cambridge, MA.

Schwary, R. L. (Producer), & Redford, R. (Director). (1980). *Ordinary people* [Motion picture]. United States: Paramount Pictures.

Shames, J., Treger, I., Ring, H., & Giaquinto, S. (2007). Return to work following traumatic brain injury: Trends and challenges. *Disability and Rehabilitation, 29*(17), 1387–1395.

Sherer, M., Bergloff, P., High, W. Jr., & Nick, T. G. (1999). Contribution of functional ratings to prediction of long-term employment outcome after traumatic brain injury. *Brain Injury, 13*(12), 973–981.

Sherer, M., Evans, C. C., Leverenz, J., Stouter, J., Irby, J. W., Jr., Lee, J. E., et al. (2007). Therapeutic alliance in post-acute brain injury rehabilitation: Predictors of strength of alliance and impact of alliance on outcome. *Brain Injury, 21*(7), 663–672.

Sherer, M., Hart, T., Nick, T. G., Whyte, J., Thompson, R. N., & Yablon, S. A. (2003). Early impaired self-awareness after traumatic brain injury. *Archives of Physical Medicine and Rehabilitation, 84*, 168–176.

Sherer, M., Oden, K., Bergloff, P., Levin, E., & High, W. M., Jr. (1998). Assessment and treatment of impaired awareness after brain injury: Implications for community reintegration. *NeuroRehabilitation, 10*(1), 25–37.

Sheridan, V. S., Cimini, M. E., Talbot, C., Huey, A., Schade, J., & Watson, R. A. (Eds.). (2009). *National trade and professional association of the United States* (44th ed). Washington, DC: Columbia Books.

Sherwin, E., Whiteneck, G., Corrigan, J., Bedell, G., Brown, M., Abreu, B., et al. (2006). Domains of a TBI minimal data set: Community reintegration phase. *Brain Injury, 20*(4), 383–389.

Sigurdardottir, S., Andelic, N., Roe, C., & Schanke, A.-K. (2009). Cognitive recovery and predictors of functional outcome 1-year after traumatic brain injury. *Journal of the International Neuropsychological Society, 15*, 740–750.

Silver, J. M., Arciniegas, D. B., & Yudofsky, S. C. (2005). Psychopharmacology. In J. M. Silver, T. W. McAllister, & S. C. Yudofsky (Eds.), *Textbook of traumatic brain injury* (pp. 609–639). Washington, DC: American Psychiatric Publishing.

Silverstein, S. (1964). *The giving tree.* New York: Harper & Row.

Silverstein, S. (1981). *The missing piece meets the big O.* New York: Harper & Row.

Simon, R. (2002). *Riding the bus with my sister: A true life journey.* Boston: Houghton-Mifflin.

Simpson, G., & Long, E. (2004). An evaluation of sex education and information resources and their provision to adults with traumatic brain injury. *Journal of Head Trauma Rehabilitation, 19*(5), 413–428.

Simpson, G., & Tate, R. (2007). Suicidality in people surviving a traumatic brain injury: Prevalence, risk factors and implications for clinical management. *Brain Injury, 21*(13–14), 1335–1351.

Simpson, G., Winstanley, J., & Bertapelle, T. (2003). Suicide prevention training after traumatic brain injury: Evaluation of a staff training workshop. *Journal of Head Trauma Rehabilitation, 18*(5), 445–456.

Sinnakaruppan, I., & Williams, D. M. (2001). Family carers and the adult head-injured: A critical review of carers' needs. *Brain Injury, 15*(8), 653–672.

Skeel, R. L., & Edwards, S. (2009). The assessment and rehabilitation of memory impairments. In B. Johnstone & H. H. Stonnington (Eds.), *Rehabilitation of neuropsychological disorders: A practical guide for rehabilitation professionals* (2nd ed., pp. 47–70). New York: Psychology Press.

Skovholt, T., Grier, T., & Hanson, M. (2001). Career counseling for longevity: Self-care and burnout prevention strategies for counselor resilience. *Journal of Career Development, 27*(3), 167–176.

Slick, D., Hopp, G., Strauss, E., Thompson, G. B. (2005). *Victoria Symptom Validity Test: Professional manual*. Lutz, FL: Psychological Assessment Resources.

Smith, C. (2008). Performing my recovery: A play of chaos, restitution, and quest after traumatic brain injury. *Forum: Qualitative Social Research, 9*(2), 1–17.

Snead, S. L., & Davis, J. R. (2002). Attitudes of individuals with acquired brain injury towards disability. *Brain Injury, 16*(11), 947–953.

Snow, P., Douglas, J., & Ponsford, J. (1998). Conversational discourse abilities following severe traumatic brain injury: A follow up study. *Brain Injury, 12*(11), 911–935.

Snyder, P. J., Nussbaum, P. D., & Robins, D. L. (Eds.). (2006). *Clinical neuropsychology: A pocket handbook for assessment* (2nd ed.). Washington, DC: American Psychological Association.

Sobell, L. C., & Sobell, M. B. (2005). Identification and assessment of alcohol abuse. In G. P. Koocher, J. C. Norcross, & S. S. Hill III (Eds.), *Psychologists' desk reference* (2nd ed., pp. 71–76). New York: Oxford University Press.

Sohlberg, M. M. (2000). Assessing and managing unawareness of self. *Speech and Language, 21*, 135–151.

Sohlberg, M. M., & Mateer, C. A. (1989). Training use of compensatory memory books: A three stage behavioral approach. *Journal of Clinical and Experimental Neuropsychology, 11*(6), 871–891.

Sohlberg, M. M., & Mateer, C. A. (2001). *Cognitive rehabilitation: An integrative neuropsychological approach*. New York: Guilford Press.

Sohlberg, M. M., McLaughlin, K. A., Todis, B., Larsen, J., & Glang, A. (2001). What does it take to collaborate with families affected by brain injury?: A preliminary model. *Journal of Head Trauma Rehabilitation, 16*(5), 498–511.

Solomon, C. R., & Scherzer, B. P. (1991). Some guidelines for family therapists working with the traumatically brain injured and their families. *Brain Injury, 5*(3), 253–266.

Sparadeo, F. R. (1993). Substance use: A critical training issue for staff in brain injury rehabilitation. In C. J. Durgin, N. D. Schmidt, & L. J. Fryer (Eds.), *Staff development and clinical intervention in brain injury rehabilitation* (pp. 189–205). Gaithersburg, MD: Aspen.

Spiers, H. J., & Maguire, E. A. (2007). Neural substrates of driving behaviour. *NeuroImage, 36*(1), 245–255.

Springsteen, B. (2009). Working on a dream. On *Working on a dream* [CD]. New York: Columbia Records/Sony BMG.

St. Claire, S. (1996). A letter from your brain. Retrieved July 19, 2008, from *www.waiting.com/letter.html*

Steadman-Pare, D., Colantonio, A., Ratcliff, G., Chase, S., & Vernich, L. (2001). Factors associated with perceived quality of life many years after traumatic brain injury. *Journal of Head Trauma Rehabilitation, 16*(4), 330–342.

Steel, P. (2007). The nature of procrastination: A meta-analytic and theoretical review of quintessential self-regulatory failure. *Psychological Bulletin, 133*(1), 65–94.

Stein, D. G., & Hoffman, S. W. (2003). Concepts of CNS plasticity in the context of brain damage and repair. *Journal of Head Trauma Rehabilitation, 18*(4), 317–341.

Stern, D. (1985). *The interpersonal world of the infant.* New York: Basic Books.

Stern, J. M. (1985). The psychotherapeutic process with brain injured patients: A dynamic approach. *Israeli Journal of Psychiatry and Related Sciences, 22*(1–2), 83–87.

Strauss, E., Sherman, E. M. S., & Spreen, O. (2006). *A compendium of neuropsychological tests: Administration, norms, and commentary* (3rd ed.). New York: Oxford University Press.

Stroebe, M., & Schut, H. (1999). The dual process model of coping with bereavement: Rationale and description. *Death Studies, 23*(3), 197–224.

Strom, T. Q., & Kosciulek, J. (2007). Stress, appraisal and coping following mild traumatic brain injury. *Brain Injury, 21*(11), 1137–1145.

Strozier, C. B. (2001). *Heinz Kohut: The making of a psychoanalyst.* New York: Farrar, Straus & Giroux.

Strupp, H. H. (1980). Success and failure in time-limited psychotherapy: Further evidence (comparison 4). *Archives of General Psychiatry, 37*(8), 947–954.

Stuss, D. T. (1991). Disturbance of self-awareness after frontal system damage. In G. P. Prigatano & D. L. Schacter (Eds.), *Awareness of deficit after brain injury: Clinical and theoretical issues* (pp. 63–83). New York: Oxford University Press.

Stuss, D. T., & Benson, D. F. (1984). Neuropsychological studies of the frontal lobes. *Psychological Bulletin, 95*(1), 3–28.

Stuss, D. T., & Benson, D. F. (1986). *The frontal lobes.* New York: Raven Press.

Stuss, D. T., Gow, C. A., & Hetherington, C. R. (1992). "No longer Gage": Frontal lobe dysfunction and emotional changes. *Journal of Consulting and Clinical Psychology, 60*(3), 349–359.

Sundet, K., Goffeng, L., & Hofft, E. (1995). To drive or not to drive: Neuropsychological assessment for driver's license among stroke patients. *Scandinavian Journal of Psychology, 36*, 47–58.

Sutherland, O., & Couture, S. (2007). The discursive performance of the alliance in family therapy: A conversation analytic perspective. *Australian and New Zealand Journal of Family Therapy, 28*(4), 210–217.

Sveen, U., Mongs, M., Roe, C., Sandvik, L., & Bautz-Holter, E. (2008). Self-rated competency in activities predicts functioning and participation one year after traumatic brain injury. *Clinical Rehabilitation, 22*(1), 45–55.

Svendsen, H. A., & Teasdale, T. W. (2006). The influence of neuropsychological rehabilitation on symptomatology and quality of life following brain injury: A controlled long-term follow-up. *Brain Injury, 20*(12), 1295–1306.

Swift, W. J., & Wonderlich, S. (1993). House of games: A cinematic study of countertransference. *American Journal of Psychotherapy, 47*(1), 38–57.

Swindoll, C. (n.d.). Attitude. Retrieved September, 2, 2008, from *faculty.kutztown.edu/friehauf/attitude.html*

Tadir, M., & Stern, J. M. (1985). The mourning process with brain injured patients. *Scandinavian Journal of Rehabilitation Medicine Supplement, 12*, 50–52.

Tafarodi, R. W., & Ho, C. (2006). Implicit and explicit self-esteem: What are we measuring? *Canadian Psychology, 47*(3), 195–202.

Tamietto, M., Torrini, G., Adenzato, M., Pietrapiana, P., Rago, R., & Perino, C. (2006). To drive or not to drive (after TBI)?: A review of the literature and its implications for rehabilitation and future research. *NeuroRehabilitation, 21*, 81–92.

Tantam, D. (2003). The flavour of emotions. *Psychology and Psychotherapy: Theory, Research and Practice, 76*, 23–45.

Tate, R. L. (1997). Beyond one-bun, two-shoe: Recent advances in the psychological rehabilitation of memory disorders after acquired brain injury. *Brain Injury, 11*(12), 907–918.

Tate, R. L., & Broe, G. A. (1999). Psychosocial adjustment after traumatic brain injury: What are the important variables? *Psychological Medicine, 29*(3), 713–725.

Taylor, L. A., Kreutzer, J. S., Demm, S. R., & Meade, M. A. (2003). Traumatic brain injury and substance abuse: A review and analysis of the literature. *Neuropsychological Rehabilitation, 13*(1–2), 165–188.

Teitelbaum, S. (1991). Countertransference and its potential for abuse. *Clinical Social Work Journal, 19*(3), 267–277.

Testa, J. A., Malec, J. F., Moessner, A. M., & Brown, A. W. (2006). Predicting family functioning after TBI: Impact of neurobehavioral factors. *Journal of Head Trauma Rehabilitation, 21*(3), 236–247.

Testani-Dufour, L., Chappel-Aiken, L., & Gueldner, S. (1992). Traumatic brain injury: A family experience. *Journal of Neuroscience Nursing, 24*(6), 317–323.

Thaxton, L., & Myers, M. A. (2002). Sleep disturbances and their management in patients with brain injury. *Journal of Head Trauma Rehabilitation, 17*(4), 335–348.

Toglia, J., & Kirk, U. (2000). Understanding awareness deficits following brain injury. *NeuroRehabilitation, 15*(1), 57–70.

Tomas, R. (2007). Little wonders. On *Meet the Robinsons soundtrack* [CD]. Burbank, CA: Walt Disney Records.

Tombaugh, T. (1996). *Test of Memory Malingering.* North Tonawanda, NY: Multi-Health Systems.

Tomberg, T., Toomela, A., Ennok, M., & Tikk, A. (2007). Changes in coping strategies, social support, optimism and health-related quality of life following traumatic brain injury: A longitudinal study. *Brain Injury, 21*(5), 479–488.

Tomberg, T., Toomela, A., Pulver, A., & Tikk, A. (2005). Coping strategies, social support, life orientation and health-related quality of life following traumatic brain injury. *Brain Injury, 19*(14), 1181–1190.

Trahan, E., Pepin, M., & Hopps, S. (2006). Impaired awareness of deficits and treatment adherence among people with traumatic brain injury or spinal cord injury. *Journal of Head Trauma Rehabilitation, 21*(3), 226–235.

Turkstra, L. S., & Flora, T. L. (2002). Compensating for executive function impairments after TBI: A single case study of functional intervention. *Journal of Communication Disorders, 35*(6), 467–482.

Turner-Stokes, L., & MacWalter, R. (2005). Use of anti-depressant medication following acquired brain injury: Concise guidance. *Clinical Medicine, 5*(3), 268–274.

Tyerman, A., & Booth, J. (2001). Family interventions after traumatic brain injury: A service example. *NeuroRehabilitation, 16*(1), 59–66.

U.S. Department of Education. (2004). *Building the legacy: IDEA 2004.* Retrieved June 2, 2009, from *idea.ed.gov*

U.S. Department of Justice. (2005). *A guide to disability rights laws.* Retrieved October 25, 2008, from *www.ada.gov/cguide.htm*

Uomoto, J. M. (2004). The contribution of the neuropsychological evaluation to traumatic brain injury rehabilitation. In M. J. Ashley (Ed.), *Traumatic brain injury: Rehabilitative treatment and case management* (pp. 581–611). Boca Raton, FL: CRC Press.

Vaishnavi, S., Rao, V., & Fann, J. R. (2009). Neuropsychiatric problems after traumatic brain injury: Unraveling the silent epidemic. *Psychosomatics, 50*(3), 198–205.

Van Denburg, T. F., & Kiesler, D. J. (2002). An interpersonal communication perspective on resistance in psychotherapy. *Journal of Clinical Psychology/In Session, 58*(2), 195–205.

Vasques, M. J. T., Bingham, R. P., & Barnett, J. E. (2008). Psychotherapy termination: Clinical and ethical responsibilities. *Journal of Clinical Psychology, 64*(5), 653–665.

Verburg, G., Borthwick, B., Bennett, B., & Rumney, P. (2003). Online support to facilitate the reintegration of students with brain injury: Trials and errors. *NeuroRehabilitation, 18*, 113–123.

Verhaeghe, S., Defloor, T., & Grypdonck, M. (2005). Stress and coping among families of patients with traumatic brain injury: A review of the literature. *Journal of Clinical Nursing, 14*(8), 1004–1012.

Vickery, C. D., Gontkovsky, S. T., & Caroselli, J. S. (2005). Self-concept and quality of life following acquired brain injury: A pilot investigation. *Brain Injury, 19*(9), 657–665.

Vickery, C. D., Gontkovsky, S. T., Wallace, J. J., & Caroselli, J. S. (2006). Group psychotherapy focusing on self-concept change following acquired brain injury: A pilot investigation. *Rehabilitation Psychology, 51*(1), 30–35.

Vickery, C. D., Sherer, M., Evans, C. C., Gontkovsky, S. T., & Lee, J. E. (2008). The relationship between self-esteem and functional outcome in the acute stroke-rehabilitation setting. *Rehabilitation Psychology, 53*(1), 101–109.

Vincent, S. (1972). Oooh child [Recorded by The Five Stairsteps]. On *Greatest hits* [Album]. New York: Buddah.

Wagner, A. K., Hammond, F. M., Sasser, H. C., & Wiercisiewski, D. (2002). Return to productive activity after traumatic brain injury: Relationship with measures of disability, handicap, and community integration. *Archives of Physical Medicine and Rehabilitation, 83*, 107–114.

Walker, W. C., Marwitz, J. H., Kreutzer, J. S., Hart, T., & Novack, T. A. (2006). Occupational categories and return to work after traumatic brain injury: A multicenter study. *Archives of Physical Medicine and Rehabilitation, 87*, 1576–1582.

Walker, A. J., Onus, M., Doyle, M., Clare, J., & McCarthy, K. (2005). Cognitive rehabilitation after severe traumatic brain injury: A pilot programme of goal planning and outdoor adventure course participation. *Brain Injury, 19*(14), 1237–1241.

Ward, D. E. (1984). Termination of individual counseling: Concepts and strategies. *Journal of Counseling and Development, 63*(1), 21–25.

Warden, D. L., & Labbate, L. A. (2005). Posttraumatic stress disorder and other anxiety disorders. In J. M. Silver, T. W. McAllister, & S. C. Yudofsky (Eds.), *Textbook of traumatic brain injury* (pp. 231–243). Washington, DC: American Psychiatric Publishing.

Warren, E. S. (2005). Future colleague or convenient friend: The ethics of mentorship. *Counseling and Values, 49*(2), 141–146.

Warriner, E. M., & Velikonja, D. (2006). Psychiatric disturbances after traumatic brain injury: Neurobehavioral and personality changes. *Current Psychiatry Reports, 8*, 73–80.

Warschausky, S., Kaufman, J., & Stiers, W. (2008). Training requirements and scope of practice in rehabilitation psychology and neuropsychology. *Journal of Pediatric Medicine: An Interdisciplinary Approach, 1*, 61–65.

Waska, R. (2006). The analyst as translator: Failures and successes. *Psychoanalytic Social Work, 13*(1), 43–65.

Watson, M. J. (2007). Feasibility of further motor recovery in patients undergoing physiotherapy more than 6 months after severe traumatic brain injury: An updated literature review. *Physical Therapy Reviews, 12*(1), 21–32.

Webster, G., Daisley, A., & King, N. (1999). Relationship and family breakdown following brain injury: The role of the rehabilitation team. *Brain Injury, 13*(8), 593–603.

Wechsler, D. (2008). *Wechsler Adult Intelligence Scale—Fourth Edition: Administration and scoring manual.* San Antonio, TX: PsychCorp/Pearson.

Wechsler, D. (2009). *Wechsler Memory Scale—Fourth Edition: Manual.* San Antonio, TX: Pearson.

Wedcliffe, T., & Ross, E. (2001). The psychological effects of traumatic brain injury on the quality of life of a group of spouses/partners. *South African Journal of Communication Disorders, 48*, 77–99.

Wehman, P., Targett, P., Yasuda, S., & Brown, T. (2000). Return to work for individuals with TBI and a history of substance abuse. *NeuroRehabilitation, 15*(1), 71–77.

Weiner, S. (1997). The actor–director and patient–therapist relationships: A process comparison. *American Journal of Psychotherapy, 51*, 77–85.

Weinstein, E. A. (1991). Anosognosia and denial of illness. In G. P. Prigatano, & D. L. Schacter

(Eds.), *Awareness of deficit after brain injury: Clinical and theoretical issues* (pp. 240–257). New York: Oxford University Press.

Weintraub, J., Louis, R., Smith, B. (Producers), & Avildsen, J. (Director). (1984). *The karate kid* [Motion picture]. United States: Columbia Pictures.

Wells, R., Dywan, J., & Dumas, J. (2005). Life satisfaction and distress in family caregivers as related to specific behavioral changes after traumatic brain injury. *Brain Injury, 19*(13), 1105–1115.

Whitehouse, A. M. (1994). Applications of cognitive therapy with survivors of head injury. *Journal of Cognitive Psychotherapy: An International Quarterly, 8*(2), 141–160.

Wilde, O. (1998). *The picture of Dorian Gray*. Calgary, Alberta, Canada: Broadview Press. (Original work published 1891)

Wilkinson, S. (2000). Is 'normal grief' a mental disorder? *Philosophical Quarterly, 50*(202), 289–303.

Willemse-van Son, A. H. P., Ribbers, G. M., Verhagen, A. P., & Stam, H. J. (2007). Prognostic factors of long-term functioning and productivity after traumatic brain injury: A systematic review of prospective cohort studies. *Clinical Rehabilitation, 21*, 1024–1037.

Willer, B., & Corrigan, J. D. (1994). New concepts: Whatever it takes: A model for community-based services. *Brain Injury, 8*(7), 647–659.

Williams, B. Y. (2004). The friend who just stands by. In J. Cotner (Ed.), *Looking for God in all the right places: Prayers and poems to comfort, inspire, and connect humanity* (p. 125). Chicago: Loyola Press.

Williams, J. M. (1991). Family reaction to head injury. In J. M. Williams & T. Kay (Eds.), *Head injury: A family matter* (pp. 81–99). Baltimore: Brookes.

Williams, W. H., Evans, J. J., & Fleminger, S. (2003). Neurorehabilitation and cognitive-behaviour therapy of anxiety disorders after brain injury: An overview and a case illustration of obsessive–compulsive disorder. *Neuropsychological Rehabilitation, 13*(1–2), 133–148.

Wilson, B. A., Baddeley, A., Evans, J., & Shiel, A. (1994). Errorless learning in the rehabilitation of memory impaired people. *Neuropsychological Rehabilitation, 4*(3), 307–326.

Wilson, B. A., & Kapur, N. (2008). Memory rehabilitation for people with brain injury. In D. T. Stuss, G. Winocur, & I. H. Robertson (Eds.), *Cognitive neurorehabilitation: Evidence and application* (2nd ed., pp. 522–540). New York: Cambridge University Press.

Winkler, D., Unsworth, C., Sloan, S., & Caplan, B. (2006). Factors that lead to successful community integration following severe traumatic brain injury. *Journal of Head Trauma Rehabilitation, 21*(1), 8–21.

Winwood, S. (1982). Valerie. On *Talking back to the night* [Album]. New York: Polygram Records.

Wise, K., Ownsworth, T., & Fleming, J. (2005). Convergent validity of self-awareness measures and their association with employment outcome in adults following acquired brain injury. *Brain Injury, 19*(10), 765–775.

Wiseman-Hakes, C., Stewart, M. L., Wasserman, R., & Schuller, R. (1998). Peer group training of pragmatic skills in adolescents with acquired brain injury. *Journal of Head Trauma Rehabilitation, 13*(6), 23–38.

Wolberg, L. R. (1967). *The technique of psychotherapy: Part one* (2nd ed.). New York: Grune & Stratton.

Wolf, E. S. (1988). *Treating the self: Elements of clinical self psychology*. New York: Guilford Press.

Wood, R. L., Liossi, C., & Wood, L. (2005). The impact of head injury neurobehavioural sequelae on personal relationships: Preliminary findings. *Brain Injury, 19*(10), 845–851.

Woodruff, L., & Woodruff, B. (2007). *In an instant: A family's journey of love and healing*. New York: Random House.

Worthington, A. D., Matthews, S., Melia, Y., & Oddy, M. (2006). Cost–benefits associated with social outcome from neurobehavioural rehabilitation. *Brain Injury, 20*(9), 947–957.

Worthington, A., & Waller, J. (2009). Rehabilitation of everyday living skills in the context of executive disorders. In M. Oddy & A. Worthington (Eds.), *The rehabilitation of executive disorders: A guide to theory and practice* (pp. 195–210). New York: Oxford University Press.

Yalom, I. D. (1975). *The theory and practice of group psychotherapy* (2nd ed.). New York: Basic Books.

Yalom, I. D. (1980). *Existential psychotherapy.* New York: Basic Books.

Yalom, I. D. (2002). *The gift of therapy: An open letter to a new generation of therapists and their patients.* New York: HarperCollins.

Yamagami, T. (1998). Psychotherapy, today and tomorrow: Status quo of behavior and cognitive therapy and its efficacy. *Psychiatry and Clinical Neurosciences, 52*(Suppl.), S236–S237.

Ylvisaker, M., & Feeney, T. (2000). Reconstruction of identity after brain injury. *Brain Impairment, 1*(1), 12–28.

Ylvisaker, M., Hanks, R., & Johnson-Greene, D. (2002). Perspectives on rehabilitation of individuals with cognitive impairment after brain injury: Rationale for reconsideration of theoretical paradigms. *Journal of Head Trauma Rehabilitation, 17*(3), 191–209.

Ylvisaker, M., Jacobs, H. E., & Feeney, T. (2003). Positive supports for people who experience behavioral and cognitive disability after brain injury: A review. *Journal of Head Trauma Rehabilitation, 18*(1), 7–32.

Ylvisaker, M., Todis, B., Glang, A., Urbanczyk, B., Franklin, C., DePompei, R., et al. (2001). Educating students with TBI: Themes and recommendations. *Journal of Head Trauma Rehabilitation, 16*(1), 76–93.

Zafonte, R. D., Cullen, N., & Lexell, J. (2002). Serotonin agents in the treatment of acquired brain injury. *Journal of Head Trauma Rehabilitation, 17*(4), 322–334.

# Index

281